T0246334

Reproductive Donation

Reproductive donation is the most contentious area of assisted reproduction. Even within Europe there are wide variations in what is permitted in each country. This multidisciplinary book takes a fresh look at the practices of egg, sperm and embryo donation and surrogacy, bringing together ethical analysis and empirical research. New evidence is offered on aspects of assisted reproduction and the families these create, including non-traditional types. One of the key issues addressed is should children be told of their donor origin? If they do learn the identity of their donor, what kinds of relationships may be forged between families, the donor and other donor sibling families? Should donation involve a gift relationship? Is intra-familial donation too close for comfort? How should we understand the growing trend for 'reproductive tourism'? This lively and informed discussion offers new insights into reproductive donation and the resulting donor families.

MARTIN RICHARDS is Emeritus Professor of Family Research in the University of Cambridge Centre for Family Research, which he founded, and directed until 2005. His research concerns the psychosocial aspects of new reproductive and genetic technologies and the social and ethical issues that deployment of new technologies may raise. He publishes widely in academic journals. His books include: *The Troubled Helix: Social and Psychological Implications of the New Human Genetics*, edited with Theresa Marteau (1996); *The Limits of Consent: a Socio-Ethical Approach*, edited with John McMillan *et al.* (2009); *Regulating Autonomy: Sex, Reproduction and Families*, edited with Shelley Day-Slater *et al.* (2009); and *Birthrights or Rites*, edited with Fatemeh Ebtehaj *et al.* (2011).

GUIDO PENNINGS is Professor of Ethics and Bioethics at Ghent University where he is also the Director of the Bioethics Institute Ghent (BIG). He mainly publishes on ethical problems associated with medically assisted reproduction and genetics including sex selection, gamete donation, stem cell research, fertility preservation and preimplantation genetic diagnosis. In addition, he is Affiliate Lecturer in the Faculty of Politics, Psychology, Sociology and International Studies at Cambridge University and Guest Professor on 'Ethics in Reproductive Medicine' at the Faculty of Medicine and Pharmaceutical Sciences of the Free University Brussels.

JOHN B. APPLEBY is currently a Wellcome Trust PhD student in Bioethics at the Centre for Family Research and a member of Corpus Christi College at the University of Cambridge.

Reproductive Donation

Practice, Policy and Bioethics

Edited by

Martin Richards
Centre for Family Research, University of Cambridge

Guido Pennings
Bioethics Institute Ghent, Ghent University

John B. Appleby
Centre for Family Research, University of Cambridge

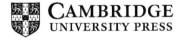

CAMBRIDGE
UNIVERSITY PRESS

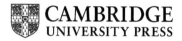

CAMBRIDGE
UNIVERSITY PRESS

Shaftesbury Road, Cambridge CB2 8EA, United Kingdom

One Liberty Plaza, 20th Floor, New York, NY 10006, USA

477 Williamstown Road, Port Melbourne, VIC 3207, Australia

314–321, 3rd Floor, Plot 3, Splendor Forum, Jasola District Centre, New Delhi – 110025, India

103 Penang Road, #05–06/07, Visioncrest Commercial, Singapore 238467

Cambridge University Press is part of Cambridge University Press & Assessment, a department of the University of Cambridge.

We share the University's mission to contribute to society through the pursuit of education, learning and research at the highest international levels of excellence.

www.cambridge.org
Information on this title: www.cambridge.org/9781107007772

© Cambridge University Press & Assessment 2012

First published 2012

A catalogue record for this publication is available from the British Library

Library of Congress Cataloging-in-Publication data
Reproductive donation: practice, policy, and bioethics / [edited by] Martin Richards, Guido Pennings, John Appleby.
   p.;   cm.
Includes bibliographical references and index.
ISBN 978-1-107-00777-2 (hbk.) – ISBN 978-0-521-18993-4 (pbk.)
I. Richards, Martin, 1940 Jan. 26– II. Pennings, Guido. III. Appleby, John, 1984– [DNLM: 1. Reproductive Techniques, Assisted–ethics. 2. Directed Tissue Donation. 3. Family Relations–legislation & jurisprudence. 4. Reproductive Techniques, Assisted–legislation & jurisprudence. 5. Surrogate Mothers–legislation & jurisprudence. 6. Tissue Donors. WQ 208]
   176–dc23
   2012011806

ISBN   978-1-107-00777-2   Hardback
ISBN   978-0-521-18993-4   Paperback

Contents

List of contributors   *page* vii
Acknowledgements   ix

1   Introduction   1
    MARTIN RICHARDS, GUIDO PENNINGS
    AND JOHN B. APPLEBY

2   The biology of donation   13
    MARTIN H. JOHNSON

3   Ethics for reproductive donation   30
    ROBERT KLITZMAN

4   Parenthood – whose right is it anyway?   51
    ANJA KARNEIN

5   Reproductive donation: global perspectives
    and cultural diversity   70
    ZEYNEP B. GÜRTIN AND EFFY VAYENA

6   UK and US perspectives on the regulation
    of gamete donation   90
    THERESA GLENNON

7   Gamete and embryo donation: a legal
    view from Spain   112
    YOLANDA GARCÍA-RUIZ AND DIANA GUERRA-DIAZ

8   The legal and ethical regulation of
    transnational donation   130
    GUIDO PENNINGS AND ZEYNEP B. GÜRTIN

9   Balancing ethical criteria for the recruitment
    of gamete donors   150
    GUIDO PENNINGS, EFFY VAYENA
    AND KAMAL AHUJA

10   Challenges in intra-family donation   168
     EFFY VAYENA AND SUSAN GOLOMBOK

11   ARTs and the single parent   189
     SUSANNA GRAHAM AND ANDREA BRAVERMAN

12   Reproductive donation and justice for gay
     and lesbian couples   211
     JOHN B. APPLEBY, SARAH JENNINGS
     AND HELEN STATHAM

13   Is disclosure in the best interests of children
     conceived by donation?   231
     JOHN B. APPLEBY, LUCY BLAKE AND
     TABITHA FREEMAN

14   Identifiable donors and siblings: implications
     for the future   250
     TABITHA FREEMAN, JOHN B. APPLEBY
     AND VASANTI JADVA

15   Ethical issues in embryo donation   270
     FIONA MACCALLUM AND HEATHER WIDDOWS

16   Reproduction through surrogacy: the UK and
     US experience   289
     ANDREA BRAVERMAN, POLLY CASEY
     AND VASANTI JADVA

17   Some conclusions regarding the interaction of
     normative and descriptive elements in
     reproductive donation   308
     GUIDO PENNINGS

     Index   311

Contributors

KAMAL AHUJA The London Women's Clinic

JOHN B. APPLEBY Centre for Family Research, University of Cambridge

LUCY BLAKE Centre for Family Research, University of Cambridge

ANDREA BRAVERMAN Department of Obstetrics and Gynecology, Robert Wood Johnson Medical School

POLLY CASEY Centre for Family Research, University of Cambridge

TABITHA FREEMAN Centre for Family Research, University of Cambridge

YOLANDA GARCÍA-RUIZ Facultad de Derecho, Universidad de Valencia

THERESA GLENNON Beasley School of Law, Temple University

SUSAN GOLOMBOK Centre for Family Research, University of Cambridge

SUSANNA GRAHAM Centre for Family Research, University of Cambridge

DIANA GUERRA-DIAZ Instituto Valenciano de Infertilidad (IVI) Barcelona

ZEYNEP B. GÜRTIN Centre for Family Research, University of Cambridge

VASANTI JADVA Centre for Family Research, University of Cambridge

SARAH JENNINGS Centre for Family Research, University of Cambridge

MARTIN H. JOHNSON Department of Physiology, Development and Neuroscience, University of Cambridge

ANJA KARNEIN Institute for Political Science, Goethe-Universität Frankfurt

ROBERT KLITZMAN Columbia University College of Physicians and Surgeons

FIONA MACCALLUM Department of Psychology, University of Warwick

GUIDO PENNINGS Bioethics Institute Ghent (BIG), Ghent University

MARTIN RICHARDS Centre for Family Research, University of Cambridge

HELEN STATHAM Centre for Family Research, University of Cambridge

EFFY VAYENA Institute of Biomedical Ethics, University of Zurich

HEATHER WIDDOWS Department of Philosophy, University of Birmingham

Acknowledgements

This book grew from a workshop that was supported by a Wellcome Trust Biomedical Ethics Enhancement Award to Professor Susan Golombok and others in the Centre for Family Research, University of Cambridge. We are grateful to the Wellcome Trust for making this project possible.

The editors would like to express their thanks for the assistance of a number people, not least to the authors of the chapters for their forbearance and compliance with editorial demands, and to Abby Scott, Hita Hirons, Jill Brown and Frances Murton for all their work. The grant holders of the Wellcome Enhancement Award who played a vital role in the planning of the project are Susan Golombok, Tabitha Freeman, Vasanti Jadva, Helen Statham and Zeynep B. Gürtin. And our thanks to the discussants for their contributions to our workshop, Irenee Daly, John Parsons and Wannes Van Hoof.

1   Introduction

Martin Richards, Guido Pennings and John B. Appleby

This volume offers a survey of the practices of reproductive donation and a discussion of the social and ethical issues that these may raise. Our focus is on collaborative, or third-party reproduction. Here a child is not conceived through sexual intercourse by the parents, but rather the conception is likely to take place in a clinic with others involved in providing the eggs, sperm, embryo or sometimes the uterus in which the fetus grows. Typically in collaborative reproduction, roles are separated, so that these third-party progenitors do not become parents and usually play no part in the lives of the children they help to create. Indeed, it is often the case in collaborative reproduction that the children are unaware of the part that others have played. Within the technologies and practices of assisted reproduction, a child can have up to five progenitors: a social mother, a social father, a biological father (sperm provider), a biological mother (egg provider) and a surrogate (gestational) mother.[1]

There are a number of different reasons why people may turn to collaborative reproduction. It can provide a means of overcoming infertility. So where, for example, a man's sperm is defective or not produced in sufficient quantity, or a woman no longer has viable eggs because of her age, gametes (egg or sperm) from a third party can provide a substitute. Without such collaborative reproduction, their only other possibility

---

[1] This list is likely to be extended very soon to include mitochondrial mothers. Techniques have been developed to transfer a nucleus between eggs. This can be used to avoid the transmission of mitochondrial disease by a mother to her children. The nucleus of a donor egg is replaced by the nucleus from an egg from the mother who suffers from mitochondrial disease. The hybrid egg is then fertilized in vitro and the resulting embryo is placed in the mother with mitochondrial disease. Normally mitochondria are transferred from mother to child in the body of the egg (cytoplasm), not in the nucleus, so that through the use of nuclear transfer between eggs the child will have healthy mitochondria from the woman who provided the egg but nuclear genetic material from the mother. In the UK this technique has been used experimentally but it has yet to be approved for use in fertility clinics.

of having a child would be to adopt. The main difference, obviously, is that an adopted child is not a blood relative of either parent.

Some people may use egg or sperm donation as a way of avoiding the transmission of a genetic disease to children. There are ways of achieving this that avoid the use of collaborative reproduction, such as prenatal diagnosis and termination of affected pregnancies or pre-implantation genetic diagnosis and embryo selection. However, these alternatives are not always applicable and they may also be rejected by the would-be parents for moral and psychological reasons. Nevertheless, the use of egg or sperm donation for this purpose is becoming rare.

There is an important underlying factor in couples' choice of procedures in assisted reproduction: using gametes from others is usually a last resort that is only contemplated where there is no possibility of a couple having 'their own' child conceived with their own gametes. This has driven the uptake of new (expensive and invasive) techniques in the treatment of male infertility. Intra-cytoplasmic sperm injection (ICSI) is a procedure in which a single sperm, which may be surgically extracted from the testes, is injected into an egg to effect in vitro fertilization and so avoid problems with low sperm counts or non-motile sperm. ICSI was first used in Britain in 1992 and records show that as the use of ICSI increased, the use of sperm donation declined. In 1992 there were 25,000 donor insemination clinic treatments. By 2002 this had fallen to about 5,000 but by then there were over 15,000 ICSI procedures carried out (HFEA, 2006).

But while the use of sperm from others for treatment of infertility may have declined, it has become increasingly important in a number of countries, including the UK and USA, for baby-making by those who do not have an appropriate reproductive partner. This includes single women (Graham and Braverman, Chapter 11) and lesbian couples (Appleby, Jennings and Statham, Chapter 12). Gay men, of course, need a woman to carry the pregnancy as well as an egg donor. While the same woman can do both, many gay couples in the USA seem to prefer to separate these two roles and use in vitro fertilization (IVF) with an egg donor and surrogate mother, rather than insemination of the surrogate mother.

Surrogacy comes in two forms, often referred to as full or partial (Braverman, Casey and Jadva, Chapter 16). Full, or gestational, surrogacy is where IVF is used with the gametes of the commissioning parents – or a donor(s) – and the resulting embryo is placed in the surrogate mother, who carries the pregnancy and hands over the baby after the birth. In partial, or genetic, surrogacy the surrogate's own egg is used and the pregnancy is usually achieved by artificial insemination. Unlike full surrogacy and sperm donation, egg or embryo donation require the use of IVF to achieve a pregnancy and that technique is but a generation old, with its beginning marked by the birth of the first IVF baby in July 1978 (Edwards and Steptoe, 1980).

With the involvement of third parties, collaborative reproduction is disruptive of the social order of sexual reproduction and it has often been seen as transgressive (Haimes, 2000). Today in many countries and jurisdictions some or all of the practice of third-party reproduction is subject to restrictive regulation or is completely outlawed (Gürtin and Vayena, Chapter 5). There are those who object to the complicated relationships that are created and claim that the well-being of children can only be assured by banning all forms of reproduction that result in children growing up apart from both their biological parents (Karnein, Chapter 4).

Concerns and controversy are often focused on questions of legal and social parentage in collaborative reproduction and the status of the third parties in relation to the parents and resulting children. There is also the issue of the character of the transaction between provider and user of the gametes or embryos. Throughout this book we refer to reproductive 'donation'; however, we are not always discussing gifts. In some societies sperm and eggs are bought from the providers and sold to users, and surrogate mothers are paid for their services. But in other parts of the world there is at least an ideal that gametes (like any other part of the body) are beyond commerce and should only change hands as part of a virtuous gift relationship. If there is payment, regulations often limit this to the reimbursement of expenses (Pennings, Vayena and Ahuja, Chapter 9).

There are international declarations and directives that prohibit commercial trade in gametes or embryos (and other human tissue). The European Union Tissues and Cells Directive (2004) requires voluntary donation without money changing hands except payments that are 'strictly limited to making good the expenses and inconveniences of donation'. While some bioethicists write of the perils of commercialization and commodification, others contest the whole concept of market inalienability. Much more could be said about the gift relationship (Titmuss, 1971) and commercialization, but here we will follow common usage and, throughout the book, the term 'donation' will refer to the process by which sperm, eggs and embryos are provided for users regardless of whether this is an altruistic gift or a commercial sale.

Another major ethical issue that runs through many considerations of reproductive donation concerns the welfare of the children who may result: should these children be told of the manner of their conception?

Do children have a right to know? What are the consequences of secrecy or disclosure? Should children know the identity of their donor parent? Should it be possible for them to meet and perhaps form a social relationship? And does the same go for donor siblings who may be born in other families who have used the same donor? A couple of decades ago secrecy was the general rule and it was argued that this would protect the welfare of children. Sometimes, of course, children who are not told of their origins may discover this – perhaps through another family member who knows what has gone on. In addition, today there is a growing trend to end anonymity in donation and provide systems through which adult children of donation can discover the identity of their donor parents.

The technique of DNA paternity testing, combined with access to large databases, has raised a new possibility of identifying an 'anonymous' sperm donor. In 2004 a 15-year-old American teenager who had discovered he was a donor child tracked down his donor (Motluk, 2005). He sent a sample of his DNA to a commercial firm (Family Tree DNA) for analysis and to see if anyone on their database might share his paternal blood line. There were two matches and both people had the same surname – so it was likely that this would be his father's name. From his mother, he learnt the date and place of birth of his anonymous donor father. Using another online search company, he was able to purchase a list of all those born in the same locality on the same date. One of these had the same surname as his two DNA matches. Within ten days, he had made contact with his donor.

Today there are also websites where donor families and donors can post details that can be used to identify families who have used the same donor as well as the donors themselves (Freeman, Appleby and Jadva, Chapter 14). In the USA linking is usually done through the unique numbers that are assigned to donors and that are known to recipients. However, discussions are underway about the possibility of setting up new databases that hold DNA from donors and recipients, which would allow direct linking without the use of any other information from either party. So people are finding new ways of unravelling the secrets of collaborative reproduction. Today, the notion of an 'anonymous' donor must be regarded as an increasingly provisional category.

History may often help to illuminate the present and so we will turn briefly to the history of artificial insemination. It is a history which is not only significant for the continuing resistance to any acceptance of reproductive practices which include third parties, but one which also included rather different interpretations of these practices than those found today. Significant objections to artificial insemination were often based on the relationship between the parents and the donor rather than the manner of conception itself.

There are accounts of the medical use of artificial insemination from the eighteenth century in Britain. By the end of the nineteenth century, at least a few doctors in France, the USA, Britain and doubtless elsewhere were treating problems of male infertility using either husband's sperm (so called homologous insemination) or occasionally donor sperm (heterologous insemination). In 1887 this had provoked a *non licence* from the Sacred Congregation of the Holy Office of the Vatican (Schellen, 1957; Bartholomew, 1958; Pfeffer, 1993). But there were also those who saw that reproduction that did not involve a sexual relationship could be put to new social purposes.

In Australia, Marion Louisa Piddington proposed 'scientific' or 'celibate motherhood' through artificial insemination by donor (AID) for widows and single women unable to find husbands because of the casualties of the First World War, which were particularly heavy for the Australian army (Louis, 1916; Curthoys, 1989; Richards, 2008). The plan included establishing a governmental 'Eugenic Institute' to run the scheme, selecting desirable superior donors and providing the mothers with an allowance to support them through the child-rearing years. The Institute would hold records of donors and births, and the 'scientific children' would require the permission of the Institute to marry to avoid the possibility of intermarriage of donor siblings – a possibility that continues to trouble some detractors of secret artificial insemination (AI) to the present day. In a society where the Catholic Church had a strong influence, the proposal found little support. But one who did offer support was a Sydney doctor, Henry Waterman Swan (one of a handful in Australia at the time who provided AID for his patients), who wrote an anonymous pamphlet, 'Facultative Motherhood without Offence to Moral Law: Every Woman's Right to Motherhood' (Wyndham, 2003). But while this doctor might have believed that AID would remove the moral offence of single motherhood, few others accepted the argument and were very critical of what the press called the 'conscription of the virgins' (Wyndham, 2003). Interestingly similar suggestions were made in Britain after the Second World War. C. O. Carter, who ran one of the first genetic clinics in the UK, suggested that 'there will be a number of young widows of a good type who have only been able to have one or two children before their husbands were killed' who should use AID to expand their families. (Carter, 1945: 130). The USA National Research Foundation for Eugenic Alleviation offered a kind of reproductive lease lend to Britain with a proposal for clinics in London where American semen from prime donors could be available to British women (Pfeffer, 1993).

In the 1930s a number of eugenicists familiar with AI – not least from its wide use in agriculture – saw the potential for eugenic enhancement of 'test tube babies', as some called them (Rohleder, 1934), who were conceived without the complications of a sexual relationship. Brewer (1935: 122–3) suggested 'generation without antecedent sexual union', or 'eutelegenesis', could be applied to human populations 'by using the germ cells of a few highly selected males to impregnate the general body of females. Such a process might produce a great and rapid improvement in the hereditary qualities of the race.' The proposed scheme would enrol volunteers. 'Eugenic advance must be the voluntary adventure of free men and women or nothing' (Brewer, 1935: 124).

An American Nobel Prize-winning geneticist, Hermann Muller (1935), made similar proposals. Like Brewer, Muller thought that positive eugenics need not wait for the development of techniques for ectogenesis (in vitro fertilization) and eutelogenesis (AID) would be a good start. While Brewer's proposal led to little more than some anxious discussion within the UK Eugenics Society, Muller's proposal did lead to the setting-up of a sperm bank, but not for another forty-five years (Richards, 2008). The Californian Hermann J. Muller Repository for Germinal Choice opened its doors for business in 1980. This was a sperm bank that offered sperm from selected males (including a few Nobel Prize winners) to selected couples. This 'genius factory' traded for nineteen years, over which time some 215 babies were born (Plotz, 2005).

Aside from these eugenic proposals, the practice of AI grew very slowly in Britain between the First and Second World War. There was a handful of doctors who offered AID to infertile couples, and, possibly, the occasional 'bachelor mother'. Some people encouraged infertile couples to do it for themselves. Marie Stopes, the birth control and sex education pioneer, told wives whose husbands might be sterile to 'avoid expensive doctors ... and arrange the whole matter with [their] husband and do it [themselves]'. They were advised to enlist the help of their husband's best friend or a relative as a donor and were given detailed instruction on self-insemination (Richards, 2008). This shows that the use of intrafamilial donors, although still considered problematic at present, is not a new idea (Vayena and Golombok, Chapter 10). One medical practitioner who ran a clinic for the treatment of sterility in Exeter in the 1930s found that about a quarter of those whose husbands were sterile would opt for AID and about two thirds of these were successfully inseminated (Church of England, 1948).

In 1948 an expert advisory committee set up by the Archbishop of Canterbury reported and called for the criminalization of AID (the practice of artificial insemination by husband, or AIH, was found acceptable) (Church of England, 1948), but these recommendations were never acted on. Indeed, as the availability of illegitimate babies for adoption decreased in the post-war years, there was more interest in AID from infertile couples. But while there continued to be a few clinics that offered it (outside the National Health Service), official attitudes were slow to change. In 1960 a UK Government Departmental Committee (Feversham, 1960) recommended that while AIH was acceptable, it was suggested that AID should be strongly discouraged 'as it may well disturb the harmony of society': 'We think the fact that through the need for secrecy the donor must donate in complete ignorance of the identity of the recipient of his seed indicates a lack of responsibility on his part.' However, by 1968 the Minister of Health had agreed that both AID and AIH should be available to patients in the National Health Service. Another important landmark was the Family Law Reform Act of 1987, which made AID recipients and their partners legal parents and removed all rights and duties of fatherhood from sperm donors. This also covered egg and embryo donation, which became available in the late 1980s. In 1990 there was the Human Fertilisation and Embryology Act, which regulated assisted reproduction, including donation, under the Human Fertilisation and Embryology Authority. In the early 1990s, over 40 per cent of children conceived in fertility clinics (the majority being for-profit clinics in the private sector rather than the National Health Service) were the results of donor treatment and this was mostly sperm donation (e.g. 1993: 2,283 sperm, 169 egg and 35 embryo donations). At the beginning of the twenty-first century, that proportion had dropped sharply – only 10 per cent in 2006, despite the increase in treatments for single women and lesbian couples, and by then egg donation was almost as common as sperm donation (2006: 693 sperm, 562 egg and 74 embryo donations) (HFEA, 2006).

Of course, every country has its own history of assisted reproduction (Glennon, Chapter 6; García-Ruiz and Guerra-Diaz, Chapter 7). AID developed earlier and more widely in the USA than in the UK. By 1941 a US survey of doctors claimed that at least 9,580 American women had been impregnated by artificial means (Seymour and Koerner, 1941). In 1948, the year in which the UK Archbishop's Committee had advised criminalization, AID made its first appearance on the big screen in America in a movie entitled *Test Tube Baby*[2], which told the story of

---

[2] The title comes from the title of a book published in 1934 (Rohleder, 1934). The term became widely used especially in the USA as a term for AID. But following the birth of the first IVF baby in 1978 the phrase resurfaced as a description – probably intended to be pejorative – of IVF children.

a successful use of AID by an infertile couple. At the time there were many reports in the press about test tube babies. It has been argued that the increasing use of AID was associated with the developing autonomy of women, which was related to their efforts to gain control over their bodies through the separation of sex and procreation by the use of artificial methods of birth control. This, combined with the historical circumstances of the Second World War, acted to weaken moral inhibitions regarding AI. Despite continuing uncertainties about the legal status of AI children and parents, physicians involved in infertility treatment took a major role in encouraging the use of AI (Bernstein, 2002).

The USA also pioneered the commercial cryobanking of sperm with the first sperm bank opening in 1972. By 1992 this was a $164 million a year industry dominated by a few very large operators (Mamo, 2005). These companies offered extensive catalogues giving detailed descriptions and photos of donors, which may now be viewed online. Two types of donors are offered: identity release and anonymous. Donors are carefully screened and are typically contracted for 9 months or 1 year, over which time they are expected to donate weekly. They are only paid for donations that reach specified quality standards. Because of the difficulty of freezing, eggs are not banked, but companies offer similar catalogues with donor characteristics. Only when an egg donor has been selected (and usually would have met the customer) is the process of ovulation induction started and eggs later collected.

To conclude this brief history, we will present a comparison of the reports of the two UK expert committees that investigated artificial insemination in 1948 and 1984, as these represent not simply the changing moralities of these two periods, but also the different ways in which collaborative reproduction was seen and the rather different anxieties it raises. These committees were very similar in their composition, both made up of expert professionals: medics, Christian theologians, lawyers, social workers, but significantly in the case of the later committee, a biological scientist. The 1948 committee was appointed by the Archbishop of Canterbury and chaired by the Lord Bishop of London, J. W. C. Wand (Church of England, 1948), while the later one was a government committee chaired by an academic philosopher Mary Warnock (Warnock, 1984). Both sought evidence rather widely from professional bodies, practitioners and interested parties. But while Wand was confined to artificial insemination, Warnock's brief was wider, to cover all of assisted reproduction, which by then, of course, included IVF, as well as sperm, embryo and egg donation (the first live birth from egg donation had taken place in Australia by the time the report was written) and embryo research. While Wand declared that AID for single women was beyond their remit (but nevertheless reported that 'problems of the gravest possible character would inevitably arise in the case of insemination of unmarried women'), Warnock's committee stated explicitly that access to treatment should not be based exclusively on the legal status of marriage. Wand concluded (with one dissenting voice) that 'the evils necessarily involved in artificial insemination (donor) are so grave that early consideration should be given to the framing of legislation to make the practice a criminal offence'. Warnock did set some limits, but basically constructed a detailed specification for the provision of fertility treatment within a legally regulated system. Indeed, such a system was set up under the terms of the 1990 Human Fertilisation and Embryology Act with a quango (the Human Fertilisation and Embryology Authority) in control, licensing both the commercial clinics and those of the National Health Service. Both reports list pros and cons for AI, but while Wand considers eugenic implications, Warnock is silent on eugenic matters. Warnock provides only a brief dismissal of Wand's major preoccupation and reason for criminalization: the issue of adultery. A contemporary reader might wonder what adultery has to do with collaborative reproduction. However, Wand considered the issues of AIH/D in terms of a view of reproduction as the coming together of bodies and so the relationship of those persons. Thus AID is symbolically the coming together of donor and recipient. We may contrast that with the Warnock symbolism of gametes fusing, which is represented as the image of a human egg – detached from any body or person, in vitro – surrounded by sperm, one of which will penetrate the egg and effect fertilization.

The Wand committee expressed 'profound compassion [for] married women who long for children'. Indeed, they received 'eloquent testimony from a number of married couples to their joy in the new baby and the increased happiness of their marriage'.

However, ends cannot justify means and their final conclusion was that AID was not morally acceptable:

Artificial insemination with donated semen involves a breach of the marriage. It violates the exclusive union set between husband and wife. It defrauds the child begotten, and deceives both his putative kinsmen and society at large. For both donor and recipient the sexual act loses its personal character and becomes a mere transaction. For the child there must always be a risk of disclosure, deliberate or unintended, of the circumstances of his conception. We therefore judge artificial insemination with donated semen to be wrong in principle and contrary to Christian standards (1948: 58).

For the Wand Committee, there were both legal and moral issues of adultery. Lawyers on the Committee were of 'no doubt at all that the act of both a married "donor" and a married recipient constitute adultery', following UK (*Russell* v. *Russell*, 1924) and Canadian (*Orford* v. *Orford*, 1921) jurisprudence.

Unlike the Wand committee, there were those who saw the process of reproduction separate from that of sexual connection. Indeed, for them that was exactly the point. For example, it was no accident that a radical like Piddington, who argued for 'scientific motherhood' by way of AID, was also a feminist birth control and sex education activist. She saw that sexual relationships could be separated from procreation, not simply in practice by the use of birth control, but also in terms of a symbolic scientific understanding of conception. So she saw AID, not as a conjugal act of intercourse, but as a means of conception – so it could provide a path to motherhood 'without sin'. In a similar way later eugenicists, such as Brewer, regarded it as a way to improve the race without compromising marriage or marriage choice.

The subject of investigation for the Warnock committee was the 'alleviation of infertility' and the means by which this might be achieved. The committee was able to give short shrift to the adultery argument – helped no doubt by judges who had some time earlier in a Scottish case (*MacLennan* v. *MacLennan*, 958) decided that AID, even in the absence of the husband's knowledge and consent, did not constitute adultery:

Some go so far as to suggest that the introduction of a third party into the marriage means that AID is in fact comparable to adultery, and that it violates the exclusive physical union of man and wife, and represents a break in the marriage vows ... [But] AID involves no personal relationship between the mother and donor at all, and the identity of the true father of the AID child will normally be unknown to the mother, and unascertainable by her. In most cases it can be assumed that the mother's husband is willing from the start to treat any resulting child as his own and merely as an accepted 'child of the family' (Warnock, 1984: 20–1).

So for the Warnock committee there is no relationship between donor and recipient: instead a need for 'absolute anonymity' that protects 'all parties not only from the legal complications but also from emotional difficulties'. But the report does recommend that 'at the age of 18 the child should have access to basic information about the donor's ethnic origin and genetic health', but not, of course, the donor's name. There is also concern for the welfare of the children and the Committee concluded that practice should not be 'left in a legal vacuum'. They recommend that the donor should have no parental rights in relation to the child and that these should pass to the recipient and her partner.

In general, through its history, sperm donation has started with a simple, coherent framework that has gradually evolved into a more complex structure of rules. The earlier idea was the complete assimilation of the act within the nuclear family. Secrecy and anonymity were part of the original structure. With such rules there was a reduction of the person from a sperm donor to a sperm. Sperm was the drug that would cure infertility. The sperm donor, as a person, was erased and separated from the recipient family. More recently, some people have felt that this position is untenable, not least because this position seems to ignore the rights of the children. As a consequence, modifications to the rules imply cracks in the earlier wall between donor and recipients. By lifting the veil of secrecy, the parents accept the existence of a person whose actions have led to the conception of their child. By allowing the identification of donors and known donation, the donor can even be contacted either by the recipients or the child. We are at present in this phase of transition and relatively little is known about where this might lead us. Will children be happier when they can contact their donor? How will donors react to a belated request for contact? Will we be able to construct a coherent framework that includes these new requests while respecting people's views on how social and genetic parenthood should balance? This book offers a view on this changing landscape and a road map that may be useful for navigation.

REFERENCES

Bartholomew, G. W. (1958). 'The development of artificial insemination'. *Eugenics Review*, 49, 187–95.

Bernstein, G. (2002). 'The socio-legal acceptance of new technologies: a close look at artificial insemination'. *Washington Law Review*, 77, 1035–58.

Brewer, H. (1935). 'Eutelegenesis'. *Eugenics Review*, 37, 121–6.

Carter, C. O. (1945). 'Artificial insemination'. Letter. *British Medical Journal*, 1, 130.

Church of England (1948). *Artificial Human Insemination. The Report of a Commission Appointed by His Grace the Archbishop of Canterbury*. London. SPCK (Wand Report).

Curthoys, A. (1989). 'Eugenics, feminism and birth control: the case of Marion Piddington'. *Hecate*, 15, 79–87.

Edwards, R. G. and Steptoe, P. C. (1980). *A Matter of Life: The Story of a Medical Breakthrough*. London: Hutchinson.

Feversham, Earl of (1960). *Report of the Departmental Committee on Human Artificial Insemination*. Cmnd. 1105. London: HMSO.

Haimes, E. (2000). '"Everybody's got a dad ... ". Issues for lesbian families in the management of donor insemination'. *Sociology of Health and Illness*, 22, 477–99.

Human Fertilisation and Embryology Authority (HFEA) (2006). *Unpublished Statistics*. London: HFEA.

Louis [M. L. Piddington] (1916). *Via Nuova, or Science and Maternity*. Sydney: Dymock's Book Arcade.

Mamo, L. (2005). 'Biomedicalizing kinship: sperm banks and the creation of affinity-ties'. *Science as Culture*, 14, 237–64.

Motluk, A. (2005). 'Tracing dad online'. *New Scientist*, 5, Nov. 6.

Muller, H. J. (1935). *Out of the Night*. London: Gallancz.

Pfeffer, N. (1993). *The Stork and the Syringe*. Oxford: Polity Press.

Plotz, D. (2005). *The Genius Factory*. London: Simon and Schuster.

Richards, M.P.M. (2008). 'Artificial insemination and eugenics: celibate motherhood, eutelegenesis and germinal choice'. *Studies in the History and Philosophy of Biology and Biomedical Science*, 39, 211–21.

Rohleder, H. (1934). *Test Tube Babies: A History of the Artificial Impregnation of Human Beings*. New York: Penurge Press.

Schellen, A. (1957). *Artificial Insemination in the Human*. Amsterdam: Elsevier.

Seymour, F. I. and Koerner, A. (1941). 'Artificial insemination: present status in United States as shown by recent survey'. *Journal of the American Medical Association*, 116, 2747–9.

Titmuss, R. M. (1971). *The Gift Relationship. From Human Blood to Social Policy*. London: Allen and Unwin.

Warnock, M. (1984). *Report of the Committee of Inquiry into Human Fertilisation and Embryology*. Cmnd. 9314. London: HMSO.

Wyndham, D. (2003). *Eugenics in Australia: Striving for National Fitness*. London: The Galton Institute.

CASES

MacLennan v. *MacLennan*, 1958 Sc 105-1958
Orford v. *Orford*, 1921 DLR 251-1921
Russell v. *Russell*, 1924 AC 689-1924

LEGISLATION

UK

Family Law Reform Act 1987
Human Fertilisation and Embryology Act 1990

EUROPE

Directive 2004/23/EC of the European Parliament and of the Council of 31 March 2004 on setting standards of quality and safety for the donation, procurement, testing, processing, preservation, storage, and distribution of human tissues and cells. Official Journal of the European Union, L 102/48.

2 The biology of donation

Martin H. Johnson

Introduction

It is commonly asserted that new technologies drive political, social and ethical changes. However, such influences are rarely unidirectional (Theodosiou and Johnson, 2011); indeed, historically the technologies and practices of sperm donation were themselves much influenced by social, ethical and political considerations. However, the advent of in vitro fertilization technology undoubtedly provided a powerful stimulus to sperm, embryo and egg donation, and the nature of many of the ethico-socio-political issues generated were themselves resolved or changed by the further refinements of single sperm injection, and the capacity to freeze and store gametes and embryos. Whether these technologies can or should be applied or not, and if so how, is of course much influenced by socio-ethical factors. This chapter examines some of the basic medico-scientific issues as a background to the complex and bidirectional interactions with ethics that follow.

Infertility and sterility

Fecundity is a measure of reproductive potential, and where that potential is zero, the individual (or couple, or population) is said to be sterile. In contrast, fertility is a measure of reproductive outcome and is usually expressed in terms of children born per woman, per couple or per population unit. Infertility is a measure of the failure to produce children, and is variously defined as occurring after a specified period of time – for example one or two years of attempts. Infertility may result from sterility but not necessarily so; a sole individual or two of the same sex will be infertile however long they try for children, but need not be sterile. This distinction has led to the concepts of medical and social infertility, and both are the subjects of this volume.

In considering the biology of donation, the 'stuff' of donation – the eggs, sperm and embryos – forms the meat of the chapter. Then an attempt is made to distinguish myths from risks.

The 'stuff' of donation

Reproductive donation can theoretically take a variety of forms. The donated tissues could be gametes (that is, spermatozoa, and eggs – or oocytes), embryos, blastomeres (that is, the component cells of one embryo which can contribute to a second embryo to form a chimaera), uteri (as in surrogacy) or embryonic stem cells (ESCs) – both as ESCs or as gametes derived in vitro from them. Subcellular 'donation' is also possible, for example of organelles such as mitochondria, nuclei or centrioles, or of genes or cytoplasm. Currently, clinical practice focuses on gametes, embryos and uteri, or more strictly 'uterine time and space'. However, even within this restricted domain, a variety of donation practices exist. Amongst these practices is the storage and use of cryopreserved (frozen) donated material. Given the increasingly intertwined relationship between donation and cryostorage, the principles of the latter are considered first. Then donation of sperm, embryos and eggs are considered in turn, followed by consideration of underlying biological issues for 'uterine donation' in surrogacy. This chapter ends with a look at scientific risks and myths.

Cryopreservation and donation

Cryopreservation forms an integral element in most medically assisted gamete and embryo donations and in surrogacy (Shufaro and Schenker, 2010). Cryopreservation allows long-term storage with minimal degradation of the biological samples. The lower the temperature of storage, the less degradation will occur, just as deep-frozen food keeps longer than refrigerated food. In practice, clinical storage at -196°C is achieved by immersion in liquid nitrogen (liquid phase storage) or in the vapour above it (gas phase storage). The fundamental problem for cryostorage is the avoidance of irreversible damage during freezing and thawing. Because biological tissues consist mainly of water, ice crystals will form during freezing and, due to the peculiar property of water, which on freezing forms ice crystals that occupy a larger volume than the liquid water from which they were made, cell disruption and lysis occur. An additional hazard is that as ice forms, the salts in the tissue fluids are excluded from the crystals and so become very concentrated and cause osmotic damage to cells.

This problem has been circumvented by use of biologically effective cryoprotectants that act as a form of 'anti-freeze'. Natural cryoprotectants are present in organisms exposed to sub-zero temperatures, but for freezing in liquid nitrogen higher levels of chemical cryoprotectants, such as glycerol or dimethylsulphoxide (DMSO), are used. Two approaches to the use of cryoprotectants are available. Conventionally they were added to cells in increasing concentrations allowing time for equilibration and then slowly cooled in a controlled freezing apparatus. This procedure can bring its own potential problems as the prolonged exposure to cryoprotectant at higher temperatures may itself have damaging effects, and so protocols for their equilibration must be carefully determined, largely empirically. Recently, an alternative approach has been used that relies on ultra-rapid cooling of cells or tissues so that the water transforms into a glassy state, a process known as 'vitrification' (Bhat *et al.*, 2005). This process is usually used in conjunction with high levels of cryoprotectant, but the rapidity of freezing means that damage due to cryoprotectant is, theoretically at least, less likely.

When cryopreserving large numbers of cells, such as the many spermatozoa in a semen sample, some loss of cells through toxicity or freezing is compatible with biological functionality of the sample. However, with eggs and embryos, where a single cell or few cells are present, such losses cannot be tolerated. Moreover, eggs and early embryos present special problems in that the cells are much larger than sperm cells and large cells are more difficult to freeze as the equilibration of the cryoprotectant between the inside and outside of the cell takes longer.

Cryopreserved tissues can, in principle, be stored indefinitely, although where regulations exist, limits of 5–10 years are common. No effects of duration of freezing on fertility outcomes have been reported (Riggs *et al.*, 2008).

Gametes and embryos

Spermatozoa Semen may be inseminated into the vagina, or spermatozoa, after being washed free of seminal fluid, may be inseminated vaginally into the cervix (intra-cervical insemination: ICI) or uterus (intra-uterine insemination: IUI). Surgical insemination, together with eggs, into the Fallopian tube (or oviduct) is called gamete intra-Fallopian transfer (GIFT). Sperm may also be injected directly into an egg in vitro (intra-cytoplasmic sperm injection: ICSI), or may be used outside the body to inseminate eggs as with in vitro fertilization (IVF). Embryos resulting from either ICSI or IVF are cultured in vitro for 2 to 5 days and then transferred to uteri.

Of the above techniques, only vaginal insemination does not require medical assistance, and may be supported through self-help organizations, commercial firms and websites that exist for this non-medical practice (e.g. Clarke and Saffron, 2006). Donation, other than by vaginal insemination of fresh semen, is considered part of the range of assisted reproductive technologies (ARTs) and maybe regulated as such. While use of spermatozoa by insemination has a long history (see Richards, Pennings and Appleby, Chapter 1), the first reports of successful use in IVF to establish full-term pregnancies dates from 1978 (Edwards and Steptoe, 1978) and for ICSI from 1992 (Palermo *et al.*, 1992).

Spermatozoa may be recovered by masturbation, or surgically by aspiration from, or microsurgical dissection of, either the testis (testicular sperm extraction: TESE), or epididymis (percutaneous or micro-epididymal sperm aspiration: PESA or MESA), or may be recovered from the urine in cases of retrograde ejaculation (in which sperm ejaculate into the bladder) or male sexual dysfunction. Where sperm are relatively abundant and motile they are used for IUI or IVF and usually, for donation, after cryopreservation. Donations of high-quality sperm can be used in IUI, IVF or ICSI, but for any donation where the number, maturity or motility of spermatozoa are poor (for example, use of a relative's sperm), they are usually used fresh in an ICSI procedure because cryostorage is not consistently successful (AbdelHafez *et al.*, 2009). However, the problem of cryopreserving small numbers of male germ cells is becoming an issue clinically, either because of the few sperm recoverable by TESE/PESA so as to avoid repeat biopsy (AbdelHafez *et al.*, 2009) or of immature germ cells from boys undergoing chemotherapy with the aim of subsequently generating sperm ex vivo (Wyns *et al.*, 2010).

Cryopreservation is used for various reasons: for convenience; to quarantine the semen (defined as the spermatozoa plus associated fluids) in case it carries infectious agents (such as HIV, hepatitis viruses and cytomegalovirus); to provide the opportunity for repeated or multiple use of the same donor; and in advance of cancer (and other) therapies that use potentially damaging spermotoxic drugs, radiation or surgery.

The main adverse medical outcome from spermatozoal donation is the risk of transmission of infection or genetic defects in inadequately screened donors/samples, or from contamination introduced during handling or cryopreservation (Bielanski and Vajta, 2009) and storage (Tomlinson and Sakkas, 2000). There is a small but significant risk of side-effects from the procedures involved in IVF or ICSI, such as ovarian hyperstimulation

Table 1 *Official outcome data for the UK and USA. These crude data ignore age variations in women receiving treatment and also multiple births − see published sources for richer details.*

Type of donation: UK*	No. IVF treatment cycles initiated	Live births/cycle initiated
Fresh *donor* eggs/embryos	1,748	26%
Frozen *non-donor* embryos	8,541	30%
Donor sperm	3,876	11%
Type of donation: USA**	No. IVF cycles in which 0 transfer occurred	Live births/embryo transfer
Fresh *donor* eggs/embryos	10,349	55%
Frozen *donor* embryos	7,056	32%
Fresh *non-donor* embryos	82,347	36%
Frozen *non-donor* embryos	23,133	30%

*UK National returns for 2007 from Human Fertilisation and Embryology Authority at www.hfea.gov.uk/.
** USA Federal data for 2007 from Centers for Disease Control and Prevention at www. cdc.gov/art/ARTReports.htm. Donor Insemination (DI) is not recorded.

syndrome and increased risk of birth defects. Undoubtedly the most problematic medical outcome from using any of these procedures is the increased risk of a multiple pregnancy. Some outcome rates for medically assisted donation by different routes are summarized in Table 1.

Embryos Embryo donation has become a realistic and routine clinical procedure only since the advent of IVF in 1978, the first reported case being that by Trounson *et al.* (1983) using fresh embryos – although the trisomy 21 pregnancy was lost spontaneously at 10 weeks, and the study was criticized as being unethical on account of the donor being 42 years old and infertile (Edwards and Steptoe, 1983). Prior to 1983 there was considerable discussion about the ethico-legal status of embryo transfer (see for example Craft and Yovich, 1979; Cusine, 1979). However, IVF is not strictly essential for donation, as indicated by a human pregnancy following recovery by uterine lavage of embryos generated by fertilization in vivo followed by transfer to an infertile recipient (Buster *et al.* 1983, 1985; Bustillo *et al.*, 1984).

Use of fresh embryos for transfer brought problems of possible cross-infection, and also the requirement to synchronize the cycles of donor and recipient. The freezing of embryos, with their subsequent thawing and transfer to achieve a clinical pregnancy, was described for animals by Whittingham *et al.* (1972) and for humans by Trounson and Mohr (1983) and Zeilmaker *et al.* (1984).

Studies of the obstetric outcome of the use of cryopreserved early cleavage embryos do not indicate any increase in preterm birth or low birth-weight compared with children born after fresh cycles. Most studies report comparable neonatal malformation rates between frozen and fresh IVF/ICSI cycles. Limited outcome data are available for vitrification of early cleavage stage embryos and blastocysts, as well as for slow freezing of blastocysts. Long-term follow-up studies of children born after embryo cryopreservation are lacking (Wennerholm *et al.*, 2009).

Eggs (oocytes)   Egg donation is indicated where a woman is unable to produce healthy eggs of her own, whether due to age, to previous chemotherapy, to ovarian dysgenesis, dysfunction or absence, or for genetic/chromosomal/infection reasons. Donation can be absolute or via egg-sharing in which one woman receives a free or reduced cost IVF treatment cycle in return for donating some of her eggs to a second woman, who pays for both treatment cycles (Johnson, 1999). The earliest suggestion we have found that egg donation (and indeed cryopreservation) might be clinically useful is a letter to *The Lancet* from Craft and Yovich (1979; see also Pembrey, 1979), which is ambiguous about whether they have actually offered or tried it – possibly for legal reasons. Thereafter egg donation appears in the literature from about 1982 (Craft *et al.*, 1982).

Until recently, only fresh eggs were used, which meant that supplies were very limited and synchronization of treatment cycles between donor and recipient was required, thereby limiting the opportunities for egg donation and increasing the risk of infection transmission. The cryopreservation of eggs in a state that reliably preserves their fertility has lagged far behind that of spermatozoa and embryos – a situation that arises because egg freezing poses particular problems.

First, whereas sperm are usually abundant and can suffer some losses, and eight-cell embryos can survive the loss of one or two cells, each egg is a single cell, so its death is a 100 per cent loss. Second, unfertilized eggs are ovulated partway through an arrested cell division with their chromosomes sitting on a very thermolabile structure called a spindle. Both cooling and cryoprotectants have been shown to affect spindle structure in ways that lead to the dispersal of chromosomes, potentially resulting in chromosomal anomalies in any embryos that result from the fertilization of those oocytes that survive the freezing process (Pickering *et al.*, 1990). Third, the zona pellucida, an acellular membrane that surrounds the egg and through which the spermatozoa must penetrate if fertilization is to occur, is hardened and rendered impenetrable by cooling and thawing (Johnson *et al.*, 1988; Vincent *et al.*, 1990), unless preventative strategies are adopted or ICSI is used to bypass the zona (George *et al.*, 1993). Moreover, human eggs seem particularly sensitive to such damage (Pickering *et al.*, 1990, 1991) compared with mouse eggs, which some years ago were successfully frozen, thawed, fertilized and transferred to uteri to produce viable pregnancies at equivalent rates to control eggs (George *et al.*, 1994). Thus, despite sporadic claims to successful pregnancies after egg-freezing from the late 1980s (Chen, 1988), until recently human eggs have proved resistant to consistently successful freezing. The past twenty years has witnessed slowly improving post-thaw viability, chromosomal normality, fertilizability and rates of blastocyst development (Gook *et al.*, 1994; Cobo *et al.*, 2001; Rienzi *et al.*, 2004), which were followed by claims to pregnancies (Porcu *et al.*, 2000; Quintans *et al.*, 2002; Borini *et al.*, 2004). Modifications to these slow-freeze protocols for eggs have incrementally improved implantation and pregnancy outcomes (De Santis *et al.*, 2007; Bianchi *et al.*, 2007). More recently, egg vitrification has been reported to result in faster spindle recovery post-thaw than slow-freeze protocols (Ciotti *et al.* 2009; Noyes *et al.*, 2010b), and case reports of births after egg vitrification have been reported (Kuleshova *et al.*, 2002; Oakes *et al.*, 2008).

Three studies have now compared fertilization, development, implantation and pregnancy outcome rates for slow-frozen or vitrified oocytes with those for non-frozen matched controls (Cobo *et al.*, 2008; Grifo and Noyes, 2010; Nagy *et al.*, 2009). While numbers are small (20–23 frozen oocyte cycles per study), comparability of outcomes is claimed. No increased population incidence of low birth weight or congenital abnormalities has been found after use of frozen oocytes (Chian *et al.*, 2008; Noyes *et al.*, 2009). Taken together, these outcomes have led to a plea that oocyte freezing no longer be regarded as an experimental treatment (Noyes *et al.*, 2010a). While this may be the case for experienced clinics, and warranted for women for whom no other option for preserving or promoting fertility is available, the variability in outcomes among clinics may make a clinic-by-clinic approach to the more general use of egg freezing advisable.

Surrogacy – donation of uterine use

Surrogacy involves the 'donation' of her uterus by a women (the surrogate) to carry a pregnancy for 'commissioning' couples lacking a uterus anatomically or functionally or for health reasons. Surrogacy may be *traditional* (also called straight surrogacy), in which the surrogate uses her own egg with sperm from a commissioning couple's male partner. Such a form of surrogacy is used if there is no commissioning female partner (two gay men for example) or where the female does not have her own eggs. Traditional surrogacy can be achieved non-medically by intercourse or artificial insemination, but often is medically facilitated for health reasons (see Braverman, Casey and Jadva, Chapter 16).

Medical intervention is required for *gestational* (or host) surrogacy in which an embryo created from the commissioning couple's gametes is placed in the uterus of the surrogate. The biological issues concerning the donation of the uterus concern primarily the age of the surrogate and the impact this might have on her capacity to initiate and carry the pregnancy to term successfully. These issues are most likely to come into play when older women act as surrogates for younger family members. It is perfectly possible for older women to carry a pregnancy to term, but the incidence of prematurity, low birth weights, perinatal death and congenital abnormalities increases (Pasupathy *et al.*, 2011; Salem Yaniv *et al.*, 2011).

Novelty, myths and risks

When moving from experiments on humans to use of experimental therapies, the ethico-legal landscape changes. Experiments on humans are governed by a number of international treaties mostly arising from the Nuremburg trials (see Klitzman, Chapter 3), whereas experimental therapies are governed primarily by the ethics of the doctor–patient relationship. Broadly, for experimental therapies to be ethical, the doctor must be convinced that net benefit will accrue to the patient, who must give informed and competent consent to these novel treatments. In the early days of ART, the hurdle of net benefit was set high for novel interventions to relieve infertility (Johnson *et al.*, 2010). However, that hurdle has been lowered with the greater familiarity with ARTs, with a wider range of novel therapies, and given the heterogeneous socio-religious locations in which these new therapies are practised (see Chapters 4–8).

Novelty is associated with public hope but also anxiety, both often fanned by disproportionate media coverage of inflated claims or of a few problematic outcomes, respectively. Outcomes must be monitored and acted upon if we are to avoid the thalidomide and diethylstilboestrol tragedies of the 1960s, as well as the various problems arising for some women from oral contraception. A careful assessment of risks and benefits should be undertaken in advance and throughout the early phases of novel treatment use, and the basis of individual variations in responsiveness to different treatments that characterize human needs to be understood and managed. In this section some of these issues are addressed from a biological perspective for both existing and potential donation practices.

Cryopreservation and long-term follow-up

The absence of long-term follow-up studies of children born after embryo cryopreservation was noted earlier, although neonatal outcomes are reassuring (Wennerholm et al., 2009). Similarly, there is no suggestion of any major adverse events arising from use of cryopreserved spermatozoa (Lansac and Royere, 2001). For eggs, proceeding with care seems to be the appropriate course for the immediate future.

Are pregnancies from egg and embryo donation at increased risk of miscarriage?

Following in vivo fertilization, the fetus shares half its genes with its mother. However, after egg or embryo donation (including gestational surrogacy), the genetic disparity between mother and fetus will be much greater. Recent evidence suggests that for some women this increased disparity might be problematic. Thus, several common disorders of pregnancy, such as recurrent miscarriage, pre-eclampsia and fetal growth restriction, seem to be associated with poor invasion of the maternal uterine lining by the trophoblast cells early in pregnancy. Trophoblast tissue is the major cell type of fetal origin in the placenta, and the effectiveness of its invasion is in turn affected by interactions between the trophoblast cells and maternally derived immune cells called uterine natural killer (uNK) cells. Key interactions between uNKs and the trophoblast cells are mediated by interacting molecules on their surfaces – specifically between trophoblast HLA-C molecules and killer Ig-like receptors (KIRs) on the uNK cells. In the general population there are many genetic variants of both KIR and the HLA-C molecules. This variation seems to be important for reproductive outcome, because certain combinations of maternal KIR and fetal HLA-C are associated with an increased risk of pre-eclampsia and recurrent miscarriage. In particular, it is one type of paternally derived HLA-C variant (C2) that is problematic in a subset of women with certain KIRs (AA genotype). Clearly, the chances of both the paternal and maternal HLA-C type being 'wrong' will be there when donated eggs and embryos are used. These data raise the possibility that the incidence of pre-eclampsia and miscarriage may be higher after donation for a subgroup of women (Hiby *et al.*, 2010). A genetic study of pregnancies resulting from egg or embryo donation needs to be performed to see if indeed this hypothesis is correct. If this does turn out to be true, then HLA-C/KIR typing of the donors and recipients may be indicated in order to minimize the risk. Such a screening process is premature until the outcome of further research is known.

Subcellular donation?

Various forms of donation involving subcomponents of the egg have been discussed and/or attempted in animals and humans. Basically they reduce to two broad categories: *cytoplasmic*, including mitochondria, and *nuclear*, including the nuclear genetic complement – also called 'cloning'. Both types of donation are most usually justified clinically in terms of helping avoid the transmission of certain mitochondrial diseases, and discussion here will be largely restricted to this aspect.

Mitochondria constitute a major energy-generating component of the body's tissues. They are small intra-cellular cytoplasmic organelles, and each cell has many of them. Each mitochondrion carries its own DNA (mtDNA) in a single small chromosome, and each of these mtDNAs can be mutated independently, thereby generating a genetically heterogeneous population of mitochondria in the cytoplasm of each cell (called heteroplasmy). Some of these mutations affect mitochondrial function adversely, and if the balance of mitochondria in a cell or tissue tips too far towards malfunction, distressing pathologies can become evident (Schapira, 2006). Mitochondrial genetic disease can be transmitted to children, but only via the mother through her egg cytoplasm. This maternal transmission arises because the egg synthesizes large numbers of mitochondria, while the sperm does not contribute any to the embryo (Aiken *et al.*, 2008). Thus, if a woman is known to carry a high proportion of abnormal mitochondria with a high risk of transmitting them to her children, she may want to have a 'mitochondrial donation'. This can in principle be achieved either by injecting some cytoplasm from a 'healthy' egg into her eggs, or by transferring a nucleus from one of her eggs into the cytoplasm of an enucleated 'healthy' egg.

Cytoplasmic transfer was used in 1997 in an attempt to overcome the supposed cytoplasmic deficiencies in the eggs of older women with recurrent implantation failure (Cohen *et al.*, 1997). By 2001 over thirty births had been reported worldwide, and evidence that injected mtDNA could be detected in at least some of these offspring was presented (Barritt *et al.*, 2001). However, worries were expressed about both the safety and efficacy of this approach (Malter and Cohen, 2002; Brown *et al.*, 2006), the US Federal Drug Administration intervened, and the programme has ceased (Malter, 2011).

The alternative strategy, namely transferring the nuclear material from the egg of an affected woman into the enucleated egg cytoplasm of an unaffected woman has not, to my knowledge, been attempted. However, this strategy did successfully overcome mtDNA mutations in mice (Sato *et al.*, 2005), and a research licence to examine this question in humans was granted in the UK by the Human Fertilisation and Embryology Authority (HFEA) in 2005. Some of the more practical and ethical issues with both of these approaches are considered in more detail by Bredenoord *et al.* (2008) and Fulka *et al.* (2009).

What are the genetic risks of consanguinity?

Fear of consanguinity has influenced regulatory responses to use of (especially male) donors' gametes in some jurisdictions, usually through attempts to restrict the number of offspring resulting from a single donor and/or the provision of registers so that donor offspring can check for relatedness to a potential partner. In population genetics, consanguinity (or in-breeding) refers to any departure from non-random mating patterns, that is mating with an individual who is genetically more similar to you than if you mated at random in the population. It follows that there are degrees of consanguinity depending on how many ancestors in common a couple has. There is a strong socio-cultural element to the acceptability of consanguineous relationships. Generally speaking, European and North American Christian-based cultures frown on them, whereas many Middle Eastern and Asian countries encourage them. These cultural differences affect the relative acceptability of gamete donation (see B. Gürtin and Vayena, Chapter 5). Incest is a socio-legal term used to describe proscribed sexual relationships.

Offspring of consanguineous unions may be at an increased risk for pregnancy loss and/or genetic disorders if autosomal recessive gene mutations are inherited from a common ancestor. When the biological relationship between the couple is close, the probability that their offspring will inherit identical copies of a detrimental recessive gene increases. Thus, half-siblings share 1/4 of their genes, so the chance of receiving two copies of an autosomally recessive gene, and so manifesting a genetic condition, is 1/8. Of course, if there is more than one autosomal recessive gene in the family line, the risk of a genetic disorder goes up accordingly. There may also be an increased risk of disorders with an underlying multifactorial genetic basis, but that is less clearly established. Thus, it is difficult to generalize about the consequences for donor offspring of consanguinity. Epidemiological data are hard to come by because the social stigma attached to incest means that there are difficulties in ascertainment (see Bittles, 2001; Bennett *et al.*, 2002).

Donation of 'artificial gametes' made from stem cells?

Stem cells are pluripotent, self-renewing cells that arise during normal development, and can also be induced in vitro. Stem cells may be fully competent and able to generate a complete individual, such as embryonic stem cells (ESCs) or induced stem cells (ISCs), or show tissue-restricted developmental potential, such as germ-line, spermatogenic or oogenic stem cells. The recent surge of interest in stem cell biology has resulted in several claims to have developed gamete-like cells in vitro from human and animal stem cells, some of which, in animals, have been used successfully in fertilization to produce live young – albeit with massive pregnancy losses and little long-term survival (see Zhou *et al.*, 2010 for review). However, the success rates are currently very low and the procedures highly experimental. Were they to improve for humans, they might reduce the demand for donation. Thus, chemical transformation of any somatic cell from the body of an infertile man or woman to make ISCs, or transfer of an infertile patient's somatic cell nucleus to an enucleated egg followed by production of ESCs, could be followed by the differentiation from the SCs of sperm or eggs in vitro to replace the missing gametes. Such a scenario is unlikely to work for some genetic forms of infertility, but would be of use for those who have lost functional gametes through accident, disease or age. It is, however, unlikely to work for gay or lesbian couples hoping to make 'opposite-sex' gametes from ISCs of one of the partners. This is because, in lesbian couples, the presence of two X chromosomes seems to be incompatible with sperm formation, while for gay couples, the absence of two X chromosomes seems to be incompatible with egg cell development.

However, such therapies seem a long way off, so donation is likely to be needed for some time yet!

REFERENCES

AbdelHafez, F., Bedaiwy, M., El-Nashar, S. A., Sabanegh, E., *et al.* (2009). 'Techniques for cryopreservation of individual or small numbers of human spermatozoa: a systematic review'. *Human Reproduction Update*, 15, 153–64.

Aiken, C. E. M., Cindrova-Davies, T. and Johnson, M. H. (2008). 'Temporal and tissue variations in mitochondrial DNA levels from fertilisation to birth in the mouse are associated with oxidative stress'. *Reproductive BioMedicine Online*, 17, 806–13.

Barritt, J. A., Brenner, C. A., Malter, H. E. and Cohen, J. (2001). 'Mitochondria in human offspring derived from ooplasmic transplantation'. *Human Reproduction*, 16, 513–16.

Bennett, R. L., Hart, K. A., O'Rourke, E., Barranger, J. A., *et al.* (2002). 'Genetic counseling and screening of consanguineous couples and their offspring: recommendations of the National Society of Genetic Counselors'. *Journal of Genetic Counseling*, 11, 97–119.

Bhat, S. N., Sharma, A. and Bhat, S. V. (2005). 'Vitrification and glass transition of water: insights from spin probe ESR'. *Physical Review Letters*, 2, 95(23): 235702 (epub only).

Bianchi, V., Cottichio, G., Distratis, V., Di Giusto, N., *et al.* (2007). 'Differential sucrose concentration during dehydration (0.2 Mol/L) and rehydration (0.3 Mol/L) increases the implantation rate of frozen human oocytes'. *Reproductive BioMedicine Online*, 14, 64–71.

Bielanski, A. and Vajta, G. (2009). 'Risk of contamination of germplasm during cryopreservation and cryobanking in IVF units'. *Human Reproduction*, 24, 2457–67.

Bittles, A. (2001). 'Consanguinity and its relevance to clinical genetics'. *Clinical Genetics*, 60, 89–98.

Borini, A., Bonu, M. A., Coticchio, G., Bianchi, V., *et al.* (2004). 'Pregnancies and births after oocyte cryopreservation'. *Fertility and Sterility*, 82, 601–5.

Bredenoord, A. L., Pennings, G. and de Wert, G. (2008). 'Ooplasmic and nuclear transfer to prevent mitochondrial DNA disorders: conceptual and normative issues'. *Human Reproduction Update*, 14, 669–78.

Brown, D. T., Herbert, M., Lamb, V. K. Chinnery, P. F., *et al.* (2006). 'Transmission of mitochondrial DNA disorders: possibilities for the future'. *The Lancet*, 368, 87–9.

Buster, J. E., Bustillo, M. and Thorneycroft, I. (1983). 'Non-surgical transfer of an in-vivo fertilised donated ovum to an infertility patient'. *The Lancet*, 321, 816–7.

Buster, J. E., Bustillo, M., Rodi, I. A., Cohen, S. W., *et al.* (1985). 'Biologic and morphologic development of donated human ova recovered by non-surgical uterine lavage'. *American Journal of Obstetrics and Gynecology*, 153, 211–7.

Bustillo, M., Buster, J. E., Cohen, S. W., Thorneycroft, I. H., *et al.* (1984). 'Nonsurgical ovum transfer as a treatment in infertile women. Preliminary experience'. *Journal of the American Medical Association*, 251, 1171–3.

Chen, C. (1988). 'Pregnancies after human oocyte cryopreservation'. *Annals of the New York Academy of Sciences*, 541, 541–9.

Chian, R. C., Huang, J. Y., Tan, S. L., Lucena, E., *et al.* (2008). 'Obstetric and perinatal outcome in 200 infants conceived from vitrified oocytes'. *Reproductive Biomedicine Online*, 16, 608–10.

Ciotti, P. M., Porcu, E., Notarangelo, L., Magrini, O., *et al.* (2009). 'Meiotic spindle recovery is faster in vitrification of human oocytes compared to slow freezing'. *Fertility and Sterility*, 91, 2399–407.

Clarke, V. and Saffron, L. (2006). 'Challenging preconceptions about lesbian parenting: Victoria Clarke in conversation with Lisa Saffron'. *Lesbian & Gay Psychology Review*, 7, 78–85. Available at: http://eprints.uwe.ac.uk/11728/.

Cobo, A., Rubio, C., Gerli, S., Ruiz, A., *et al.* (2001). 'Use of fluorescence in situ hybridization to assess the chromosomal status of embryos obtained from cryopreserved oocytes'. *Fertility and Sterility*, 75, 354–60.

Cobo, A., Kuwayama, M., Perez, S., Ruiz, A., *et al.* (2008). 'Comparison of concomitant outcome achieved with fresh and cryopreserved donor oocytes vitrified by the CryoTop method'. *Fertility and Sterility*, 89, 1657–64.

Cohen, J., Scott, R., Schimmel, T., Levron, J., *et al.* (1997). 'Birth of infant after transfer of anuclear donor oocyte cytoplasm into recipient eggs'. *The Lancet*, 350, 186–7.

Craft, I. and Yovich, J. (1979). 'Implications of embryo transfer'. *The Lancet*, 314, 642–3.

Craft, I., McLeod, F., Bernard, A., Green, S., *et al.* (1982). 'Birth following oocyte and sperm transfer to the uterus'. *The Lancet*, 320, 773.

Cusine, D. J. (1979). 'Some legal implications of embryo transfer'. *The Lancet*, 314, 407–8.

De Santis, L., Cino, I., Rabelloti, E., Papaleo, E., *et al.* (2007). 'Oocyte cryopreservation: clinical outcome of slow-cooling protocols differing in sucrose concentration'. *Reproductive Biomedicine Online*, 14, 57–63.

Edwards, R. G. and Steptoe, P. C. (1978). 'Birth after the reimplantation of a human embryo'. *The Lancet*, 312, 366.

(1983). 'Pregnancy in an infertile patient after transfer of an embryo fertilised in vitro'. *British Medical Journal*, 286, 1351.

Fulka, H., Langerova, A., Barnetova, I., Novakova, Z., *et al.* (2009). 'How to repair the oocyte and zygote?' *Journal of Reproduction and Development*, 55, 583–7.

George, M. A., Johnson, M. H. and Vincent, C. (1993). 'Use of fetal bovine serum to protect against zona hardening during preparation of mouse oocytes for cryopreservation'. *Human Reproduction*, 7, 408–12.

George, M. A., Johnson, M. H. and Howlett, S. K. (1994). 'Assessment of the developmental potential of frozen-thawed mouse oocytes'. *Human Reproduction*, 9, 130–6.

Gook, D. A., Osborn, S. M., Bourne, H. and Johnston, W. I. (1994). 'Fertilization of human oocytes following cryopreservation: normal karyotypes and absence of stray chromosomes'. *Human Reproduction*, 9, 684–91.

Grifo, J. A. and Noyes, N. (2010). 'Delivery rate using cryopreserved oocytes is comparable to conventional in vitro fertilization using fresh oocytes: potential fertility preservation for female cancer patients'. *Fertility and Sterility*, 93, 391–6.

Hiby, S. E., Apps, R., Sharkey, A. M., Farrell, L. E., *et al.* (2010). 'Maternal activating KIRs protect against human reproductive failure mediated by fetal HLA-C2'. *The Journal of Clinical Investigation*, 120, 4102–10.

Johnson, M. H. (1999). 'The medical ethics of paid egg sharing in the UK'. *Human Reproduction*, 14, 1912–8.

Johnson, M. H., Pickering, S. J. and George, M. A. (1988). 'The influence of cooling on the properties of the zona pellucida of the mouse oocyte'. *Human Reproduction*, 3, 383–7.

Johnson, M. H., Franklin, S. B., Cottingham, M. and Hopwood, N. (2010). 'Why the Medical Research Council refused Robert Edwards and Patrick Steptoe support for research on human conception in 1971'. *Human Reproduction*, 25, 2157–74.

Kuleshova, L., Gianaroli, L., Magli, C., Ferraretti, A., *et al.* (2002). 'Birth following vitrification of a small number of human oocytes: case report'. *Human Reproduction*, 14, 3077–9.

Lansac, J. and Royere, D. (2001). 'Follow-up studies of children born after frozen sperm donation'. *Human Reproduction Update*, 7, 33–7.

Malter, H. E. (2011). 'Fixing oocytes? A bovine model provides new hope'. *Reproductive Biomedicine Online*, 22, 229–31.

Malter, H. E. and Cohen, J. (2002). 'Ooplasmic transfer: animal models assist human studies'. *Reproductive Biomedicine Online*, 5, 26–35.

Nagy, Z. P., Chang, C. C., Shapiro, D. B., Bernal, D. P., *et al.* (2009). 'Clinical evaluation of the efficiency of an oocyte donation program using egg cryo-banking'. *Fertility and Sterility*, 92, 520–6.

Noyes, N., Porcu, E. and Borini, A. (2009). 'Over 900 oocyte cryopreser-vation babies born with no apparent increase in congenital anomalies'. *Reproductive Biomedicine Online*, 18, 769–76.

Noyes, N., Boldt, J. and Nagy, Z. P. (2010a). 'Oocyte cryopreservation: is it time to remove its experimental label?' *Journal of Assisted Reproduction and Genetics*, 27, 69–74.

Noyes, N., Knopman, J., Labella, P., McCaffrey, C., *et al.* (2010b). 'Oocyte cryopreservation outcomes including pre-cryo and post-thaw meiotic spin-dle evaluation following slow cooling and vitrification of human oocytes'. *Fertility and Sterility*, 94, 2078–82.

Oakes, M. B., Gomes, C. M., Fioraventi, J., Serafini, P., *et al.* (2008). 'A case of oocyte and embryo vitrification resulting in clinical pregnancy'. *Fertility and Sterility*, 90, 2013.

Palermo, G., Joris, H., Devroey, P. and Van Steirteghem, A. C. (1992). 'Pregnancies after intracytoplasmic injection of single spermatozoon into an oocyte'. *The Lancet*, 340, 17–18.

Pasupathy, D., Wood, A. M., Pell, J. P., Fleming, M., *et al.* (2011). 'Advanced maternal age and the risk of perinatal death due to intrapartum anoxia at term'. *Journal of Epidemiology and Community Health*, 65, 241–5 (epub ahead of print 18 August 2010).

Pembrey, M. (1979). 'Embryo transfer in prevention of genetic disease'. *The Lancet*, 314, 802.

Pickering, S. J., Braude, P. R., Johnson, M. H., Cant, A., *et al.* (1990). 'Transient cooling to room temperature can cause irreversible disruption of the meiotic spindle in the human oocyte'. *Fertility and Sterility*, 54, 102–8.

Pickering, S. J., Braude, P. R. and Johnson, M. H. (1991). 'Cryoprotection of human oocytes: inappropriate exposure to DMSO reduces fertilization rates'. *Human Reproduction*, 6, 142–3.

Porcu, E., Fabbri, R., Damiano, G., Giunchi, S., *et al.* (2000). 'Clinical experience and applications of oocyte cryopreservation'. *Molecular and Cellular Endocrinology*, 169, 33–7.

Quintans, C. J., Donaldson, M. J., Bertolino, M. and Pasqualini, R. (2002). 'Birth of two babies using oocytes that were cryopreserved in a choline based freezing medium'. *Human Reproduction*, 17, 3149–52.

Rienzi, L., Martinez, F., Ubaldi, F., Minagi, M. G., *et al.* (2004). 'Polscope analysis of meiotic spindle changes in living metaphase II human oocytes during the freezing and thawing procedures'. *Human Reproduction*, 19, 655–9.

Riggs, R., Mayer, J., Dowling-Lacey, D., Chi, T. F., *et al.* (2008). 'Does storage time influence postthaw survival and pregnancy outcome? An analysis of 11,768 cryopreserved human embryos'. *Fertility and Sterility*, 93, 109–15.

Salem Yaniv, S., Levy, A., Wiznitzer, A., Holcberg, G., *et al.* (2011). 'A significant linear association exists between advanced maternal age and adverse perinatal outcome'. *Archives of Gynecology and Obstetrics*, 283(4), 755–9 (epub 8 April 2010).

Sato, A., Kono, T., Nakada, K., Ishikawa, K., *et al.* (2005). 'Gene therapy for progeny of mito-mice carrying pathogenic mtDNA by nuclear transplantation'. *Proceedings of the National Academy of Sciences USA*, 102, 16765–70.

Schapira, A. H. V. (2006). 'Mitochondrial disease'. *The Lancet*, 368, 70–82.

Shufaro, Y. and Schenker, J. G. (2010). 'Cryopreservation of human genetic material'. *Annals of the New York Academy of Sciences*, 1205, 220–4.

Theodosiou, A. A. and Johnson, M. H. (2011). 'The politics of human embryo research and the motivation to achieve PGD'. *Reproductive BioMedicine Online*, DOI, 22, 457–4710.

Tomlinson, M. and Sakkas, D. (2000). 'Is a review of standard procedures for cryopreservation needed? Safe and effective cryopreservation – should sperm banks and fertility centres move toward storage in nitrogen vapour?' *Human Reproduction*, 15, 2460–3.

Trounson, A. and Mohr, L. (1983). 'Human pregnancy following cryo-preservation, thawing and transfer of an eight-cell embryo'. *Nature*, 305, 707–9.

Trounson, A., Leeton, J., Besanko, M., Wood, C., *et al.* (1983). 'Pregnancy established in an infertile patient after transfer of a donated embryo fertilised in vitro'. *British Medical Journal*, 286, 835–8.

Vincent, C., Pickering, S. J. and Johnson, M. H. (1990). 'The hardening effect of dimethylsulphoxide on the zona pellucida requires the presence of an oocyte and is associated with a reduction in the number of cortical granules present'. *Reproduction*, 89, 253–9.

Wennerholm, U-B., Soderstrom-Anttila, V., Bergh, C., Aittomaki, K., *et al.* (2009). 'Children born after cryopreservation of embryos or oocytes: a systematic review of outcome data'. *Human Reproduction*, 24, 2158–72.

Whittingham, D. G., Leibo, S. P. and Mazur, P. (1972). 'Survival of mouse embryos frozen to –196 degrees and –269 degrees C'. *Science*, 178, 411–4.

Wyns, C., Curaba, M., Vanabelle, B., Van Langendonckt, A., *et al.* (2010). 'Options for fertility preservation in prepubertal boys'. *Human Reproduction Update*, 16, 312–28.

Zeilmaker, G. H., Alberda, A. T., van Gent, I., Rijkmans, C. M., *et al.* (1984). 'Two pregnancies following transfer of intact frozen-thawed embryos'. *Fertility and Sterility*, 42, 293–6.

Zhou, G. B., Meng, Q. G. and Li, N. (2010). 'In vitro derivation of germ cells from embryonic stem cells in mammals'. *Molecular Reproduction and Development*, 77, 586–94.

3   Ethics for reproductive donation

Robert Klitzman

The growing use of assisted reproductive technologies (ART) poses a myriad of ethical dilemmas that clinicians, gamete donors and recipients, policy makers and others confront each day around the world. These dilemmas underlie the development and implementation of a range of institutional, professional and public policies. But various stakeholders view, interpret and respond to these conundrums in different ways that must be taken into account, and that generate numerous social science research questions.

In recent years, scholars and others have increasingly sought to build bridges between bioethics and social science (Ives, 2008; Ives and Draper, 2009). These efforts stem in part from heightened awareness of the fact that philosophical approaches to bioethics can be abstract in ways that make them difficult to apply in 'real world' settings. In addition, bioethics seeks to examine the ethical, legal and social implications of advances in biotechnology, necessitating multidisciplinary approaches, and posing questions as to how such integration can, or should best occur (Strech, Synofzik and Marckmann, 2008).

This book attempts to both engage in, and comment upon, these intersections between bioethics and social science, illustrating how these two sets of disciplinary realms can enrich each other, through complementary and integrative approaches and insights.

This chapter examines, first, several broad, underlying ethical principles, and then explores how these interface with social science in key areas of reproductive donation that subsequent chapters probe in further depth.

As we will see, psychology, sociology and other social sciences can elucidate how and why ethical principles get interpreted and applied in different contexts, and what these variations reveal about broader philosophical and sociological issues. Countries approach ARTs differently due to their history, culture and other characteristics. To understand how these various forces shape ethical discourse, and the weighing of competing ethical arguments, is extremely valuable in understanding the nature of, and interactions between, these ethical principles. The discussions here can thus illuminate not only these ethical issues, but also the cultural 'meanings' of these controversies, and larger issues involved. For instance, ethicists may be using concepts (e.g. of 'donor–patient relationships' or 'good parenting') that are insufficiently based on the social realities. Hence, resultant ethical analyses may inadequately address the ethical dilemmas involved (Hedgecoe, 2004) in ways that social science can identify.

Bioethicists must frequently weigh potential risks against potential benefits, and psychosocial research can also inform these efforts by shedding light on the actual risks and benefits. Importantly, social science can assess whether concerns about possible risks are legitimate or unsubstantiated.

Clear answers may not be possible for all of the ethical questions posed by ART, but researchers in psychology and other social sciences can clarify how health care providers, egg and sperm donors and recipients, policy makers and others in fact view and approach these dilemmas, what difficulties they encounter and what assistance (e.g. guidelines or education) might be helpful.

Still, as we will see, in the end, empirical data cannot always determine policy. Profound questions about the fair allocation of resources, for instance, may be involved, requiring value judgements that the polity as a whole (e.g. through its elected representatives or courts) must make.

What are the underlying ethical principles and where do they come from?

Historically, several key sets of medical ethics have been formulated. Each of these documents articulates principles that jointly form a framework for approaching issues and controversies now posed by ARTs. The basic underlying principles involved may appear deceptively simple. Indeed, it is the conflict that can emerge between them, and the definitions, interpretations and applications of each, that can create significant difficulties. Due to their importance for the subsequent discussions in this volume, several aspects of these sets of guidelines are quoted at length here.

Dating from the fifth century BC, the Hippocratic Oath stipulates 'never do harm to anyone', and '[a]ll that may come to my knowledge in the exercise of my profession or in daily commerce with men, which ought not to be spread abroad, I will keep secret and will never reveal'(North, 2002).

In the mid-twentieth century, following the atrocities of the Holocaust, in which the Nazis routinely conducted fatal experiments at concentration camps without the participants' consent, the Nuremberg Tribunal issued a document adding key principles in medical research (United States Department of Health and Human Services, 1949). This code includes the statements:

- 'The voluntary consent of the human subject is absolutely essential.'
- 'During the course of the experiment the human subject should be at liberty to bring the experiment to an end if he has reached the physical or mental state where continuation of the experiment seems to him to be impossible.'

Subsequently, the continued rise of medical research led the World Medical Association in 1964 to issue the Helsinki Declaration, which it subsequently revised in 1975, 1983, 1989, 1996, 2000, 2002, 2004 and 2008 (The World Medical Association, 2008). This document currently consists of thirty-five paragraphs, including:

- 'It is the duty of the physician to promote and safeguard the health of patients.'
- 'The health of my patient will be my first consideration.'
- 'A physician shall act in the patient's best interest when providing medical care.'
- 'In medical research involving human subjects, the well-being of the individual research subject must take precedence over all other interests.'

Yet well-publicized lapses of medical ethics continued to occur. In 1974, following the egregious ethical lapses in the Tuskegee syphilis study, the United States Congress passed the National Research Act, which mandated the development of an ethical code, which was subsequently published as the Belmont Report. This report presented four key principles: autonomy, beneficence, nonmaleficence and justice (The National Commission for the Protection of Human Subjects of Biomedical and Behavioral Research, 1979), presenting definitions of each of these terms:

- **Respect for Persons:** 'Respect for persons incorporates at least two ethical convictions – that individuals should be treated as autonomous agents, and that persons with diminished autonomy are entitled to protection.'

- **Beneficence:** 'one should not injure one person regardless of the benefits that might come to others ... The obligations of beneficence affect both individual investigators and society at large ... members of the larger society are obliged to recognize the longer term benefits and risks that may result.'
- **Nonmaleficence:** Ethics involves not only promoting the good, but also avoiding harm, which can in practice represent separate goals. Ethically, clinicians and policy makers seek not only to help patients (e.g. provide care), but prevent harm (e.g. prevent practices that may foster eugenics and injustice). As we will see, social science research can elucidate when, how, and to what degree these goals occur in actual situations.
- **Justice:** 'Who ought to receive the benefits of research and bear its burdens? This is a question of justice, in the sense of "fairness in distribution" or "what is deserved". An injustice occurs when some benefit to which a person is entitled is denied without good reason or when some burden is imposed unduly ... What considerations justify departure from equal distribution? ... There are several widely accepted formulations of just ways to distribute burdens and benefits: (1) to each person an equal share, (2) to each person according to individual need, (3) to each person according to individual effort, (4) to each person according to societal contribution, and (5) to each person according to merit.'

The Belmont Report also lays out other concepts that are involved in the implementation of these principles through informed consent:

- **Voluntariness:** 'This element of informed consent requires conditions free of coercion and undue influence ... Undue influence, by contrast, occurs through an offer of an excessive, unwarranted, inappropriate or improper reward or other overture in order to obtain compliance. Also, inducements that would ordinarily be acceptable may become undue influences if the subject is especially vulnerable.'
- **The Systematic Assessment of Risks and Benefits:** 'It is commonly said that benefits and risks must be "balanced" and shown to be "in a favorable ratio". The metaphorical character of these terms draws attention to the difficulty of making precise judgments. Only on rare occasions will quantitative techniques be available for the scrutiny of research protocols.'

Importantly, this brief historical overview suggests that formulations and clarifications of ethical principles have continued to evolve as science and technology advance, presenting new, unforeseen situations and challenges. ART presents one such area in which biomedical developments pose new, unforeseen dilemmas, requiring further analyses and articulations of principles.

One can ask from where these varied ethical codes originate. The Hippocratic Oath starts with the statement 'I swear by Apollo, the healer', invoking religious authority. The Nuremberg Code, developed by lawyers at the trials, has a firm moral foundation, but in fact no governmental authority. The Helsinki Declaration was issued by the World Medical Association, of which many physicians are not members. The Belmont Report, though mandated by the US Congress, does not itself constitute law. Thus, none of these statements are law per se, and their authority remains unclear. This limitation causes many problems, since providers and others may then choose not to follow them. Nonetheless, these guidelines set clear and recognized standards, and hopefully inform as much as possible the legislation that policy makers develop and implement. Still, adherence to, and implementation, interpretation and application of, these principles varies widely. As we will see, how and why these variations occur, and with what implications, poses critical questions for social scientists and others to address.

Critical questions arise of whether these principles are universal, and if so, which, how and why. Human rights are by definition presumed to be universal, but these questions persist, along with debates as to whether all individuals, regardless of their country or culture, have certain rights.

In 1948 the United Nations General Assembly adopted the Universal Declaration of Human Rights (The General Assembly of the United Nations, 1948), but, despite their membership in the UN, certain countries have violated it. Concerning health, Article 25 of this document states:

- '(1) Everyone has the right to a standard of living adequate for the health and well-being of himself and of his family, including food, clothing, housing, and medical care and necessary social services, and the right to security in the event of unemployment, sickness, disability, widowhood, old age, or other lack of livelihood in circumstances beyond his control.'
- '(2) Motherhood and childhood are entitled to special care and assistance. All children, whether born in or out of wedlock, shall enjoy the same social protection.'

Yet while this statement upholds a right to medical care 'adequate for ... health and well–being', ambiguities persist as to how much care is 'enough' and who should pay for it. Questions remain, too, concerning where human rights come from, and how strong and binding they are – particularly in certain countries, given limited resources and competing priorities and rights.

Historically, several broad approaches to moral theory have also been employed, and are worth mentioning here. Consequentialism weighs moral decisions based on their consequences. The most well-known type of consequentialism – utilitarianism, first articulated by Jeremy Bentham (1823) and John Stuart Mill (1863) – argues, in essence, that decisions should be made such that they yield 'the greatest good for the greatest number'. Yet critics have pointed out several problems with this approach (Beauchamp and Childress, 1994). For instance, notions of 'good' can be defined in various ways, to include pleasure vs. loftier values such as health and autonomy. In each of these cases these goods can in fact be difficult to measure, and can at times conflict. Importantly, this theory can also permit the good of the majority to outweigh the rights of the minority.

In contrast, deontology (from the Greek 'deon', meaning 'duty') emphasizes making ethical decisions based not only on the consequences, but also on the importance of underlying moral duties, values and obligations in and of themselves. Immanuel Kant (1989) described key aspects of this approach, arguing that humans have a 'categorical imperative' to act in ways that would follow universal laws or duties. He argued that individuals must not treat others only as a means to an end, but should be valued for their own intrinsic worth as humans. Yet as Beauchamp and Childress (1994) and others point out, deontology, too, has several limitations, in that obligations to other individuals can themselves conflict (i.e. what one owes to a spouse vs. to a child), and in practical situations the consequences of actions can be significant and not easily ignored. A parent may feel a duty to protect a child from harm, and hence not to disclose that the child was created using donor gametes. Yet the consequence of that decision can be that this child, if later learning this information, may feel betrayed.

A third approach to moral theory, known as virtue ethics, focuses on virtues and moral character, arguing that possessing these traits results in moral decisions and actions. This approach, dating from Plato (1955), and Aristotle (1962), emphasizes the need to pursue a well-lived life, and considers questions of what sort of person we should each be, and how such moral character might be developed through education. Yet this approach has limitations as well. For instance, it does not yield clear principles of conduct per se, or address how conflicts between virtues (e.g. benevolence toward a spouse *vs.* benevolence toward a child) should be resolved, or from where these aspects of character in fact derive (Hursthouse, 2010).

These three approaches might lead to similar decisions. For instance, one could argue that a parent should tell a child who was created through donor gametes that this technology was used because such disclosure will have good consequences (e.g. the avoidance of feelings of betrayal later in life), or because there is a duty of disclosure (e.g. to help, and avoid harming, a child) or because disclosure reflects virtue and moral character (i.e. honesty, benevolence and charity).

These approaches to moral theory have been explored and debated for millennia, in ways that lie beyond the scope of the present chapter. Yet these matters surface in new ways in discussions about ARTs and donation, and may be helpful in attempting to frame and understand the complex and at times competing issues that these technologies pose.

For example, with regard to ART, specific questions emerge as to whether individuals have a right to services (i.e. for the costs of these services to be covered), and if so, how much, and why. One could argue that 'infertility' is a disease that requires treatment. Yet the desire to have children may be seen as extending beyond a basic need and standard of 'adequate well-being'. Moreover, other options (e.g. adoption) exist. Hence, arguably, limited health care resources should thus be used for other diagnoses (e.g. life-threatening disease) instead. However, debates arise, too, concerning positive and negative human rights – the former referring to rights to welfare and services, and the latter referring to rights to be left alone (Vasquez *et al.*, 1990). Individuals who can pay for ART services (e.g. single mothers by choice) may invoke negative rights, and argue that the state does not have a right to interfere in their decisions.

New conceptions of humans, families and the self pose underlying challenges, too, of whether we need to rethink several issues concerning rights. For instance, as we demystify genetics and sex within the contexts of health care systems and markets, some critics may argue that commodification occurs, whereby eggs are treated as economic commodities in a way that inappropriately disrespects them. Questions remain as to whether and when such commercialization is inevitable and/or acceptable.

Questions surface as to whether parenthood is a right, and if so, what that right means, whether it should ever be limited in any way and if so, when, how and by whom. If it should be based on the ability to be a loving and compassionate parent, quandaries emerge of whether health care providers or others should attempt to assess this characteristic a priori, and if so, how.

Arguments persist as to whether ethics is universal or relative, yet such a simple dichotomy may be overly simplistic. Rather, as explored throughout this book, critical tensions require close analysis – for example, how ethical principles get interpreted and applied in different contexts, and why, and what these varying interpretations may suggest. Specifically, the chapters that follow here shed light on how historical, political, cultural, social and economic factors shape ethical discourse and weighings of competing ethical concerns in different contexts. For example, in debates about compensation to gamete donors, important questions arise involving not only the ethical issues, but also the cultural 'meanings' of eggs, sperm, sex, sexuality and reproduction. In the field of bioethics as a whole, scrutiny of such comparative cultural contextual analyses are vital, and this volume can thus contribute to this discourse.

Bringing together ethic and science in the context of reproductive donation

In a diverse civil society, many of the issues surrounding reproductive donation will generate disagreements, and lack clear answers. But clarifying how health care providers, researchers and policy makers do and should approach these conundrums can nonetheless be very helpful. Individuals may claim moral status for arguments (e.g. that gays and lesbians should not be parents because they would harm their children) that social science research can counter by demonstrating incorrect premises and logic.

The present chapter aims not to resolve all of these questions, but to lay them out as a starting point for ongoing analyses throughout the rest of this volume. As we will see, in drawing on ethical principles in an array of situations involving ART, several critical challenges emerge that social science research can probe, enriching our understandings in numerous ways.

Egg donation

Egg donation poses a range of moral questions, such as how to balance the autonomy and rights of the donor vs. the recipient vs. the unborn child. The donor faces potential risks – both known and unknown. She may experience ovarian hyperstimulation syndrome (The Practice Committee of the American Society for Reproductive Medicine, 2008a, 2008b), and if she has donated eggs too frequently in the past, may potentially encounter difficulty conceiving a child in the future if she so desires. Yet additional data need to be collected to clarify how often these complications in fact occur.

Ethical questions surface, too, as to whether the donors have any rights to see, or help raise the child. They may decide that because they are biologically linked to the child, they should be socially linked as well. Yet the egg recipient also has rights, and may feel that she alone is 'the mother', and thus has the right to ban any contact between the child and the donor.

Additional questions emerge here as to the rights of the child – for example, if it is in the best interest of the child to know of, and/or be able to contact, the egg donor, and if so, when. A utilitarian approach would suggest that these decisions about anonymity vs. disclosure be made in a way that ensures the greatest good for the greatest number. Hence, the fact that offspring may be harmed by not knowing their biological parents should perhaps trump egg recipients' fears that these children would feel less close to them as a result. Susan Golombok and colleagues are now investigating whether, when and how disclosure occurs, and what effects result (see Appleby, Blake and Freeman, Chapter 13 and Freeman, Appleby and Jadva, Chapter 14). Social science research can thus potentially help by informing decisions on whether such contact is in fact desired, beneficial and/or harmful, and when, how and to what extent. Social science research can probe, too, how much anonymity in fact exists, and how it is now perceived and/or expected in the era of the Internet, with Google and Facebook providing pictures and other information about people over which these individuals may have little control.

Egg donation raises concerns as well regarding justice, and the potential spectre of eugenics. In the recruitment of donors, it is possible that women of certain ethnic or racial backgrounds or with certain educational test scores (Levine, 2010) may be more or less sought and/or compensated than others. Policy makers and providers then face questions of whether to permit these differentials – whether these discrepancies represent legitimate extensions of individual autonomy (i.e. egg recipients are willing to pay more), or unfairness, and how one should decide.

ART can also generate new forms of kinship that need to be explored – for example, what the nature of the familial, social and moral bonds are within these new kinds of families. For instance, donation decisions may have potential benefits and harms for biological 'half-siblings' of children created through ART. Thus, psychosocial studies are needed to explore the experiences of these biological offspring in learning that they in fact have half-siblings, and when it is best for parents to disclose this information.

Concerns also arise as to whether payment for eggs represents commodification. Here, questions surface of how much 'respect' is necessary and/or desired, what a 'lack' of respect would mean, and who/what the subject(s) of this respect would be. Defining 'commodification', 'lack' and 'respect' is not necessarily an easy task in the debate surrounding ARTs.

Relatedly, several countries permit 'egg-sharing', whereby a couple undergoing in vitro fertilization (IVF) can choose to donate their excess embryos to another patient at the same clinic in exchange for reductions in the costs of undergoing IVF themselves. This practice can generate embryos for use without 'paying' for them directly. However, an implicit price – the reduction in fee – is thus nonetheless affixed to them, raising concerns about commodification. This practice generates dilemmas of how much of a discount to provide, and whether the 'quality' of the embryos matter, and if so, how and why. For instance, it is not known whether an embryo created through the gametes of individuals both of whom hold doctoral degrees, or are of particular ethnic or religious groups that are perceived as 'desirable', should ever be more expensive than another embryo. Quandaries appear as to whether these practices 'disrespect' embryos, and constitute de facto 'sale'. Studies are needed to understand the current market, what problems exist and whether these practices legitimately raise eugenics concerns.

Sperm donation

Sperm donation poses intricacies concerning the rights of the donor (to remain anonymous) vs. that of the child (to find out the genetic father's medical history and/or identity). Moreover, if the donor and child eventually do meet, it is uncertain what rights and responsibilities they each have to the other, and whether either can claim a right to resources from the other. The possibility of siblings, as adults, not knowing their biological relationship, and having children together, could cause harm through inbreeding. A donor sibling 'registry' can prevent that possibility. But an individual conceived through donor sperm may not know of this donation, or wish to be part of the registry. It is not apparent whether such registration and listing should be required, or how such possibilities of harm should be weighed against requirements that all such offspring check the registry before procreating. Individuals might be concerned that registries may not be entirely confidential and that discrimination will result. These arenas, too, require further empirical exploration and scholarship.

Embryo donation

With embryo donation, heated controversies exist about the amount and type of 'respect' that an embryo, as a potential human being, is due. In the USA and several other pluralistic Western countries, views on this issue range widely. Leaders of the Roman Catholic Church argue that life begins at conception, and many citizens believe that embryos should receive the same respect as human beings.

Some conservative critics argue that since the buying and selling of human beings is prohibited, the exchange of cash for embryos should be banned as well. Others argue that embryos deserve respect, but are not morally equivalent to a living human being, and hence that embryo donors may be compensated for their time and burden.

Questions arise, too, concerning re-donation of embryos. A couple may produce embryos, but use only a few, and donate the extras to another couple. This second couple may then implant only one or two, and wish to donate the remainder to a third couple, posing questions of whether this second couple is in fact entitled to do so – that is, who 'owns' these embryos. Legal definitions of property and ownership become problematic since the 'property' can become a human being. Surveys of views and attitudes of the public, and of potential donors and recipients, can potentially inform decisions by both clinicians and policy makers in these realms.

Not only the donation, but the longer term storage and use of embryos pose difficulties. Clinics often end up storing many unused embryos. Frequently, couples initially pay the costs of this storage, but at a certain point stop doing so, and fail to respond to clinic requests to either pay or agree to have these embryos discarded. Clinics must then decide whether to cover the storage costs themselves, or to dispose of the cells. Generally, at least in the USA, clinics have struggled, opting to date to not discard the cells, given the moral sensitivities involved, and the fact that some conservative religious groups may see such disposal as akin to murder. Clinics thus confront dilemmas concerning the scope and limitations of conflicting definitions of 'respect' and 'justice'. Fears of litigation also lead many clinics to continue to store these cells ad infinitum. Surveys of how the couples who produced these embryos in fact feel about these issues can help guide discussions of these areas.

Surrogacy

Surrogacy presents potential conflicts regarding the rights of surrogates vs. future parents vs. unborn children. Ordinarily, surrogates and the future parents sign legal contracts that these future parents, and not the surrogate mother, will be responsible for the child once he or she is born. But on occasion surrogates have insisted on keeping the child – either after, or in the absence of, such a contract – prompting court battles. Questions emerge of whether a surrogate has a right to change her mind – whether she can, after carrying the fetus for nine months and undergoing the complications of pregnancy, decide that she wants to keep or help raise the child. The legal contract may stipulate that she cannot change her mind, but it is not clear that that is wholly fair. Many other types of contracts permit reneging, though often at a cost. If the surrogate has had an extremely difficult pregnancy, endangering her life, additional dilemmas emerge as to whether she should then have more of a right to keep or interact with the child. One might argue that surrogacy contracts should permit such changes if a cost is paid. Yet research is needed to investigate legal cases that have occurred in various countries, and ways these suits have been resolved.

Intrafamilial donation

While donation always requires balancing the rights of the donor, the recipient and the child within families, the first two of these three individuals may have different rights than if they were unknown to each other. Family members confront questions of how much responsibility they have to donate eggs or sperm, if asked, to each other, and whether the moral claims of family ever obligate such donation, and if so, when and to what degree. Individuals may feel pressured or coerced to donate to a family member. Alternatively, siblings may feel hostile, or competitive with each other, and thus not want to donate. Providers must then decide whether to speak to these potential donors, and if so, what to say. If a family member does agree to donate, he or she may then have to decide to what extent to do so. A sister may try to donate once, unsuccessfully, and be unclear if she is morally obligated to try a second time.

In addition, since the donor will already have a relationship to both the child (e.g. as an 'aunt', 'uncle' or 'cousin') and the recipient, questions surface of whether the donor has more of a prerogative to interact with the child, and if so, how much and when. Presumably, the donor will not be receiving payment. But whether he or she then has a justified claim to be more involved with the child, or accrue other benefits, and if so, what, is unclear. Social science can shed light on how members of families in which donation has and has not occurred view and experience these complexities.

Infertile couples

With infertile couples questions emerge as to the extent of their right to have a child if they cannot wholly afford the costs out-of-pocket, and these expenses must be borne partly by others (e.g. governmental or private insurance). Should all infertile couples be entitled to health insurance coverage for the costs of as much infertility treatment as they want; and if not, where and how should limits be placed? In the USA individual states vary widely: from mandating that private insurance companies cover one cycle of IVF for all infertile couples, to requiring that such couples 'have access' to such services (without requiring insurance companies to pay for these), to having no such requirement. Nations vary widely in these regards as well. While Israel covers relatively high amounts of IVF costs, many other countries cover little, if any. No country can readily offer as much health care as its citizens may want or need. How then should limited resources be distributed? Here, tensions emerge between perceived 'rights' to have a child vs. questions of perceived distributive justice – that is, how a pool of insurance monies should be distributed among those covered. How rights to have a child should be weighed against other health care needs (e.g. for all medications) remains unknown.

Insurers – whether governmental or private – that decide to cover infertility services then encounter dilemmas of how much, for whom and how to decide this. Insurers may opt to cover only one cycle of IVF, for which the odds of success are generally only 25 to 40 per cent. Quandaries emerge of whether insurers should be mandated to cover second cycles as well, and whether all patients should receive the same amount of ART services, or certain patients should receive more or less because of particular characteristics. For instance, one could argue that 25-year-olds should receive less coverage than 35-year-olds, since the former presumably have a longer period of time to try to get pregnant without medical intervention. Infertile couples may also argue that they want to have more than one child, and should receive sufficient services to do so. These and other questions may need to be revisited over time as the success rates of various interventions improve. Different countries may also approach these issues very differently based on relative resources, and cultural values placed on having children vs. stigma from being childless.

Political responses may vary, based on several factors. In some states in the USA patient advocates have managed to find a 'champion' among elected officials – often a fellow infertility patient – to push for mandated coverage. Anecdotally, such efforts appear to have been more successful in relatively 'liberal' rather than 'conservative' states, but not always.

Social science research is needed to examine how state and national governments differ in their coverage, what historical, political, economic, social and psychological factors may account for these differences, and whether attempts to expand coverage have been successful, and if so, how.

Single parents

With regard to single parents by choice, these ethical issues take different forms as well. Here, the rights of the parent can potentially clash with those of the yet unborn child. Specifically, since the child would have only a single parent to rely on, if that adult is impaired in ways that can impede parenting skills (e.g. having a serious life-threatening illness, ongoing substance abuse or a major psychiatric disorder), dilemmas may emerge – whether the rights of the parent to have a child conflict with the rights of the child to have a 'good enough' parent and home environment. Whether clinicians should ever make these decisions, and how, are unclear. While a current significant psychiatric impairment may prompt a provider not to offer ART, other situations can be more ambiguous. For instance, if a parent has a past history of major depression or substance abuse, but no symptoms at that moment, it is unclear whether this past history should ever affect the provider's approach and decision in any way, and if so, when, to what degree and how. If the right to parenthood is based on the ability to be a loving and compassionate parent, questions then arise of whether ART providers or others should attempt to assess this characteristic a priori. One could argue that such screening would be unjust since a couple having a child 'naturally' without the use of ART is not similarly evaluated in any way. Yet ART providers have professional ethical obligations to yet unborn children. Future studies can assess the effects of singlehood or other characteristics of parents on child development, and potentially help enlighten any policies that may prove to be based on faulty assumptions.

Reproduction for gays and lesbians

Additional issues arise with the use of assisted reproduction for gays and lesbians, either as individuals or members of a couple. Religious conservatives have argued that gays and lesbians would harm their children, and thus should not be parents (BBC News, 2007). Yet, importantly, social science research by Susan Golombok (Golombok and Tasker, 1994) and others have revealed that these assumptions are incorrect. Moreover, gays and lesbians who seek ART are not, by definition, biologically 'infertile'. Yet, as Chapter 12 suggests, they may be 'structurally' infertile. Still, they are generally not eligible for reimbursement by insurers who cover many other types of patients. This discrepancy appears unjust. Single gay men or lesbians may also face obstacles in ART services due to prejudice from certain providers in ways that also need to be investigated.

Transnational donation

Reproductive tourism has been rapidly spreading, with patients traveling to other countries for ART. Patients journey to and from both developed and developing countries, creating four broad patterns: going from a developed to a developed country, a developed to a developing country, a developing to a developed country, and a developing to a developing country. In each of these scenarios the issues can vary. The use of egg donors and surrogates from the developing world pose concerns about possible coercion and exploitation. The amounts of money received for such services in the West (i.e. $5,000–$10,000 for egg donation and $15,000–$35,000 for surrogacy (Schreiner, 2010)) are of far greater value in the developing world, where per capita GDP is far less. Hence, if a surrogate in the developing world receives only one quarter of what her counterpart in the West would receive, that amount could easily still constitute two entire years of salary. In poorer countries women may thus become pressured by their husbands, or by perceived needs to care for children, to become egg donors or surrogates. Clinics have already been established in India for women who 'rent their wombs' to Westerners. 'Reproductive imperialism' or 'reproductive colonialism' may thus occur, whereby women in wealthier countries take advantage of women in poorer countries.

Yet proponents of transnational donation may reply that these activities are fair if women in the developing world are adequately informed of the risks and benefits of engaging in these services – that is, that such 'work' does not differ from employment in, for instance, a factory that makes products used in the West. Observers who are wary of reproductive tourism may respond that donation can involve unknown risks to these women's bodies. Yet a critic might counter that working in a factory can also pose unknown physical harms (e.g. exposure to toxic substances). Experiences and long-term outcomes of such reproductive tourism require serious study. Social science can shed light on the experiences of surrogates in the developing world – for example, whether they (vs. their husbands) are able to control funds received, and what long-term psychological, social and biomedical problems may ensue.

Questions are also raised as to the responsibilities of the health care system in the visited country to provide additional medical services, if needed, to foreign visitors using ARTs in that country. If a woman from one country undergoes IVF elsewhere, and as a result develops acute complications, necessitating emergency hospitalization, it is not clear who should pay the consequent medical costs – for example, whether she should be solely responsible. If she cannot afford these costs, questions of justice emerge as to whether the health care system of the host country should always pay, and if so, how much, and whether such coverage may facilitate reproductive tourism more than is otherwise optimal. Social scientists can explore how often and what kinds of problems in coverage emerge in order to inform policy discussions of these problems.

The fact that the living conditions in the developing world may be less conducive to health than in the West raises concerns, too. Egg donors or surrogates in the developing world may encounter environmental stressors (poor nutrition or exposures to infectious diseases) that can harm the future child. Patients who go to the developing world for fertility treatment to save money may receive inferior care, and they or their future children may develop medical complications that health systems in their home country then have to treat, adding to costs in these home countries. These possibilities may support provision of additional ART in westernized countries to prevent these longer term problems.

As suggested above, these phenomena are of mounting importance, but have received little attention. Empirical investigations are important to gauge the nature and frequency of medical complications among all of the parties involved in transnational reproduction, what problems in service delivery in fact arise and how these are addressed.

Factors involved

Clearly, individual countries view and address these ethical issues differently, based on historical, cultural, social, political, economic and other factors. Scholarship is needed to understand more fully why even in the West, with many shared political, ethical and cultural ideals, policies vary widely in whether they permit or prohibit certain practices (e.g. surrogacy, anonymous sperm donation or compensation for egg donation), thereby interpreting, applying and weighing competing ethical principles differently. Such scholarship can enrich the bioethics literature by shedding light on how bioethical principles are viewed and weighed, and are ambiguous and/or open to debate, in ways that philosophers have not fully addressed. Social science research that provides descriptions of lived experiences of the various parties involved in ART transactions (e.g. recipients, donors, offspring, siblings and providers) can reveal additional ethical conflicts that they may confront that have not been addressed by bioethicists.

Within the field of bioethics as a whole, the roles of broader comparative cultural contexts, particularly those of non-Western countries, need much more exploration. At root, some would argue, are questions of whether ethics is universal or relative. In many ways, that dichotomy is too simplistic. Rather, to understand how different stakeholders in different cultures view, experience and address ethical conflicts is crucial. For instance, the chapter on the relatively large egg donation business in Spain suggests that the growth of this industry can be explained as part of the political and cultural context, post-Franco. Between Western and non-Western cultures, views and approaches toward rights and ethics can differ markedly. For instance, even in the West, the notion that children have certain rights is relatively new. The US government did not regulate the minimum age and maximum hours of employment for children until 1938 (Child Labor Public Education Project, 2010).

Implications

For social science

As suggested above, the issues in this and subsequent chapters highlight a wide range of issues that psychologists, other social scientists and bioethicists can address in ways that mutually enrich each other's work. Some critics perceive tensions between ethical analyses that seek to understand 'what ought to be', and empirical bioethics that can describe 'what is'. Yet empirical bioethics can cover both domains, and be both normative and descriptive. Empirical research can elucidate how individuals in fact make ethical decisions, but inform bioethics in other ways as well. For example, social science can provide data on whether potential benefits and harms that ethicists posit in fact exist, and if so, how frequently, when and to what degree. Studies can also grasp how different groups of stakeholders – prospective parents, gamete donors, physicians, policy makers and the public at large – each view and experience these complex issues in a variety of cultural contexts, and define and balance key ethical terms (e.g. 'justice', 'coercion', 'exploitation', 'respect', 'autonomy' and 'rights'). Researchers can probe how donors and recipients of gametes each perceive and understand or misunderstand the risks and benefits involved, what psychological, social, familial and other factors shape these perspectives, and how these various groups each resolve these ethical conundrums.

Empirical studies can also reveal ethical conflicts that arise in the daily lives and experiences of clinicians, patients, parents, family members and others, but have received little, if any, systematic attention. Such research can also demonstrate unintended consequences of ethical decisions or policies. For instance, given that the risks of egg donation are not fully known, empirical research is crucial to elucidate whether the relatively high amounts of compensation do indeed 'blind' young women to the potential risks, and if so, when; whether this compensation disproportionately attracts poorer women; and what and how potential donors are selected by clinics, agencies and prospective recipients. Comparative studies of government policies can assist diverse political entities in learning from each other, in determining how best to address these complex tensions and trade-offs.

For ethics and policy

These analyses are key, too, for better understanding issues in ethics more fully – for example, the ways in which complex cultural, social, political, economic, medical and other factors shape how individuals and institutions interpret and weigh principles. The discussions in this book illuminate the range of ways in which ethical terms are defined and applied. For instance, notions of 'right' emerge in many of the chapters here, and in qualitative research in these realms. But individuals invoke this term in varying manners that can be elucidated, and powerfully inform policy makers and scholars across several disciplines.

For policy makers, social science can answer questions (e.g. about psychological and other harms), but in the end cannot always determine policy. Rather, questions concerning allocations of resources may ultimately involve value judgements that the polity as a whole (e.g. through elected representatives or courts) must decide.

Public policy can be a crude instrument of change. Regulations based on ethical principles can have unintended consequences that social science can assess in individuals' daily lives. Nevertheless, the analyses in this and subsequent chapters can illustrate the breadth of policy responses, and help frame ethical conflicts in ways that can foster the development and implementation of appropriate legislation. For instance, policy makers may weigh justice less than autonomy in some, but not other decisions in ways that can be further investigated.

Conclusions

In deciding how to proceed in these complex arenas, reliance on principles alone goes only so far, at which point, empirical research is needed to understand the dilemmas that arise, and how these should most appropriately be addressed. At these junctures, integration of ethical principles and social science is critical. This chapter has presented a broad overview and framework of issues that subsequent chapters here will probe in far more depth. Not all of these questions will have ready answers, but articulation of the tensions, and of areas in which evidence is available and/or lacking, can hopefully help guide clinicians, patients, family members, policy makers, scholars and others.

With rapidly advancing reproductive and other technologies, these issues will continue to evolve, generating new dilemmas. Researchers are collecting more data on more patients over longer periods of time, shifting understanding of the risks and benefits of ART. Social scientists are illuminating the behaviours, decisions and experiences of key stakeholders, providing insights into how these individuals comprehend and address complex choices. Ethicists are further refining, interpreting and applying principles to meet these evolving needs in diverse contexts. Clearly, medical science, social science and ethics shape each other in multiple ways that need to be understood in order to ensure the appropriate use of these new and powerful technologies in our varied worlds.

REFERENCES

Aristotle (1962). *Nichomachean Ethics*. M. Ostwald (trans. and ed.). Indianapolis: Bobbs-Merrill.

BBC News (2007). 'Catholic threat on gay rights law' (online). Available at: http://news.bbc.co.uk/2/hi/6289301.stm (accessed 17 December 2010).

Beauchamp, T. L. and Childress, J. F. (1994). *Principles of Biomedical Ethics*. New York: Oxford University Press.

Bentham, J. (1823). *An Introduction to the Principles of Moral Legislation* (e-book). Oxford University Press. Available at: http://openlibrary.org (accessed 15 December 2010).

Child Labor Public Education Project (2010). 'Child labor in U.S. history' (online). Available at: www.continuetolearn.uiowa.edu/laborctr/child_labor/about/us_history.html (accessed 16 December 2010).

Golombok, S. and Tasker, F. (1994). 'Children in lesbian and gay families: theories and evidence'. *Annual Review of Sex Research*, 4, 73–100.

Hedgecoe, A. M. (2004). 'Critical bioethics: beyond the social science critique of applied ethics'. *Bioethics*, 18, 120–43.

Hursthouse, R. (2010). 'Virtue Ethics', in E. N. Zalta (ed.), *The Stanford Encyclopedia of Philosophy* (Winter 2010 Edition) (online). Available at: http://plato.stanford.edu/entries/ethics-virtue/ (accessed 16 December 2010).

Ives, J. (2008). 'Encounters with experience: empirical bioethics and the future'. *Health Care Analysis*, 16, 1–6.

Ives, J. and Draper, H. (2009). 'Appropriate methodologies for empirical bioethics: it's all relative'. *Bioethics*, 23, 249–58.

Kant, I. (1989). *Foundations of the Metaphysics of Morals*. 2nd edn. New York: Prentice Hall.

Levine, A. D. (2010). 'Self-regulation, compensation, and the ethical recruitment of oocyte donors'. *Hastings Center Report*, 40, 25–36.

Mill, J. S. (1863). *Utilitarianism* (e-book). London: Parker, Son, and Bourn. Available at: http://openlibrary.org (accessed 15 December 2010).

The National Commission for the Protection of Human Subjects of Biomedical and Behavioral Research (1979). *The Belmont Report: Ethical Principles and Guidelines for the Protection of Human Subjects of Research* (online). Available at: http://ohsr.od.nih.gov/guidelines/belmont.html (accessed: 3 August 2010).

North, M. (trans.) (2002). 'The Hippocratic Oath'. *National Library of Medicine, National Institute of Health* (online). Available at: www.nlm.nih.gov/hmd/greek/greek_oath.html (accessed 3 August 2010).

Plato (1955). *The Republic*. D. Lee (trans. and ed.). New York: Penguin.

The Practice Committee of the American Society for Reproductive Medicine (2008a). 'Ovarian hyperstimulation syndrome'. *Fertility and Sterility*, 90, S188–S193.

The Practice Committee of the American Society for Reproductive Medicine (2008b). 'Repetitive oocyte donation'. *Fertility and Sterility*, 90, S194–S195.

Schreiner, E. (2010). 'How much does a surrogate mother make?' *Modern Mom* (online). Available at: www.modernmom.com/article/how-much-does-a-surrogate-mother-make (accessed 16 December 2010).

Strech, D., Synofzik, M. and Marckmann, G. (2008). 'Systematic reviews of empirical bioethics'. *Journal of Medical Ethics*, 34, 472–7.

United States Department of Health and Human Services (1949). 'Nuremberg Code'. *Trials of War Criminals Before the Nuremberg Military Tribunals Under Control Council Law,* No. 10, Vol. 2, pp. 181–2 (online). Washington, DC: US Government Printing Office. Available at: http://ohsr.od.nih.gov/ guidelines/nuremberg.html (accessed 3 August 2010).

Vasquez, M., Andre, C., Shanks, T. and Meyer, M. J. (1990). 'Rights'. *Issues in Ethics,* 3. Available at: www.scu.edu/ethics/practicing/decision/rights.html (accessed 14 October 2010).

LEGISLATION

INTERNATIONAL

The General Assembly of the United Nations (1948). The Universal Declaration of Human Rights (online). Available at: www.un.org/en/documents/udhr/ (accessed 15 December 2010).

The World Medical Association (2008). WMA Declaration of Helsinki – Ethical Principles for Medical Research Involving Human Subjects (online). Available at: www.wma.net/en/30publications/10policies/b3/ index.html (accessed 3 August 2010).

USA

National Research Act 1974

4   Parenthood – whose right is it anyway?

Anja Karnein

The question of who should be parents is age-old. Until about thirty years or so ago, it was directed almost exclusively to those who could conceive without medical assistance. Today, with the advance of new technologies of assisted reproduction, the question regularly applies to many more, including all those who are infertile, do not have a partner of the opposite sex, are single or for other reasons can only reproduce with medical help. Judgements about who should be parents tend to be different depending on which of these groups one belongs to: while there are frequently very few – if any – restrictions for persons who can conceive without medical help, individuals who seek such assistance are often viewed with some suspicion with respect to a variety of features, including their sexual orientation, mental health, age or their marital and financial status.

For such unequal treatment to be justified, one would have to show that the two groups of people are indeed different in a morally relevant way, that is, with regard to their ability to parent. There are two kinds of differences that may come to mind: (a) the possibly dissimilar consequences of comparable treatment, and (b) the type of people who might be included in these groups.

Some may think that scrutinizing individuals for whether they would or would not be good parents has different effects on each of the two groups. Arguably, while denying fertile persons their right to be parents requires coercing them into not reproducing, not allowing everyone to have their own biologically related child 'merely' entails refusing a service. The reason some think this distinction is important is because they consider coercion, quite unlike the 'mere' refusal of a service, to be illegitimate in principle. However, preventing individuals who are capable of reproducing (without help) from becoming parents need not be coercive – at least not impermissibly so. We could, for instance, follow the advice of Hugh Lafollette. He points out that just as we think we can legitimately ask people to obtain a licence for driving a vehicle or for shooting a gun – both practices that are potentially dangerous to others – we would be fully justified in asking people to acquire a licence for parenting, a practice which undoubtedly is potentially harmful to others (i.e. their children) (Lafollette, 1980). This solution may have practical obstacles, but it shows that the crucial difference cannot be that one group would have to be impermissibly coerced into reproducing while the other one is merely being refused a service.

There is a second possible difference between those who can reproduce without medical assistance and those who cannot. While the former are more likely to create offspring within a traditional family context (at least to begin with), the latter sometimes seek reproductive help in different contexts.[1] Assisted reproductive technologies (ARTs) allow individuals with no partner, or at least not one of the opposite sex, or individuals who are beyond the reproductive age, to fulfil their wish for offspring.[2] The possibility of creating alternative family forms has given rise to at least two kinds of concerns. First, some are anxious about the well-being of children who grow up in single-parent households, with two parents of the same sex or with parents who are beyond the 'normal' reproductive age. Second, some oppose reproduction in non-traditional circumstances because children created with the help of ARTs will occasionally, and sometimes unavoidably, not be genetically related to those who wish to raise them. The worry here is that biological kinship might be a necessary ingredient for a healthy and loving relationship between parents and their children.

Many of the other chapters in this volume provide the empirical data needed to show that these concerns are largely unfounded. But as a theorist I want to ask whether the fact that some people want to raise children in the context of non-traditional family structures and without biological ties justifies being more critical of their parental qualities. Answering this concern will require a closer look at the criteria we use to ascertain whether someone qualifies for being a parent. The qualities that emerge will show that the features that make adults reasonably decent parents are not primarily linked to their age, their sexual orientation, their marital or their financial status. Thus, I find that there are no good reasons to deny reproductive assistance to people whose parenthood nobody would object to if they did not have to rely on medical

---

[1] Here a traditional family refers to a family in which children are conceived, carried to term and raised by both of their biological parents who permanently live together in one household.

[2] Pennings (2003) suggests that medically assisted reproduction is distinct from unassisted reproduction in another way, namely, in that the former requires the complicity of a physician, while the latter does not.

assistance.[3] Moreover, I argue that society shoulders some responsibility for materially supporting the reproductive pursuits of people requiring medical help. This argument will proceed in four steps.

I begin by exploring what people want when they express their wish to become parents and how the question of parenthood has been complicated by new technologies of assisted reproduction. I will then turn to an inquiry of what makes the 'good' of parenthood valuable for adults and continue by looking at the same question from the child's perspective. This analysis will reveal that it would be difficult to claim that the particular challenges that may arise for parents and children in non-traditional family structures or in families in which parents and children are only partially biologically connected (or not at all) are not qualitatively worse than the challenges frequently encountered in conventional parent–child relationships. The final part of the argument deals with the question of why we should be sympathetic to people's wishes to have children, never mind their own biological children, in the first place. That is an expensive undertaking which requires valuable resources that could be expended somewhere else. In response, I will provide an argument for why society ought to be held accountable for fulfilling the desire of individuals to have children if its values are partly responsible for the prevalence of these desires. Finally, I will conclude this discussion with a plea for universal access to reproduction – at least in principle.

Three forms of parenthood

Not everyone wants children and not having children is not a disease. However, for those who have the wish to raise a child it is usually not one wish among many. Frequently it is experienced as an essential ingredient for personal well-being and happiness. But what do people mean when they express a desire to be parents? To answer this question, we need a better understanding of what constitutes the 'good' of parenthood. Parenthood can be understood in three different ways. First, it can be understood biologically and be taken to refer narrowly to those people whose gametes contributed to the creation of a child. The 'good' this could be said to entail is mere biological reproduction. Some might aspire to this because they hope that living on in their

---

[3] Obviously, even if my argument succeeds, it would still be difficult to establish that everyone has a 'right' to become a parent. The services required for this are simply not enforceable. For instance, nobody can make women donate their eggs or carry another's child. But everyone can ask not to have reproductive assistance denied to them just because they are not traditional parents.

children's genes, their memory or both, will insure their immortality. But if this was all that parenthood was about then it would suffice to allow individuals to donate their sperm and egg cells. Moreover, it would also mean that no infertile person could ever properly be a parent to anyone.

Second, parenthood can be understood in purely legal terms and taken to refer to those persons who have the right to make decisions for the child. The 'good' involved in this form of parenthood consists of being recognized by society as having the authority to make all the important decisions pertaining to a child's life. It is thus an important form of social recognition. Having legal guardianship does not necessarily imply any biological relation to or any day-to-day contact with a child. In theory, it would be possible to distribute this legal form of parenthood to a number of wise persons who are given authority to make all vital decisions for all children, with others bearing them and again others raising them.

Third, parenthood can be conceived of in social terms as referring to those who are engaged in day-to-day contact with children, raising and educating them over a significant period of their lives; those people to whom the children are primarily attached. The 'good' entailed in this kind of parenthood is a particular kind of relationship. This kind of parenthood also does not necessarily depend on any biological relation to a child, nor does it imply that those who are in everyday contact with the child are those who have legal guardianship.

Traditionally, all three forms of parenthood are intimately connected to each other. Those who procreate do this with the intention not only of having a child but also with the intention of raising that child. Their authority to make all important decisions for their child is usually recognized by the state. Nevertheless, looking at these three different categories in isolation suggests that what people mostly mean when they say they want to be parents is that they desire to have a relationship with a child they can call their own. It is this aspect of parenthood that adults long for and the absence of which they mourn. The interest in legal guardianship, as important as that might be, only follows from that initial wish. The issue is more difficult when it comes to the importance of biological kinship: for some this is vitally important, so important even that they do not want children unless they are their 'own'.

To show that the relationship between parent and child does not become dysfunctional just because it takes place in non-traditional family contexts, or because there is no biological bond between them, requires looking at what it is about the parent–child relationship that makes it so desirable for some adults and to explore what could be detrimental about such a relationship from the child's perspective.

Why (some) adults want to be parents

From the perspective of adults, what is the 'good' that parenthood entails? Harry Brighouse and Adam Swift adamantly claim that parenthood, understood in the social way described above, uniquely contributes to human flourishing (Brighouse and Swift, 2006; 2009):

Parents have an interest in being in a relationship of this sort. They have a non-fiduciary interest in playing this fiduciary role. The role enables them to exercise and develop capacities the development and exercise of which are, for many, ... crucial to their living fully flourishing lives (Brighouse and Swift, 2006: 95).

The authors argue that the kind of fulfilment adults can experience by being parents is unparalleled. They name four ways in which the parent–child relationship is different from other kinds of important relationships (Brighouse and Swift, 2006). First, unlike intimate relationships between adults, that between parent and child is asymmetrical: children are wholly dependent on adults for their well-being and vulnerable to adults' decisions and choices. Second, this asymmetry is aggravated by the fact that there is no exit option for children, even if this relationship turns out to be harmful to them. This is true both legally and psychologically. Adults are (relatively speaking) much freer to quit their parental responsibilities (especially and traditionally, if they are fathers). This again is unlike intimate relationships between adults, where, even if there is some power-asymmetry, the parties involved are equally free to leave. Third, according to the authors, the quality of the intimacy is of a different sort in parent–child relationships: the love parents receive from their children is unconditional and spontaneous, beyond the children's rational control. They share their excitements and disappointments unselfconsciously with their parents and trust them entirely. Parents would have to do terrible things to undermine this trust. The authors maintain that adults do not share themselves with each other in the same way: intimacy requires a considerable act of will on the parts of adults interacting with each other. With regard to their children, parents also have to be more guarded than they would be with another adult: they have to hide the feelings of sadness, anger and frustration they might experience on account of other aspects of their lives.

The fourth aspect that Brighouse and Swift consider to be different about parent–child relationships – what they call the distinct moral quality of the relationship. Parents have to care not only for the immediate interests of children but also for the development of their capabilities. This will occasionally require parents to force children to do things they might not feel like doing (such as brushing their teeth or not eating a fifth scoop of ice cream) or to manipulate their interests (by, for instance, feeding them wholegrain pasta in the hope that they will develop a taste for wholegrain foods).

Brighouse and Swift persuasively show how the parent–child relationship is different from any other intimate relationship between adults. What they do not so successfully demonstrate, however, is how that relationship is different from an intimate relationship adults may have with their pets. That relationship is also asymmetrical, there is no exit option (for the pets) and the pets love their owners spontaneously and unconditionally. Moreover, this relationship also has the moral quality of pet owners occasionally having to coerce or manipulate their pets' immediate desires in the interest of their present and future well-being. Such a relationship can be of tremendous value to pet owners.

Surely the authors would be quick to reply that I am misconstruing their meaning: obviously the degree of self-fulfilment that lies in caring for a pet is constrained by the fact that the pets' developmental capacities are limited. That is true, of course. But this should make us relocate the emphasis a little when it comes to describing what makes the parent–child relationship uniquely valuable: it cannot only have to do with caring for a helpless child who is in need of assistance. It must also involve following the child's development, and watching children mature into independent people. The authors say as much, but do not make this aspect of the relationship essential to what makes it contribute to human flourishing. However, the slow and incremental change of the relationship is part of that: eventually it will be more reciprocal, much more like the relationship between adults. The initially spontaneous and unconditional love turns into something children can and will reflect upon and scrutinize. Parents have no guarantee that they will end up liking who their children grow into and there is no guarantee that children will end up appreciating who their parents are. Yet, it will remain true that there is no easy way out of this relationship, since it is fundamentally formative, especially perhaps for children, but also, as Brighouse and Swift are right to point out, for the parents.

So far, I am merely recommending a shift in emphasis, but generally agreeing with Brighouse and Swift that it is the relationship between parent and child that is what makes parenthood valuable and fundamentally desirable to many people. Note how this account comprehensively describes the 'good' of parenthood without any reference to biological kinship or, for that matter, to legal guardianship.[4]

Nevertheless, this cannot be the end of the story. Just because many people may have a fundamental interest in this particular kind of relationship it does not give them an entitlement to it. This is principally because there is another party involved here: children. Their interests are of vital importance. They might be of even greater importance than the interests of adults in being parents since they have no choice in the matter at all. Nobody is ever asked whether they want to be born and one enters this world unfinished and in need of help. In that way, children find themselves solely at the mercy of those willing to raise them. One might suppose that, to the extent parents perform their parental duties well, this will also be best for children. But notice the conditional nature of this sentence: 'if' parents perform their parental duties well. This raises the question of who, from those who seek the 'good' of parenthood, would be good parents. David Velleman has made a strong case for why biological kinship should be a key determining factor. A discussion of his arguments will lead to the heart of what concerns people most about several forms of assisted reproduction, especially sperm and egg donation, which may facilitate the establishment of non-traditional families with ruptured biological ties.

What children need

Velleman argues that by intentionally procreating, individuals incur the responsibility to help and assist their children in facing the challenging task lying ahead of them, namely to make something of their lives and to form an identity. This is a hazardous undertaking that requires work and effort at the best of times. 'To be born as a human being is to be handed a job of work, with a promise of great rewards for success, a threat of great harm for refusal, and a risk of similar harm for failure' (Velleman, 2008: 250). Therefore, parents must make sure that their child has the necessary capacities to succeed in life and to flourish as a human being. Velleman maintains that growing up with one's biological parents is essential in this pursuit. Estranging individuals from their

---

[4] Legal guardianship nevertheless continues to play an important role: if, irrespective of biological ties, many more people are involved in parenting, it will end up being of great significance who has the rights to make important decisions regarding education, medical procedures, etc.

ancestry may obstruct their capacity to make something of their lives. This is because as much as the challenges awaiting children upon birth are universal, they are also highly individual. Each child has to succeed within the limits of her particular genetic endowment. Velleman thinks that only those who share a particular child's biological fate can truly be of assistance here:

Most parents realize that part of their job is to help their child form realistic aspirations, folded into an identity in which it can truly flourish; and they realize that their ability to do so is greatly enhanced by their ability to recognize in the child various traits, inclinations, and aptitudes that they have seen before, either in themselves or in other members of the family (Velleman, 2008: 259).

Velleman claims that it helps parents in assisting their children to have some familiar reference point with whom to compare their children. Likewise, he believes that in order for children not to feel adrift and alienated, they need to know where they came from and where they are going. He maintains that only biological kinship allows children to feel rooted in the world by providing them with a unique and determinable place in the infinite chain of reproduction. For this reason, parental obligations are not transferrable. Velleman concludes that practices such as anonymous sperm donation constitute a moral wrong towards the children thus created because they allow individuals to defect on their parental duties. They thereby deprive future persons of an essential source of human flourishing and subject them to suffering.

Velleman's argument depends on the assumption that a particular kind of biological kinship is essential for human flourishing. He maintains that it is part of common sense to acknowledge that prospects for personhood can only be fully realized by children who are brought up by their biological parents. He cites various cases in which parentless figures have tragically struggled: Telemachus, Oedipus, Moses and Luke Skywalker. He describes the natural tendency of children who grow up in non-biologically related families to go looking for their biological ancestors. Moreover, Velleman reminds us of Aristotle's criticism of Plato's idea of communal child-raising on the grounds that biological relatives tend to recognize and single out each other in a way that no social engineering can suppress.

There is no doubt that consanguinity is important. However, I want to explore the degree to which blood is irreplaceable in family relations. To the extent blood is indeed irreplaceable, I want to challenge whether the need for consanguinity is of a kind that obliges parents to provide such biological bonds on the grounds that children cannot flourish without them.

The first question is whether there can be good parents who are not related by blood to the child they intend to raise. Velleman would have to deny this, at least if we take good parenting to mean that they manage to satisfy their children's essential needs and do not wrong them by having provoked a situation (i.e. compelling them to grow up with biologically non-related parents) in which they are bound to experience the feeling of loss. The only way to doubt this implication of Velleman's claim would be either to reject the notion that blood relation is vitally important for human flourishing or to argue that the different ingredients that make blood-ties so precious are reproducible in non-biological relationships. The former is hard to accomplish. Velleman persuasively points to the overwhelming evidence that for most people in most cultures and at most times, consanguinity has been of fundamental significance. This of course could be attributed to one grand time- and culture-spanning misconception that constantly reproduces itself (because everyone believes blood relations are so important, blood relationships become important, etc.). But even if one became convinced of the grand misconception theory, Velleman does not rest his claim on such observations. He persuasively argues that family resemblance plays a vital role in a child's identity formation and her ability to formulate realistic aspirations in life.

> To be born in a human body is ... to be susceptible to alienation from it ... A connection to biological parents helps us to cope with this aspect of our predicament. In infancy we learn to love human faces whose features will eventually be blended in the face that emerges in the mirror as we reach adulthood. We grow into a body akin to the bodies from which we came, while growing into a personality akin to the ones that animate those other bodies ... Those who do not know their parents can only wonder who they are becoming (Velleman, 2008: 260).

There is no doubt that family resemblance can be a great comfort to a child. But this is not necessarily the case, both when it comes to formulating realistic aspirations in life and to the formation of the child's identity.

With regard to forming realistic aspirations in life, Velleman thinks that resemblance will give children some sense of who they could be and what they could or could not do. If, for instance, a child has inherited one of her parent's difficulty in spelling at school, she might have a better way of dealing with her dyslexia and have no illusions about ever being a great speller. What Velleman does not consider, however, is that although such realism could save her from disappointment, it could also be sadly stymieing. It might prevent children from surprising themselves and excelling in ways they never 'realistically' thought they could. Moreover, there is also the issue of being wrong about which features one inherited from one's parents. This could occur either from fear that one may resemble a parent more than one actually does or from a wish to resemble the parent more than one actually does. The child from the example above may therefore fail to realize that she did not inherit the dyslexia and actually could be the champion of every spelling bee contest. Thus, as important as resemblance might be in individual cases for forming realistic aspirations in life, it is not clear that being realistic in this way is itself such a blessing.

With respect to the importance of resemblance for identity formation, consider Velleman's example of Luke Skywalker. It is not clear that Darth Vader would have provided the face Luke would come to love if he developed any kind of resemblance to it. In fact, the greatest fear Luke has is that he will display any of his father's features. (This would certainly dampen any aspiration he may have in life for being a benevolent and kind person with a robust sense of justice.) Two things seem to be important for resemblance to contribute to identity-formation in a good way. First, as the Luke Skywalker example illustrates, it is important that the people children resemble are people it would not be bad to be like, who have talents it would be good to have and shortcomings one can live with. Second, and perhaps even more essential, it is vital that children have positive feelings toward the people they resemble. Even if there was nothing objectionable about these people per se, children might not develop an unproblematic identity if they happen to closely resemble a relative they despise.

Velleman may even agree with all this, but also rightly points out that it is irrelevant: just because it is not always the case in biologically related families that resemblance works out in a good way does not mean that resemblance is not generally important or that no resemblance at all (as would be the case in non-biologically related families) is a desirable option.

Thus the real question is whether resemblance, even if it works out in a good way, is necessary for that part of identity-formation that involves the self-love Velleman describes. He maintains that we learn to love the faces whose features will eventually blend into our own. Recognition theory, however, has shown that it is doubtful that self-love is primarily the result of this kind of resemblance (Honneth, 1995). While it may be conducive to children's self-appreciation if they develop features of persons they love, what will ultimately be responsible for their self-appraisal is how others respond to them. What is vital for children to develop a healthy dose of self-love is their realization that others find them lovable. To expect children to slowly come to love themselves relative to how much they turn out looking like someone in the family they adore seems complicated and somewhat risky (as the examples of Darth Vader and the despised relative sought to illustrate). It is much more likely that children will find comfort and confidence in looking at a face they love and trust who lovingly smiles back at them (Honneth, 2001). Feeling alienated from their bodies is an indication that there are some aspects of their physicality that they do not accept. But there has to be a reason for them not to accept something about themselves, that is, a feeling that something is strange or different about the way they are, look or feel. This sentiment is not obviously or inevitably the result of being raised by people who are, as a mere matter of fact, different. If non-biological parents are interested enough in who their children are, who they grow into, and appreciate and respond affectionately to their particularity, then there is no reason for these children to translate their being different into a feeling of alienation.

It also must be remembered that Luke Skywalker and Moses both turn into exceptional individuals. In both cases, they might have been far less likely to develop the pride, strength and sense of justice had they been brought up by those who were biologically responsible for their existence. Luke would have grown up with a power- and hate-ridden tin-can of a father and Moses, had he lived at all, would have grown up with the humiliating experience of being raised by and belonging to a people treated as slaves. This is not to suggest that children ought to be systematically redistributed to those people who might provide them with the maximal amount of love and appreciation. Rather, it is to indicate that, in some important sense, non-biological parents are not prima facie less capable of providing for children what they most essentially need in order to flourish. If that is the case, however, then it cannot be wrong in principle to bring children into existence who will not be raised by their biological parents.

Velleman lists another important feature of consanguinity, which is not easily reproducible. According to him, biological parents are the only ones who can root a new person in life:

To be born a living thing is to be a link in that chain [of progenitors and progeny]. Not to experience oneself as located in that chain is to lack a sense of one's membership in the realm of life which is the locus of one's membership in reality (Velleman 2008: 263).

The feeling of being located in the world seems to be important for a child and Velleman suggests that an essential part of this may be a feeling of belonging to one particular, traceable bloodline. To the extent this is true it would be hard to show how non-biologically related families could fully mimic this condition in any meaningful way. It remains to be seen, however, whether feelings of kinship and belonging cannot be experienced on the basis of other kinds of bonds. At the point in a young adult's life at which knowledge of her location in the universe begins to matter, she already shares a significant amount of history and cultural values with those she grew up with. Beyond this, she will also recognize certain things about herself that she will look for and find in others with whom she will choose to associate. She will discover other people who share her tastes, her desires, her fears or her loneliness; she might come to identify with her country, religion or a particular political belief. Although maybe none of this can replace blood ties, the human ability to form deep and lasting associative connections and friendships outside the family is an indication that we are equipped to allow other kinds of bonds to compensate for the lack of biological kinship. Velleman might respond that these other kinds of association could never fully replace the 'real' thing. Even then, however, it is not so clear what kind of moral failing the non-provision of blood relationships constitutes: a regrettable but forgivable one or a moral wrong to which it would be irresponsible to subject a child. This brings me to the next step in my argument.

To make his claim that it would be wrong to set out to raise children whom one was unable to create oneself, Velleman has to show that the need to be biologically related is more significant than other needs, the satisfaction of which parents are frequently excused for not providing. There are roughly three kinds of unfavourable conditions that children can be born into or with. The first has to do with biological obstacles caused by the physical or mental constitution a child is born with, the second with adverse political, environmental or personal conditions and the third with parental character flaws.

It remains a subject of heated discussion whether people in this first category should have children, for instance when it is known that their children will be born with a severe disease or handicap that will cause them pain and suffering. Here, some people maintain, inescapable anguish may be built into the life-plan of a future person (Steinbock, 2000: 108–23). It is probably in relation to this category of unfavourable conditions that Velleman would see the greatest problems arising from lack of a biological relationship. This is because he believes that, from the outset and by the way they were conceived, children of non-biological parents are put at a disadvantage they will not be able to overcome.

Certainly, children who are not provided with their full biological ancestry may feel some amount of loss or shortcoming. Nevertheless, as the discussion above showed, provided their nurturing parents love and accept them for who they are and for how different they might be, it is not clear that their situation is one in which they inevitably will be prevented from flourishing and forced to suffer in some existential way. In other words, it is not clear that the suffering imposed by not being raised by biological parents cannot be overcome by children to some reasonable extent. Therefore, this is unlike a situation in which children might find it more difficult or impossible to compensate for how they were born. But there are at least two more categories of unfavourable conditions for children entering the world.

The second category concerns adverse circumstances potential parents might not be able to change, such as having children during times of war, in situations of hardship (financial or otherwise) or raising them in a political and cultural environment that does not recognize them or their kin as free and equal. Here we regularly consider it legitimate for children to be born, although we understand that their suffering and scarring might be substantial. The reason for this probably includes some sense that discouraging people subject to such adverse circumstances from procreating would be adding insult to injury. They are frequently not responsible for bringing these troubles about and can do nothing to change their situation. Moreover, in some places and at some times, it might be vitally important for the survival of a particular community that its members continue to have children even if they will grow up under extremely unfavourable conditions. Although this category of cases is somewhat arguable, it still shows that we do not generally think that it is wrong to bring children into the world under less than perfect circumstances.

Finally, there are parental character flaws. Usually people think that the worst parents can do to children is to abuse and neglect them. Therefore, many think that adults who know that they are prone to such behaviour ought not to have children. From here, however, the question of what kinds of shortcomings would advise against people having children grows increasingly murky. We differ on whether we think that people who have too little patience, are generally uninterested in children, prone to extreme narcissism, are immature or emotionally unstable ought to have children. Most of the time we probably think that as long as these weaknesses are kept within bounds, children of such people will make it through their childhood with scarring they can eventually be expected to live with.

But it is by no means obvious that such complacency is warranted. About thirty years ago Lafollette, whose argument has already been briefly discussed at the beginning of this chapter, commented on how strange it is that we regulate all sorts of behaviour that is potentially harmful to others by requiring licences for driving cars, shooting guns and even for practising medicine, law and psychiatry. We impose such licensing requirements although they may inconvenience and exclude some people from engaging in certain activities. But we do it out of regard for the safety of others. From this perspective it is perplexing that the one action we do not require any prior qualification for is one of the most hazardous to others: parenting. Bad or abusive parents can irreparably damage future persons' lives. According to Lafollette, adults should be required to fulfil at least the minimal requirements for being good parents, such as not having a record of abusive behaviour towards others or of paedophilia.

Lafollette's suggestion seems entirely reasonable. As already mentioned at the outset of this chapter, if we had such a licensing system there would be no reason to discriminate between people who need reproductive help and those who do not. Even if, by contrast, there was general opposition to such a licensing scheme, this would only show that there is some agreement that we should not be overly strict with individuals' reproductive choices. There would also be no reason to treat people who need reproductive assistance differently in this regard from those who do not. This is true unless, of course, the anguish and distress bestowed on children by the former could be shown to be so great that they ought to be treated differently from the others. But even to the extent there might be built-in distress of the kind suggested by Velleman for children who are born into non-traditional family structures or raised by non-biological parents, their situation is probably similar to that of children who are raised by non-ideal parents. These are parents who have too little time, too little patience, are overwhelmed by the task at hand or lack the ability to show affection. All of this might leave some wounds on children. In most of these cases, however, parents arguably score well enough on most other aspects so that we trust that their child will survive their screw-ups and flourish nevertheless. Therefore, given that we frequently do not expect parents to satisfy all of their children's needs, and the particular need to be raised by one's biological kin is arguably similar to other needs parents regularly fall short on, there is no reason to oppose the creation of offspring in non-traditional family contexts.

This suggestion runs counter to current policy regarding the provision of artificial reproductive services in several European countries.[5]

---

[5] Lesbians, for instance, are denied donor insemination in Denmark, Norway, Sweden, Iceland, Switzerland, Germany and France.

In Germany, for instance, surrogacy and egg donation are prohibited according to the Law for the Protection of the Embryo, so that it is impossible for homosexual couples to have a biologically related child. Insemination with donor sperm may only be performed by physicians. Adoption poses a further difficulty: although there is no law regulating the age before which prospective parents ought to adopt, adoption agencies prefer married heterosexual couples who are no more than forty years older than their adoptive child. None of these prohibitions, difficulties and preferences make sense if we think that the 'good' of parenthood that so many aspire to enjoying consists in a mutually beneficial relationship between adults and the children they raise. There is no reason to think that such a relationship cannot be had between children and adults who are homosexual, above the reproductive age, not married or not biologically related to the children in their care.

Thus, the only argument against allowing individuals to be parents holds regardless of whether they need assisted reproductive help or not. It would pertain to cases in which we had some indication that a particular individual is unwilling to care for a child, incapable of providing the necessary affection, or unable to refrain from abusing or neglecting the child. These considerations suggest that singles, gays, lesbians, people of advanced age and certainly all others who cannot conceive by themselves ought not to be systematically denied access to technologies of assisted reproduction.

Exculpating parents

What follows from the above analysis, is that we cannot prevent people from seeking reproductive help to have a biologically related child. What does not immediately ensue is that we have to provide financial assistance for them to do so. There are limited resources and the needs of those requiring reproductive assistance compete with other important health care necessities.

As I have mentioned before, with many individuals the wish to have their own biologically related child runs deep. There might be several reasons for this. Some might be inspired by the romantic idea that children are the culmination of two persons' love or believe that children's memories or genes contribute to their parents' immortality. Whatever anybody may think individually about the importance of raising one's own kin, there are significant social pressures as well: whereas infertility is stigmatized as a disease, childbirth is regularly celebrated. Obviously there are good reasons for societies to encourage persons to have children and to feel responsible for them. It would certainly constitute a highly conflicting narrative if it were suggested at the same time that it is a good thing to raise someone else's children. Surely, it is also this prevailing narrative about the beauty of having and caring for one's own children that influences people's choices and wishes and that causes them to suffer if they cannot fulfil this wish. Arguably, therefore, reproduction is not an exclusively private enterprise. But to the extent society is responsible for producing these deep-seated reproductive wishes, it is also responsible for fulfilling them.

Consider the following analogy to the case of child-bearing. Suppose a governmental agency had good reasons to seize people's property. To seize the property, the government requires agents to knock on people's door and take it. Only certain people qualify for the job. There is a preference for men between the ages 20 and 40. Of these eligible men, it is regularly the case that many voluntarily apply to become agents. They do this for different reasons. Some because they attach a certain value to the job, others because they feel that it is expected of them. Surely we do not think they, as agents, are responsible for the seizing of the property. Nor do those whose property is thus taken and who have to start from scratch blame the particular agent who happened to knock on their door for their predicament. They understand that the agent, by taking on his job, did not intend to affect *their* life in particular. What these agents are certainly responsible for is to execute their job well. But there is no obvious way to accomplish this: ought agents to write letters announcing their visit (if yes, how many?); ought they to knock several times; ought they to smile and be friendly when they make their demands and may they use violence? Most of these questions will be settled by some governmental policy and only to a very small degree be a matter of personal style. But whatever the policy is, agents will be required to adhere to it to some reasonable degree if they do not want to lose their job.

In many respects, child-bearing is similar. Individuals sign up to become parents, frequently out of their own volition. They subsequently take part in a process which is much larger than them, which they did not author and from which they profit only as a side-effect. Just as the agents do not receive the benefit of the property they are seizing, but only the salary they are paid for doing their job, parents may enjoy having children, but much of the benefits of reproduction are reaped by the human collective(s) they help propagate (family, society, the species as a whole). Moreover, just as no agent is responsible for the property-seizing policy and the effects this has on those deprived of their belongings, nobody in particular is responsible for the fact that birth occurs the way it does and is an ambivalent kind of blessing.[6] Birth, in this sense, merely happens to people, most literally to those it brings about but also – to some extent at least – to those who bring it about. Finally, just as the agents' performance in the analogy is judged by governmental standards, it is mostly society that defines the rules of what is required to be a good parent.

The reader is surely tempted to think that some (maybe even all) of these suggestions are preposterous. The proposition most likely to attract objection is probably the one about parents not being wholly responsible even if they intentionally initiate the existence of a new person. One might ask: how can those who intentionally procreate (or intend to have a child in vitro) and freely agree to be the ones to raise their children not be held fully responsible for their reproductive choices if it is true that anyone can decide not to become a parent (especially in cases of assisted reproduction)? Many people argue that passing up an opportunity to have a child is not a moral wrong. We generally do not blame people for deciding not to have children. At the same time: how can it not be a blameworthy omission, if it is also true that if everybody passed up on this opportunity, we, as a society, could and would not tolerate it?

Perhaps people might say it would not be a moral wrong, just imprudent for the survival of the species. Whatever our moral responsibility for insuring the survival of the species may be, societies have generally been able to trust that a sufficient number of people will decide to create families (with the exception of modern industrialized societies perhaps) so that a little free-riding could go unpunished. This is partly because there are reasons, rooted perhaps in a combination of biological and of social pressures, which facilitate such a choice. Especially with regard to social pressure, it is certainly not accidental that infertility is treated as a disease. In many cultures, infertility makes women feel less feminine and men less masculine. Some cultures and societies believe a marriage to be null and void if, after a certain period of time, the couple has not been able to have children. Therefore, at least in societies and cultures that encourage certain stereotypes about the family and about

---

[6] This appears to be like saying that because nobody is responsible for the fact that smoking causes cancer, whoever smokes is not morally responsible for the cancer for which her smoking was causally responsible. My answer to this would be yes and no. As long as people have an honest choice between whether or not to smoke, they can be held causally as well as morally responsible. If, however, there turns out to be a large corporate (in the case of smoking) or social (in the case of procreation) interest which demonstrably skews the range of options or the desirability of smoking versus not smoking or procreating versus not procreating, then I think the primary moral responsibility may jump ship.

fertility, there are good reasons to think that society has a substantial obligation to support individuals who choose to reproduce.[7] Such obligations would have to include a whole set of material and emotional assistance for parents to fulfil the duties we think they have by choosing to raise a child.

Moreover, these obligations ought also to entail a commitment to those who are not physically capable of having their own children to help them fulfil the reproductive desires their environment has instilled in them. As Velleman persuasively puts it, life is a predicament into which we were all thrown unasked. This is true of children, but it does not cease to be equally true of the adults these children grow into. They are also faced with daunting challenges and work under the pressure of having to succeed in life. As long as having children continues to be one important marker of femininity and masculinity, a society incurs the obligation to do everything possible to provide assistance. This having been said, however, two important qualifications apply: first, that such support does not wrong others and second, that it does not unduly siphon off resources that would be needed in other important areas of health care. As I have tried to show, the first concern does not hold. Practices necessary for allowing infertile couples to have children, including gamete donation, do not systematically wrong the children created this way and do not inevitably prevent them from flourishing. The second concern, about how resources are to be allotted, will continually have to be subject to democratic negotiation. This having been said, it will have to give appropriate weight to society's obligation to take responsibility for the wishes and preferences it continues to inculcate in its members.

Conclusion

I have argued that although there are differences between people who can reproduce without medical assistance and those who cannot, these differences are not morally relevant when it comes to assessing who would be a good parent. Therefore, there is no valid reason to treat these two categories of people differently. If we allow everyone who can have children without medical assistance to have them regardless of their ability, effort and desire to being parents, we should not systematically make it harder for people seeking reproductive assistance to have a child.

---

[7] The case might be different in societies, cultures or religions (i.e. Manicheans) that explicitly discourage procreation.

I then went on to show that to the extent society is responsible for individuals' wishes to have children, there is an obligation to give some material assistance to those who need reproductive help, even if the exact amount will depend on the amount of resources there are after the need for infertility treatment has been weighed against other important health care needs in the democratic process.

REFERENCES

Brighouse, H. and Swift, A. (2006). 'Parents' rights and the value of the family'. *Ethics*, 117, 80–108.
  (2009). 'Legitimate parental partiality'. *Philosophy and Public Affairs*, 37, 43–80.
Honneth, A. (1995). *The Struggle for Recognition. The Moral Grammar of Social Conflict*. Cambridge: Polity.
  (2001). 'Invisibility. On the epistemology of "recognition"'. *Aristotelian Society Supplementary*, 75, 111–26.
Lafollette, H. (1980). 'Licensing parents'. *Philosophy and Public Affairs*, 9, 182–97.
Pennings, G. (2003). 'The physician as an accessory in the parental project of HIV positive people'. *Journal of Medical Ethics*, 29, 321–4.
Steinbock, B. (2000). 'Disability, prenatal testing, and selective abortion', in E. Parens and A. Asch (eds.), *Prenatal Testing and Disability Rights*. Washington, DC: Georgetown University Press.
Velleman, J. D. (2008). 'Persons in prospect'. *Philosophy and Public Affairs*, 36, 221–88.

5 Reproductive donation: global perspectives and cultural diversity

Zeynep B. Gürtin and Effy Vayena

One of the most striking aspects of assisted reproductive technologies (ARTs) has been their rapid globalization. Although ARTs may pose a range of (financial, practical, emotional, psychological, as well as moral) challenges for both providers and users, they have ultimately been embraced by many diverse cultures. ARTs speak to the fundamental desire to become a parent, albeit in a very particular way, and as such enjoy a wide global appeal that transcends many cultural divergences. However, although ARTs may have become 'global', their practice in different parts of the world has been subject to a range of limitations, modifications and prohibitions. These context-specific 'arenas of constraint' have mediated and defined the ways in which ARTs are offered to and received by local men and women, and have set up specific relationships between technology and culture (Inhorn, 2002). Particularly during the last two decades, a wealth of research has been dedicated to documenting the processes of 'localization' by which ARTs have been reconfigured in different global contexts, including debates regarding the morality and acceptability of certain technologies, the impact of socio-economic circumstances, and the experiences of men and women undergoing infertility treatment (for a review of this literature, see Inhorn and Birenbaum-Carmeli, 2008). While this scholarship does not (yet) provide us with a comprehensive survey of practices and attitudes regarding assisted reproduction in *all* global locations, it nevertheless highlights great cultural diversity through the exploration of a range of similarities and differences, patterns and outliers. Within this broad picture of cultural diversity in ARTs, the heterogeneity regarding reproductive donation – in other words the use of donor sperm, donor eggs and surrogates – is arguably the most varied, interesting and controversial.

In this chapter we adopt a global perspective in order to highlight some of the cultural diversity that exists in the regulation, practice and attitudes surrounding reproductive donation. We begin by providing an overview of the anthropological and ethnographic data on infertility and assisted reproduction, particularly with regard to 'third-party reproductive assistance', and move on to evaluate diversity in ethical deliberations and in the approaches of three monotheistic religions (Judaism, Christianity and Islam) towards donation. Having dedicated most of the chapter to differences *between* nations or religions, we end with a discussion of diversity *within* cultures. We argue that global and cultural diversity regarding donation in assisted reproduction not only has distinct practical implications for societies, and especially for involuntarily childless men and women, but also that it produces distinct ethical dilemmas and conundrums. If we are to present meaningful empirical insights and to develop sensitive ethical analyses, it is of paramount importance to be aware of the diversity that exists.

Anthropology and ARTs

Since the birth of Louise Brown in 1978, the uptake, proliferation and promises of assisted reproduction have reignited the traditional anthropological interests in kinship and gender, albeit with a new focus and referent (Edwards *et al.*, 1999; Carsten, 2000). ARTs intersect crucial themes of kinship, gender, embodiment, religion, medicalization and lay-expert interactions, and thus enable comment on myriad social changes and phenomena such as stigmatization and modernity, kinship and marital relations. In addition to this, the involvement of 'third parties' in the process of reproduction – egg and sperm donors and surrogates – signals new social and relational choreographies, challenges and opportunities which have proved 'fertile ground' for anthropologists.

Marilyn Strathern's seminal book *Reproducing the Future: Essays on Anthropology, Kinship and the New Reproductive Technologies* (1992) articulated the cultural relevance of ARTs (particularly with the involvement of 'third-party reproductive assistance') and the novel distinctions now enabled between social and biological parents. The potential cultural impact of this 'kinship revolution' on biogenetic definitions of relatedness (Schneider, 1980) lead to a range of ethnographic studies, initially concentrated on 'Euro-American' settings (e.g. Ragoné, 1994; Franklin, 1997; Carsten, 2004), and more recently extending to an ever greater number of locations. These studies documented social changes and problematized the previously assumed paradigm of kinship as the social recognition of the actual facts of biological reproduction (Carsten, 2004). Currently, there is a growing body of rich anthropological ART literature from myriad countries and cultures, including parts of Europe (Franklin, 1997; Paxson, 2004; Konrad, 2005; Bonaccorso, 2008), East Asia (Handwerker, 2002; Pashigian, 2009; Simpson, 2004) and South

America (Roberts, 2008), as well as sustained and rigorous studies of the USA (Sandelowski, 1993; Becker, 2000; Thompson, 2005), Israel (Kahn, 2000; 2002; Birenbaum-Carmeli, 2004; Teman, 2010), India (Bharadwaj, 2003) and the Middle East (Inhorn, 2003a; Clarke, 2009; Gürtin-Broadbent, 2012). Moreover, over the past decade increasing interest in comparing and contrasting ARTs as they are practised around the world has brought together the works of various scholars in a range of edited volumes that focus on different aspects of infertility and assisted reproduction, from the consequences of childlessness (Inhorn and Van Balen, 2002) to men's gendered experiences (Inhorn *et al.*, 2009), from genetic testing (Birenbaum-Carmeli and Inhorn, 2009), to donation practices (Blyth and Landau, 2004). Indeed, particularly in the fast expanding sub-field of medical anthropology, no subject (with perhaps the exception of HIV/AIDS) has generated as much discussion nor received as much attention as assisted reproduction (Inhorn and Birenbaum-Carmeli, 2008).

Unlike perhaps the approaches of other disciplines, anthropological studies of assisted reproduction have paid close attention to the interrelation or co-constitution of technology and society, such that each simultaneously impacts and is impacted on by the other (Ong and Collier, 2005). Inhorn and Birenbaum-Carmeli (2008: 178) explain that ARTs are culturally embedded 'socio-technical products, which are shaped by human and non-human factors, including the technical features of the ARTs themselves, as well as by the economic, political, cultural and moral environs in which they unfold', and that they are 'intimately linked with power relations'. Inhorn (2003a), based on her studies of Egypt, has coined the term 'localization' to refer to the processes whereby the global technology of in vitro fertililzation (IVF) is made (and remade) culturally pertinent and appropriate in specific locations, and has pursued medical anthropologist/psychiatrist Arthur Kleinman's (1995) trope of 'local moral worlds' to reveal the accounts of social participants regarding 'what is at stake in everyday experience'. Such approaches have recently gained great popularity and indeed much of the recent medical anthropology scholarship concerned with this area has sought to articulate local morals and to elucidate processes of local application.

Why is it that ARTs are pursued in secret and imagined to confer further stigmatization on their users in some global locations, such as Egypt (Inhorn, 2003a), while in others, such as China (Handwerker, 2002) they are regarded as prized emblems of modernity and a means of creating babies that are morally and physically superior? What are the reasons that some cultures (e.g. the UK) apply symmetrical rules to the use of sperm and eggs, whereas in others (e.g. Germany, Israel) they are subject to different regulations? Why are parents of donor-conceived offspring moving towards patterns of greater disclosure in some countries (e.g. USA and UK), whereas in others donor conception remains as secret and stigmatized as ever (Gürtin, 2012)? And perhaps most fundamentally, why have ARTs led to the creation of myriad 'non-traditional' family types in some social contexts (see Graham and Braverman, Chapter 11; Appleby, Jennings and Statham, Chapter 12), yet in others have only reinforced 'traditional' family structures, exclusively assisting the reproduction of medically infertile married heterosexual couples? Examining these anthropological questions, as well as a host of 'culturally embedded' others, sheds light on the diversity of reactions, uses and consequences of assisted reproduction around the world. This tells us not only about what happens in other exotic locations, but enables us to question the taken-for-granted assumptions of our own social contexts, revealing much of what we imagine to be 'given' as in fact socially constructed. The focus of this chapter on cultural diversity therefore highlights that there is not necessarily one ethical answer or practical solution to dilemmas surrounding donation, but rather that such dilemmas must be considered in context and in relation to broader social factors.

Reproductive donation and diversity

Infertility, often defined as the inability for a reproductive-aged couple to conceive a child after a year (or longer) of regular unprotected intercourse (Zegers-Hochschild et al., 2009), is a universally occurring health problem. It is commonly accepted that infertility affects more than 80 million people worldwide, and The World Health Organisation (WHO) recognizes infertility as an unmet need in family planning in both developed and developing nations. On average one in ten couples experience primary or secondary infertility during their lifetime; however, both the prevalence of infertility and the experiences of involuntarily childless men and women are subject to great global variation (Vayena et al., 2002).

Involuntary childlessness can have many different causes, from iatrogenic infections to age-related fertility decline, and infertility may be manifested through a range of physiologically female or male factors, such as ovarian failure or sperm immotility. Some of these causes will respond to drug treatments or can be bypassed with IVF or intra-cytoplasmic sperm injection (ICSI), although in certain intractable cases it remains impossible for individuals to conceive genetically related children. Despite great techno-scientific advances, sometimes the use of 'third-party reproductive assistance' in the form of donor gametes remains the only means for a couple to achieve conception.[1] While such potential 'treatments' are increasingly regarded as an acceptable (if 'last resort') option among heterosexual couples in some cultures, in others they remain strictly prohibited, heavily stigmatized and absolutely unacceptable.

The use of reproductive donation is one of the most globally controversial aspects of ART practice. Cultural responses to the use of donor sperm or eggs ranges from complete prohibition (e.g. in most Muslim countries) to a lucrative trade in an open-market (e.g. the USA – see Glennon, Chapter 6). Not only do donor gametes sever the (imagined if not always actual) synonymy between biological and social parenthood, but they also enable novel family formations by single women and men, lesbian and gay couples (see Graham and Braverman, Chapter 11; Appleby, Jennings and Statham, Chapter 12), and facilitate previously unimagined relations between strangers (see Freeman, Appleby and Jadva, Chapter 14) and between family members (see Vayena and Golombok, Chapter 10). Indeed, many chapters in this volume detail the new opportunities, dilemmas and relationships that result from the use of donor gametes, but it is also important to reference broader debates regarding whether reproductive donation is morally and culturally acceptable. While social attitudes towards donor gametes may be difficult to compare across cultures (due to a lack of comprehensive data and circumstantial differences across contexts), it is somewhat easier to compare regulatory frameworks and rules that pertain to the practices of 'third-party reproductive assistance'. Although, even in this regard, there is no comprehensive global survey, there is enough information to highlight an extreme diversity of regulations, ranging from laissez-faire permissiveness to specific prescriptions that strictly define parameters of legally and morally permissible practice.

According to the IFFS Surveillance 07 (Jones *et al.*, 2007), which has collated information from fifty-seven nations, their mode of ART regulation can be divided into three categories: countries that govern ART practice through legal formulations; countries that only provide guidelines; and countries in which there is no governing structure imposed. Among these there are great differences in the level of permissiveness

---

[1] Donor gametes are of course also necessary to achieve conception in single women, lesbian or gay couples (as addressed in various chapters in this volume: e.g. Graham and Braverman; Jennings *et al.*). However, perhaps the issues involved in these choreographies are not most usefully conflated with the issues that pertain to fertility problems in heterosexual couples.

and the nature of prohibitions. While thirteen of the fifty-seven participating nations (including China, Turkey, Lithuania and Egypt) impose a marriage requirement for a couple to access ARTs, fifteen others (including Korea, Mexico, South Africa and Thailand) have no requirements whatsoever. Donor sperm and eggs were disallowed either by law or by guidelines in Italy, Tunisia, Turkey, Egypt, Japan, Morocco and the Philippines. Austria and Germany both disallow the use of donor sperm in IVF, but allow it for donor insemination (DI). Germany, China, Norway and Switzerland prohibit the use of donor eggs, but with the exception of Germany all of them allow sperm donation (Jones *et al.*, 2007). Moreover, among the countries that permit the use of donor gametes, there are multiple heterogeneous conditions regarding who may donate; whether they may receive remuneration; whether donors can or must be known, identifiable, or anonymous; who may receive donated gametes under what conditions; and how many children or families may be created by one donor.

The resulting picture is a dazzling panoply according to which almost every country has defined a particular and unique set of parameters for the practice of assisted reproduction. For example, in Greece gamete donations must be anonymous, whereas in Australia, the UK and the Netherlands all donors must provide identifying information. The UK currently accepts intra-familial donors, while France does not. Embryo donation and surrogacy are forbidden in Sweden and Denmark, but permitted in Finland. Donors receive variable payments in the USA, levelled reimbursement in Spain, and in the UK no remuneration beyond loss of earnings and direct expenses. The diversity evident, even in this non-exhaustive list, carries a range of ethical and practical implications and consequences for regulators and patients, such as posing challenges to donor recruitment (see Pennings, Vayena and Ahuja, Chapter 9) and driving transnational donation (see Pennings and B. Gürtin, Chapter 8). Moreover, this diversity is also indicative of underlying cultural differences, diverse reasoning processes, and the divergent prioritization of moral and ethical principles that manifest in differing approaches to donation.

However, having said this, it must also be noted that regulations cannot necessarily be seen as indicative of general 'public opinion' or of how individuals affected with infertility will choose to resolve (or not resolve) their fertility problems. For example, a recent study conducted on infertile men and women in Turkey showed that, despite the regulatory ban on all forms of third-party reproductive assistance, 23% would accept donor eggs; 15.1% would accept surrogacy; and 3.4% would accept donor sperm if it were medically indicated and available (Baykal *et al.* 2008). Moreover, as shown in a different study, there was also high acceptance of donor eggs as a medical treatment among the general Turkish population, with over half of the women and nearly two thirds of the men surveyed replying positively and stating (mistakenly) that they thought their religion, Islam, would allow it (Isikoglu *et al.*, 2006). These studies illustrate the differences in local attitudes towards eggs and sperm, yet they also demonstrate the difficulty of inferring individuals' opinions from government regulation, or indeed from the edicts of religious authorities. As in other matters, we should not be surprised to find a spectrum and diversity of opinions on questions over ARTs, nor to detect distinct differences between regulation and public discourses on the one hand, and individual opinions on the other.

Diversity in ethical deliberations regarding donation

The diversity of perception and regulation of third-party reproductive assistance reflects how differently ethical arguments are structured and deliberated within different social contexts. This plays out in two levels: the broader societal level ethics (macroethics), namely what societies define as ethically acceptable through their various processes; and at the individual level (microethics), namely the individual's own ethical judgement regarding what is or is not ethically acceptable to him or her. These two sometimes match; however, as mentioned above, often they do not. Regulations and guidelines generated by public commissions tend to address more the macroethical level of ARTs, circumscribing, however, the area within which microethics will manoeuvre (Cook *et al.*, 2003). At the macroethical level, ethical reasoning is intertwined with various other aspects in the process of policy-making (including political agendas, ideologies, religion and budgets). Presenting a policy as ethically justified is in the interest of policy makers, as it might contribute to higher acceptability and wider public agreement. However, it is of particular interest to examine how ethical arguments can be used to support very different, and even contradicting, policies. For example, why is it ethically acceptable to allow egg donation in France but not in neighbouring Switzerland or Germany? How can these diametrically opposite policies be ethically justified by the societies in question?

Looking closely at the justification of prohibitive policies reveals that the language of 'ethics' plays a prominent role in their explanation. Countries with highly restrictive policies (such as Germany and Switzerland) have structured the argument against egg donation around the issue of medical risk. Ovarian stimulation and oocyte retrieval were viewed as too risky to be allowed. The *protection* of the potential egg donor, although at first glance reflects the non-maleficence principle, also incidentally seems to support the broader Embryo Protection Act adopted by the German government in 1990. Germany's history and the political constellation at the time the Act was deliberated are undoubtedly of great relevance here (Bleiklie *et al.*, 2004). The core ethical argument for the Embryo Protection Act was respect for human dignity. Although the German law is about twenty years old, and medical risks in ovarian stimulation and oocyte retrieval have been dramatically reduced (though not eliminated) in the intervening period, no revision of the Act is currently in sight. Another justification for the prohibition was the view that social and genetic motherhood should not be separated. Since sperm donation is allowed, this reasoning implicitly argues that motherhood is more important than fatherhood and that the separation of genetic and social fatherhood is more acceptable (Schaefer, 2007). It is hard to understand the ethical basis of this argument, beyond the pure assumption that it is better for a society to maintain the more traditional family forms.

In Italy in 2004, a new highly restrictive law prohibited, amongst other aspects of ARTs, all forms of egg and sperm donation, turning Italy overnight from the 'Wild West' of European ARTs to the most prohibitive country in this region. The law was a result of year-long debates in the Italian parliament. Here, unlike in the German example, it was not the medical risks that captured the attention of regulators, but rather the (presumed) moral risks associated with reproductive donation. The justification for prohibiting gamete donation, which loudly echoes the Vatican's opinions, was structured around the protection of future children from incestuous relationships (sexual relations between children conceived using gametes from the same anonymous donor), identity problems and parental rejection by the non-biological parent, as well as the protection of society from positive eugenics through the seeking of specific traits in donors. This language of ethics and morality at the macro level did not represent the views of most Catholic Italians. As Inhorn *et al.* (2010) showed in a recent comparative study examining ART practice in Sunni Egypt, Shi'a Lebanon and Catholic Italy, the Italian law clearly diverged from the wishes of Catholic patients and physicians. In countries with less prohibitive policies, neither the concept of medical risk nor that of social or moral risk surfaced adequately to affect policies. The countries that favoured prohibitive policies regarding gamete donation have adopted a more paternalistic approach, putting forward the argument of protecting their citizens and their societies, while those who chose to allow particular forms of donation have left the decision to be made by individuals, ultimately allowing more room for the exercise of autonomy and personal decision-making.

Another illustrative example of different ethical justifications in contradicting guidelines and policies is financial remuneration for donors. In several countries paying egg or sperm donors is forbidden by law, while in the USA it is not only allowed but there is even a price recommendation by the American Society for Reproductive Medicine (according to which a justification is needed above $5,000, and above $10,000 is considered inappropriate). In European countries the basic ethical argument against the payment of donors has been that of human dignity, which disallows trading of the human body, its cells and parts. In the USA, however, it has been considered fair to compensate people for their services (in this case provision of gametes). There is a long debate on the ethics of financial compensation of gamete donors which is discussed in detail in the chapter by Pennings, Vayena and Ahuja in Chapter 9 of this volume. However, what is of interest here is the fact that different societies choose to give priority and prominence to different ethical arguments, or that they interpret differently the same principles as best fits their cultures and traditions. Health care in the USA has traditionally been driven by market forces and the culture of fee-for-service has shaped how medicine is practised. It is within that culture that a fee for the noble service of donating gametes appears ethically justifiable. In European countries, however, with a welfare approach to health care and with historical experiences that demonstrate the stakes in human dignity, financial compensation of gamete donors seems to constitute an ethical transgression, at least at the regulatory level (ESHRE Task force on Ethics and Law, 2002). The concerns over fairness here are not about depriving the donor of what she or he deserves, but rather about not creating unfair options (i.e. inducing them to sell parts of their bodies) for the financially disadvantaged.

Cultural contexts are not only shaping the ethical arguments at the macro level but even more profoundly at the individual level. Infertility patients and their doctors shape their value systems within their cultural and religious contexts, and make their decisions accordingly. Disclosure to the donor-conceived offspring provides a good example. Ethnographic studies show that in certain cultures couples have become more open to the idea of disclosing donation while in others secrecy remains of paramount importance (e.g. Inhorn and Van Balen, 2002). This may be partially explained by the different weight that individual autonomy has in the different cultural contexts in question. In many Western cultures individual rights, autonomy and self-determination are very important. In several other cultures, however, these concepts are a lot less emphasized. Instead other moral references are in place, such as the autonomy of the family or the best interest of the family, rather than the individual. In the latter cases, relational autonomy (with the emphasis on relation) will direct the decision-making process (Turoldo, 2010).

There are a range of conundrums, dilemmas and challenges that arise as a result of diversity regarding ethical deliberations on donation. These may occur: (a) at the macro level; (b) between the macro and the micro levels; or (c) at the micro level. At the macro level, for example, the use of different ethical frameworks has led to very different regulatory outcomes (see Glennon, Chapter 6; García-Ruiz and Guerra-Diaz, Chapter 7). This diversity of government regulation has led to strikingly different parameters of ART practice even among the countries of the European Union, as we have discussed above, and would make any attempt to pursue international harmonization of ART regulation almost impossible. This, when coupled with the diversity between the macro and micro levels (i.e. between the views expressed in regulation and those held by various individuals), has produced a booming market in cross-border reproductive care (see Pennings and Gürtin, Chapter 8), as persons who disagree with the ART policies of their jurisdictions demonstrate 'moral pluralism in motion' by seeking treatments elsewhere (Pennings, 2002). Diversity can also occur as a result of differences just at the micro level, such as different reasoning process or an emphasis on different ethical principles by stakeholders. For example, whether one emphasizes individual or relational autonomy can dictate whether secrecy regarding donor conception is seen as infringing the rights of an individual to know their origins or as the best solution for the family unit (see Appleby, Blake and Freeman, Chapter 13). This could also lead to irresolvable conflicts between the interests or ethical claims of different parties, such as donors, parents and offspring.

Religious perspectives on donation

Religious authorities and sensibilities may be a significant influence on the (bio)ethical reasoning of both individuals and of collective decision makers (such as governments or regulators) and are one distinct source of ethical guidance. Although Schenker rightly cautions that 'it is often difficult to dissociate the influence of distinctly religious factors from other cultural conditions' (2005: 310), he argues that there are at least three factors that determine the influence of religious viewpoints: the size of the community; the authority of religious views within the population; and the unanimity or diversity of opinion present. Developments in reproductive technologies raise novel dilemmas and questions for religions and religious authorities, which in some instances do not have clear answers or precedents that can be used as a reference. Nevertheless, the deliberations by religious authorities and the decisions they reach may be an important guide regarding which ARTs are and are not acceptable and under what conditions.

Meirow and Schenker argued that 'The practice of gamete donation is opposed by the main religions and is not usually accepted by religious infertile couples or by religious physicians' (1997: 134). Although the intervening period, of over a decade, has seen a great increase in the use of donation accompanied in many places by greater social acceptance and more relaxed attitudes, the use of assisted reproduction techniques, including 'third-party reproductive assistance', have caused great moral debates and deliberations for the world's Abrahamic religions: Christianity, Islam and Judaism.[2]

The Roman Catholic Church headed by the Vatican has one of the most restrictive attitudes towards assisted reproduction among the Christian churches, and rejects not only donation but also IVF as a treatment option, since fertilization outside of the conjugal act is seen to be deprived of its proper perfection. The use of donor gametes is prohibited on the grounds that they involve a separation between 'the goods and meanings of marriage' (Schenker, 2005). In addition, the embryo is accorded with moral status from the moment of conception and it therefore needs to be treated in a manner that respects its humanity and potential; thus cryopreservation, storage and discarding of 'spare' embryos are all morally problematic.

Unlike Catholicism, Islam not only accepts, but positively endorses and encourages, the seeking of biomedical treatment for infertility. IVF is seen by Islam as a beneficial medical treatment and (when the gametes used for fertilization belong to the heterosexual couple intending to parent) presents no significant ethical problems (Inhorn, 2002; 2003a; 2003b; Clarke, 2006a). However, there is some disagreement between the Sunni and Shi'a branches of Islam regarding the acceptability of gamete donation (Inhorn 2006a; 2006b; 2006c; 2006d; Clarke, 2007; 2009; Inhorn *et al.*, 2010).

Among the Sunni branch of Islam (to which between 80–90 per cent of all Muslims belong), there is a widely held consensus that 'medical interventions in human reproduction should restrict themselves

---

[2] The Baha'i Faith is also an Abrahamic religion, but nothing has been written about its attitudes towards ART, thus we leave it out of the present discussion.

to a husband and (one) wife couple' (Clarke, 2006b: 26). The use of third-party reproductive assistance is seen as akin to adultery or *zina*, since it leads to confusion regarding parentage and obfuscates the lines of genealogy, whose preservation is of primary religious importance. Indeed, 'Preserving the "origins" of each child – meaning its relationship to a known biological mother and father – is considered not only an ideal in Islam, but a moral imperative' (Inhorn, 2006a: 440). Thus most Islamic authorities prohibit the use of donor gametes and view this as an illegitimate form of procreation.

The Shi'a branch of Islam, however, represents a multiplicity of opinions on donation, as advanced by different religious leaders, some of which are permissive of the use of donor eggs, embryos and sperm. Some leaders have issued *fatwa* (religious edicts) condoning the use of donor gametes, based on the reasoning that such interventions do not impact lineage (Inhorn, 2006c; 2006d; Clarke, 2009). As a result of this, Shi'a Iran and multi-sectarian Lebanon have become 'pockets of permissiveness' as regards donation within a restrictive Muslim Middle East. This difference of opinion between Sunni and Shi'a Islam, as well as between the *fatwa* of different Shi'a clerics, has resulted in fascinating social choreographies, whereby desperate infertile men and women switch their allegiances to more permissive clerics, non-Muslim practitioners display *fatwa* absolving their practices on the walls of their clinics (Clarke, 2009), and Sunni couples from surrounding Middle Eastern countries engage in surreptitious reproductive trips (Inhorn, 2011; Inhorn *et al.*, 2010).

Also situated in the Middle East, Israel has a completely different attitude towards assisted reproduction from its neighbours. Although socio-economic factors and political interests undoubtedly play a part in determining national policies around reproduction, Judaism's permissiveness is also a major factor in explaining how Israel's ART industry has become so prolific, including the provision of state-funded IVF treatment for heterosexual couples, single women and lesbians until they have given birth to two live children. In opposition to both Christianity and (Sunni) Islam, which through different routes arrive at the superficially similar prohibition of third-party assisted reproduction, Judaism has generated altogether different answers to moral and ethical debates around ARTs. This includes an acceptance of the use of donor gametes as legitimate. For example, in the 1990s Rabbinic debates in Israel concentrated on the question of how to reconcile Judaism with the use of donor sperm. The three main areas of concern were: how would sperm be procured since masturbation was prohibited under Halakha (Jewish religious law); what would the relation be between a donor and a child conceived using his sperm; and what would be the status of a child conceived in this manner (Kahn, 2000). In response to these deliberations, the Orthodox Rabbinate reached an unexpected solution, concluding that where male infertility could not be cured then donor sperm may be used, providing that it came from non-Jewish donors. This advocated use of non-Jewish donors bypassed several problems: first, since not bound by Halakha, there would be no problem regarding the production of the sperm sample; second, the practice would not be considered adulterous since Halakha only recognizes relations with other Jewish persons; and third, the use of non-Jewish sperm would not compromise the resulting child's religious identity, since Judaism is inherited directly (and solely) from the mother. Kahn (2000) argues that the negation of the genetic contribution from non-Jewish donors was so comprehensive that children conceived by different women using the same donor would not even be considered as relations.

We can see that within and between three of the monotheistic religions there are different answers to the ethical debates surrounding assisted reproduction and the use of reproductive donation. However, it is also important to bear in mind that the opinions or rulings of religious authorities are not necessarily followed by all members of the religion, nor necessarily enacted as regulations at national level. In fact, it is interesting that while Muslim countries in general and the Jewish state of Israel have regulated their ART practices in accordance with religious rulings, many Christian countries have chosen to ignore such restrictions. The influence of the Catholic or other churches is only discernable in pockets of South America (Roberts, 2008) and in Italy, which recently enacted dramatic legislative changes transforming its ART industry from 'the Wild West of European assisted reproduction' to Europe's most restrictive one (Inhorn *et al.*, 2010).

Diversity within societies

Although in this chapter we have concentrated on displaying the diversity of practices and attitudes regarding ARTs and in particular 'third-party reproductive assistance' *between* different cultures, it must also be acknowledged that great diversity (at the micro level) can exist *within* cultures. This relates to a wide range of individual differences, which may for example lead some parents of donor-conceived offspring to disclose their child's method of conception, while others find such a proposal unacceptable. Though a growing body of ethnographic literature addresses cultural differences between countries, we must not fall into the trap of imagining populations as homogenous, either in their views or their behaviour. In areas such as reproduction, socio-economic status, educational level, religiosity and family history – not to mention cultural background or ethnicity – may prove important differentiators.

Particularly in 'multicultural' and 'multi-ethnic' societies, the experiences or attitudes of minority or immigrant populations towards infertility and assisted reproduction cannot necessarily be inferred from the majority's experience (Culley et al., 2009). It is reasonable to expect that minority groups in multicultural nations may have group-specific attitudes towards, and experiences of, infertility and fertility treatment that is divergent in some ways from the majority experience, or from the experience of other minority groups. Whether their attitudes closely replicate the attitudes of their culture of origin, or represent hybrid formations, will depend on the extent to which 'home' and 'host' cultural frameworks have been maintained, mixed or reconfigured through processes of acculturation and adaptation. For example, a questionnaire study comparing Turks with Turkish migrants in the Netherlands, and with Dutch men and women, found that the experience of infertility among migrants was more similar to Turkish rather than to Dutch respondents' experiences (van Rooij et al., 2007). Similarly, a qualitative study of Turkish women undergoing fertility treatment in the UK found them to have hybrid views and a range of specific interpretations of their infertility experiences, based on their status as immigrants (Gürtin-Broadbent, 2009). Culley et al. (2009) address precisely this 'blind spot' in their volume on *Marginalized Reproduction*, suggesting that whether the minority in question is South Asians in Britain, Turks in the UK or the Netherlands, or Arab Americans, specific research is required in order to learn and make visible the views and experiences of men and women in these 'subcultures'.

There is now considerable data regarding the views of British South Asians on ARTs and gamete donation, examining both public attitudes among this group and more specifically the views of infertile men and women (Culley and Hudson, 2006; 2008; 2009; Culley et al., 2006; Iqbal and Simpson, 2006; Hudson et al., 2009). British South Asians are much less likely than the British public in general to accept and approve of gamete donation, and they are specifically averse to the use of donor sperm in assisted reproduction. This is partly because some groups maintain cultural beliefs around the relative influence of the egg and the sperm on the resultant child, with the sperm being seen as more important in transmitting the family line, and partly because of the incommensurability of using donor sperm with ideas of hegemonic masculinity. In addition, the use of donor sperm may be seen to threaten the stability of marriage and the coherence of the family line, jeopardizing harmony in kinship relations. It is therefore seen as ethically problematic and something to be avoided.

Yet, despite these cultural prohibitions, it has also been found that South Asians acknowledged that donation might sometimes happen among their community, since having children is also a highly valorized social ambition. If indeed a couple were to partake in 'third-party reproductive assistance', there was agreement among research participants that they would not reveal the method of their child's conception. Community perceptions, fear of gossip, judgement and stigmatization would restrict the information that a couple might share with the family, community and donor offspring and make secrecy the most likely option. Bearing this in mind, it may be that specific research is required to provide more information regarding disclosure and child well-being or family relationships among British South Asians, as distinct from a more general British sample. However, it is also important to emphasize that 'British South Asians' themselves form a heterogeneous and diverse group that should not be essentialized. Based on their research with individuals from Indian, Pakistani and Bangladeshi origins, Culley and colleagues (2006) note that cultural understandings and experiences of infertility are mediated by gender, generation and social class, as well as by religion. It is perhaps not surprising that Muslim South Asians are most averse to the use of donor gametes, which is forbidden according to their religion, though it is doubtless important to recognize how culture and religion may or may not exert an influence. Better understanding of the diversity of views within populations is essential if medical practitioners are to avoid misunderstandings and make adequate provisions for the optimal health care of these potential patients.

Conclusion

This chapter has engaged with the anthropological perspectives on infertility and assisted reproduction from around the world, particularly as they pertain to cultural diversity regarding 'third-party reproductive assistance'. Through references to ethnographic research, ethical reasoning and religious perspectives we have presented here a highlighted tour of the diverse global attitudes, practices and regulations on gamete donation, and the differing arguments which they reference. We hope to have shown that diversity exists not only between distant geographical locations but also among close neighbours within Europe, and moreover that there is important diversity to be found even *within* cultures. The range and scope of this diversity regarding donation needs to be acknowledged as a crucial aspect of the global landscape of assisted reproduction. We therefore hope that the cultural snapshots provided here will provide a backdrop or broader context to the more detailed donation discussions that take place throughout this volume (regarding for example anonymity, remuneration and disclosure).

REFERENCES

Baykal, B., Korkmaz, C., Ceyhan, S. T., Goktolga, U. *et al.* (2008). 'Opinions of infertile Turkish women on gamete donation and gestational surrogacy'. *Fertility and Sterility*, 89, 817–22.

Becker, G. (2000). *The Elusive Embryo: How Women and Men Approach New Reproductive Technologies*. Berkeley: University of California Press.

Bharadwaj, A. (2003). 'Why adoption is not an option in India: the visibility of infertility, the secrecy of donor insemination, and other cultural complexities'. *Social Science and Medicine*, 56, 1867–80.

Birenbaum-Carmeli, D. (2004). '"Cheaper than a newcomer": on the social production of IVF policy in Israel'. *Sociology of Health and Illness*, 26, 897–924.

Birenbaum-Carmeli, D. and Inhorn, M. C. (eds.) (2009). *Assisting Reproduction, Testing Genes: Global Encounters with New Biotechnologies*. New York: Berghahn Books.

Bleiklie, I., Goggin, M. and Rothmayr, C. (2004). *Comparative Biomedical Policy; Governing Assisted Reproductive Technologies*. London: Routledge.

Blyth, E. and Landau, R. (eds.) (2004). *Third Party Assisted Conception Across Cultures: Social, Legal and Ethical Perspectives*. London: Jessica Kingsley Publishers.

Bonaccorso, M. E. (2008). *Conceiving Kinship: Family and Assisted Conception in South Europe*. New York: Berghahn Books.

Carsten, J. (2004). *After Kinship*. Cambridge University Press.

Carsten, J. (ed.) (2000). *Cultures of Relatedness: New Approaches to the Study of Kinship*. Cambridge University Press.

Clarke, M. (2006a). 'Islam, kinship and new reproductive technology'. *Anthropology Today* 22(5), 17–20.

(2006b). 'Shiite perspectives on kinship and new reproductive technologies'. *Review of the International Institute for the Study of Islam in the Modern World*, 17, 26–7.

(2007). 'Closeness in the age of mechanical reproduction: debating kinship and biomedicine in Lebanon and the Middle East'. *Anthropology Quarterly*, 80, 379–402.

(2009). *Islam and New Kinship: Reproductive Technology and the Shariah in Lebanon*. New York: Berghahn Books.

Cook, R., Dickens, B. and Fathalla, M. (2003). *Reproductive Health and Human Rights: Integrating Medicine, Human Rights and Law*. Oxford University Press.

Culley, L. and Hudson, N. (2006). 'Disrupted reproduction and deviant bodies: pronatalism and British South Asian communities'. *International Journal of Diversity in Organisations, Communities and Nations*, 5, 117–26.

Culley, L. (2008). 'Public understandings of science: British South Asian men's perceptions of third party assisted conception'. *International Journal of Interdisciplinary Social Sciences*, 2, 79–86.

(2009). 'Constructing relatedness: ethnicity, gender and third party assisted conception'. *Current Sociology*, 57, 257–75.

Culley, L., Hudson, N., Rapport, F., Johnson, M., *et al.* (2006). 'British South Asian communities and infertility services'. *Human Fertility*, 9, 37–45.

Culley, L., Hudson, N. and van Rooij, F. (eds.) (2009). *Marginalized Reproduction: Ethnicity Infertility and Reproductive Technologies*. London: Earthscan.

Edwards, J., Franklin, S., Hirsch, E., Price F., *et al.* (1999). *Technologies of Procreation: Kinship in the Age of Assisted Conception*. London: Routledge.

ESHRE Task Force on Ethics and Law (2002). 'Gamete and embryo donation'. *Human Reproduction*, 17, 1407–8.

Franklin, S. (1997). *Embodied Progress: A Cultural Account of Assisted Conception*. London: Routledge.

Gürtin, Z. B. (2012). 'Assisted reproduction in secular Turkey: regulation, rhetoric, and the role of religion', in M. Inhorn and S. Tremayne (eds.), *Islam and Reproductive Technologies*. New York: Berghahn Books.

Gürtin-Broadbent, Z. (2009). '"Anything to Become a Mother": Migrant Turkish Women's Experiences of Involuntary Childlessness and Assisted Reproductive Technologies in London', in L. Culley, N. Hudson and F. van Rooij (eds.), *Marginalized Reproduction: Ethnicity Infertility and Reproductive Technologies*. London: Earthscan.

(2012). 'IVF Practitioners as Interface Agents between the Local and the Global: The Localization of IVF in Turkey', in M. Knect, M. Klotz and S. Beck (eds.), *Reproductive Technologies as Global Form*. Berlin: Campus Verlag.

Handwerker, L. (2002). 'The Politics of Making Modern Babies in China: Reproductive Technologies and the "New" Eugenics', in M. C Inhorn and F. Van Balen (eds.), *Infertility around the Globe: New Thinking on Childlessness, Gender, and Reproductive Technologies*. Berkeley: University of California Press.

Hudson, N., Culley, L., Rapport, F., Johnson, M., *et al.* (2009). '"Public" perceptions of gamete donation: a research review', *Public Understanding of Science*, 18, 61–77.

Inhorn, M. C. (2002). 'The "Local" Confronts the "Global": Infertile Bodies and New Reproductive Technologies in Egypt', in M. C. Inhorn and F. Van Balen (eds.), *Infertility around the Globe: New Thinking on Childlessness, Gender, and Reproductive Technologies*. Berkeley: University of California Press.

(2003a). *Local Babies, Global Science: Gender, Religion, and In Vitro Fertilization in Egypt*. New York: Routledge.

(2003b). 'Global infertility and the globalization of new reproductive technologies: illustrations from Egypt'. *Social Science and Medicine*, 56, 1837–51.

(2006a). 'Making Muslim babies: IVF and gamete donation in Sunni versus Shi'a Islam'. *Culture, Medicine and Psychiatry*, 30, 427–50.

(2006b). '"He won't be my son": Middle Eastern Muslim men's discourses of adoption and gamete donation'. *Medical Anthropology Quarterly*, 20, 94–120.

(2006c). '*Fatwa*s and ARTS: IVF and gamete donation in Sunni v. Shi'a Islam'. *Journal of Gender, Race and Justice*, 9, 291–317.

(2006d). 'Islam, IVF, and everyday life in the Middle East: the making of Sunni versus Shi'ite test-tube babies'. *Anthropology of the Middle East*, 1, 37–45.

(2011). 'Globalization and Reproductive Tourism in the Muslim Middle East: IVF, Islam, and the Middle Eastern State', in C. H. Browner and C. F. Sargent (eds.), *Reproduction, Globalization, and the State: New Theoretical and Ethnographic Perspectives*. Durham, NC: Duke University Press.

Inhorn, M. C. and Birenbaum-Carmeli, D. (2008). 'Assisted reproductive technologies and culture change'. *Annual Review of Anthropology*, 37, 177–96.

Inhorn, M. C. and Van Balen, F. (eds.) (2002). *Infertility around the Globe: New Thinking on Childlessness, Gender, and Reproductive Technologies*. Berkeley: University of California Press.

Inhorn, M. C., Tjørnhøj-Thomsen T., Goldberg, H. and Mosegaard M. C. (eds.) (2009). *Reconceiving the Second Sex: Men, Masculinity, and Reproduction*. New York: Berghahn Books.

Inhorn, M. C., Patrizio P. and Serour G. I. (2010). 'Third-party reproductive assistance around the Mediterranean: comparing Sunni Egypt, Catholic Italy and multisectarian Lebanon'. *Reproductive Biomedicine Online*, 7: 848–53.

Iqbal, N. and Simpson, B. (2006). 'Kinship, Infertility and New Reproductive Technologies: a British-Pakistani Muslim Perspective', in F. Ebtehaj, B. Lindley and M. Richards (eds.), *Kinship Matters*. Oxford: Hart Publishing.

Isikoglu, M., Senol, Y., Berkkanoglu, M., Ozgur, K., *et al.* (2006). 'Public opinion regarding oocyte donation in Turkey: first data from a secular population among the Islamic world'. *Human Reproduction*, 21, 318–23.

Jones, H. W., Cohen, J., Cooke, I. and Kempers, R. (2007). 'IFFS Surveillance 07'. *Fertility and Sterility*, 87, S1–S67.

Kahn, S. M. (2000). *Reproducing Jews: A Cultural Account of Assisted Conception in Israel*. Durham, NC: Duke University Press.

(2002). 'Rabbis and Reproduction: the Uses of New Reproductive Technologies among Ultraorthodox Jews in Israel', in M. C. Inhorn and F. Van Balen (eds.), *Infertility around the Globe: New Thinking on Childlessness, Gender, and Reproductive Technologies*. Berkeley: University of California Press.

Kleinman, A. (1995). *Writing at the Margin: Discourse between Anthropology and Medicine*. Berkeley: University of California Press.

Konrad, M. (2005). *Nameless Relations: Anonymity, Melanesia and Reproductive Gift Exchange between British Ova Donors and Recipients*. New York: Berghahn Books.

Meirow, D. and Schenker, J. G. (1997). 'Reproductive healthcare policies around the world'. *Journal of Assisted Reproduction and Genetics*, 14, 133–8.

Ong, A. and Collier, S. J. (eds.) (2005). *Global Assemblages: Technology, Politics, and Ethics as Anthropological Problems*. Oxford: Blackwell.

Pashigian, M. (2009). 'Inappropriate Relations: the Ban on Surrogacy with In Vitro Fertilization and the Limits of State Renovation in Contemporary Vietnam', in D. Birenbaum-Carmeli and M. C. Inhorn (eds.), *Assisting Reproduction, Testing Genes: Global Encounters with New Biotechnologies*. New York: Berghahn Books.

Paxson, H. (2006). 'Reproduction as spiritual kin work: orthodoxy, IVF, and the moral economy of motherhood in Greece'. *Culture, Medicine and Psychiatry*, 30, 481–505.

Pennings, G. (2002). 'Reproductive tourism as moral pluralism in motion'. *Journal of Medical Ethics*, 28, 337–41.

Ragoné, H. (1994). *Surrogate Motherhood: Conception in the Heart*. Boulder: Westview Press.

Roberts, E. F. S. (2008). 'Biology, Sociality and Reproductive Modernity in Ecuadorian In-Vitro Fertilization: the Particulars of Place', in S. Gibbon and C. Novas (eds.), *Biosocialities, Genetics and the Social Sciences: Making Biologies and Identities*. New York: Routledge.

Sandelowski, M. (1993). *With Child in Mind: Studies of the Personal Encounter with Infertility*. Philadelphia: University of Pennsylvania Press.

Schaefer, L. (2007). 'Germany's egg donation prohibition is outdated, experts say'. Deutsche Welle. Available at: www.dw-world.de/dw/article/0,2999675,00.html (accessed 9 November 2010).

Schenker, J. G. (2005). 'Assisted reproductive practice: religious perspectives'. *Reproductive BioMedicine Online*, 3, 310–19.

Schneider, D. M. (1980). *American Kinship: A Cultural Account*. University of Chicago Press.

Simpson, R. (2004). 'Acting ethically, responding culturally: Framing the new reproductive and genetic technologies in Sri Lanka'. *The Asia Pacific Journal of Anthropology*, 5, 227–43.

Strathern, M. (1992). *Reproducing the Future: Essays on Anthropology, Kinship and the New Reproductive Technologies*. New York: Routledge.

Teman, E. (2010). *Birthing a Mother: The Surrogate Body and the Pregnant Self*. Berkeley: University of California Press.

Thompson, C. (2005). *Making Parents: The Ontological Choreography of Reproductive Technologies*. Cambridge, MA: MIT Press.

Turoldo, F. (2010). 'Relational autonomy and multiculturalism'. *Cambridge Quarterly of Health Care Ethics*, 19, 542–9.

Van Rooij, F. B., Van Balen, F. and Hermanns, J. M. A. (2007). 'Emotional distress and infertility: Turkish migrant couples compared to Dutch couples and couples in Western Turkey'. *Journal of Psychosomatic Obstetrics and Gynaecology*, 28, 87–95.

Vayena, E., Rowe, P. J. and Griffin, P. D. (2002). *Current Practices and Controversies in Assisted Reproduction: Report of a WHO Meeting.* Geneva: World Health Organization.

Zegers-Hochschild, F., Adamson, G. D., de Mouzon, J., Isihara, O., *et al.* (2009). 'The international Committee for Monitoring Assisted Reproductive Technology (ICMART) and the World Health Organization (WHO) Revised Glossary on ART Terminology, 2009'. *Human Reproduction*, 24, 2683–7.

LEGISLATION

GERMANY

Embryo Protection Act 1990

6 UK and US perspectives on the regulation of gamete donation

Theresa Glennon

Introduction

Assisted reproduction (AR) has dramatically changed family formation in Western countries. It has opened access not only to couples
battling infertility, but also single individuals and gay and lesbian
couples. The United States (USA) and United Kingdom (UK) have
taken sharply different regulatory paths regarding AR. While the UK
has developed comprehensive regulatory guidance for AR providers
based on the work of multidisciplinary commissions, the US legislative scheme is quite limited and fails to address many issues related
to gamete donation. It primarily relies on a market model based on
private ordering. This chapter investigates these contrasting legal
frameworks regarding gamete donation and their ethical contexts. In
conducting this evaluation, it must be kept in mind that both regulation and the absence of regulation express ethical perspectives
(Pennings, 2004).

    While both societies agree that patient autonomy is essential to fer-
tility treatment, the UK seeks to protect the autonomy of all involved
through clearly defined government legislation and guidance. It also
trumps individual autonomy where it finds that societal values, such
as human dignity, override the rights of individuals to make decisions
regarding reproduction. The USA has, for the most part, left deter-
minations regarding autonomy to the private sector – medical professionals, market providers and consumers. Most states have little or no
regulation, so assisted reproductive choices are not restricted, but there
is also less legal certainty regarding the rights of each participant in the
process.

    These contrasting approaches each have their benefits and detri-
ments. The UK's concern for donor-conceived children and antipathy
to payment for gametes emphasize human dignity, but they have led
to a serious shortage of donor gametes. This shortage fails UK residents anxious to pursue AR with donor gametes, limits patient and

donor autonomy and may fuel fertility tourism for donor gametes and surrogacy (Braverman, Casey and Jadva, Chapter 16). The UK's clear legal rules and detailed informed consent requirements permit most participants in AR to make decisions fully aware of their legal parentage consequences, but its rejection of private ordering with respect to parentage or embryo creation limits participants' decision-making authority about matters of great personal interest.

The US approach leaves all decision-making regarding payment for gametes and the interests of donor-conceived children to the private parties participating in AR, mediated through the market. Participants may enter into private agreements but do not know if those agreements will be upheld should one participant change his or her mind. Finally, by allowing markets to set prices and providing little health insurance coverage for fertility treatments, the US approach may also push those in need of fertility services to seek cheaper outlets in other countries, once again raising concerns of exploitation of residents of other countries (Audi and Chang, 2010). The globalization of the AR market means that neither country completely controls reproductive practices by its citizens (Pennings and B. Gürtin, Chapter 8). The ethics and wisdom of the regulatory approaches should be viewed in light of these global options.

Overview of gamete donation

As employed in this chapter, the term 'assisted reproduction' refers broadly to sperm and egg donation and other forms of reproductive assistance, such as in vitro fertilization (IVF). Sperm donation is a long-standing and relatively inexpensive practice. It involves the insemination of a woman with sperm from a male who is not the woman's partner. The sperm is usually ejaculated in a clinical setting, tested for safety and preserved and placed into the woman's cervix or uterus or used to fertilize an egg through the use of IVF. Sperm donation is easily performed outside the clinical setting and so is less subject than egg donation to effective regulation (Glennon, 2010).

Egg donation is more complicated for both donor and recipient. The egg provider must undergo treatment with fertility drugs to synchronize her menstrual cycle with that of the recipient and to increase the number of eggs being created in one cycle. The eggs are extracted through aspiration and used to create an embryo through IVF. They may be implanted in the intended mother or a gestational surrogate or frozen for later use. This arduous process carries some health risks for the egg provider. When completed through medical channels, sperm and egg donations are screened to protect against health risks or the passage of known genetic diseases (Glennon, 2010).

Gamete donation involves at a minimum three parties: the sperm donor, recipient woman and child. It may involve six or more participants: egg and sperm providers, gestational surrogate, two intended parents and one or more resulting children. Technological advances in gamete manipulation may further increase these numbers as it becomes possible to combine gametes from more than two individuals to create an embryo (Mundy, 2007).

Legal regulation and ethical concerns regarding gamete donation in the UK and USA

Broadly speaking, the UK extensively regulates AR while the USA has minimal regulation beyond the laboratory handling of human tissues. The UK has a highly centralized approach to regulation of fertility treatments that relies on the use of expert commissions, public comment and legislation by Parliament. The Human Fertilisation and Embryology Act of 1990 (HFE Act) set forth a scheme of regulation of AR through licensed fertility centres that may be part of the National Health Service (NHS) or privately owned and operated. The HFE Act was amended in 2004 to require that donor identity be made available to all donor-conceived offspring, and was substantially amended in 2008 (HFE Act (as amended)). Because of inadequate funding for NHS fertility treatments, a majority of British patients receive fertility treatment in private for-profit clinics, treatment they must fund themselves (Blyth *et al.*, 2003).

The HFE Act (as amended) governs all aspects of gamete donation, storage, use and resulting family relationships. It also controls other AR technologies, including IVF and surrogacy. The Act is implemented by the Human Fertilisation and Embryology Authority (HFEA), which provides interpretation and guidance to fertility clinics and controls licensing of fertility clinics. The HFE Act (as amended) requires clinics to take into account the welfare of the child being created. It also governs the types of fertility services that may be offered and restricts compensation for gamete donors and surrogates to 'reasonable expenses'. Eggs and sperm cannot be donated on a for-profit basis in the UK, although for-profit gamete banks and clinics may profit from their transfer.

In the USA fertility treatment is an entirely private venture, dominated by for-profit clinics, with the highest fees in the world for in vitro fertilization (Spar, 2006; Connolly *et al.*, 2010). Businesses providing sperm and eggs thrive and provide easy access to those who can afford their services by making their 'donors' available to consumers through internet directories. Sperm specimens can be ordered online and delivered immediately; egg donation is a more complicated process, and, accordingly, significantly more expensive (Mundy, 2007). Few states mandate health insurance coverage for fertility treatment, and even fewer policies include gamete donation (Glennon, 2010). If they do cover some gamete donations, they may limit payment to donations required for medical reasons other than the natural effect of ageing (*Doe* v. *Blue Cross Blue Shield of Massachusetts*, 2010).

Federal law focuses on safety standards for laboratory handling of human gametes and consumer information regarding the clinic success rates in treatments involving IVF (Fertility Clinic Success Rate and Certificate Act of 1992). The federal government does not track or explicitly govern most aspects of sperm donation, but since egg donation is carried out in the context of IVF, its data collection includes IVF cycles using egg donation (Glennon, 2010).

There is little regulation at the state level either. Many states define father/child relationships in the context of sperm donation to married couples; fewer define parentage after sperm donation to single women or same-sex couples. A small number define mother/child relationships in the context of egg donation with IVF or surrogacy. Only a few states restrict the use of donor gametes or surrogates, and in most states donors, surrogates and intermediaries freely enter into contracts as they see fit, though they may be uncertain about the outcome if the contract is challenged in court (Cahn, 2009).

Assisted reproduction is also regulated by state medical licensing requirements, contract, tort and criminal law (Cahn, 2009). Two US organizations have developed model legislation: the National Conference of Commissioners on Uniform State Laws proposed the Uniform Parentage Act of 2000 (UPA 2000), and the American Bar Association (ABA) proposed the Model Act on Assisted Reproductive Technology (ABA Model Act) in 2008. Their efforts have not generated widespread legislation, although the UPA 2000 has been implemented by nine states. Professional societies, such as the American Society for Reproductive Medicine (ASRM), have promulgated practice guidelines that gamete providers and clinics may follow. Practice guidelines do not have the force of law and their only remedy for a violation is removal from membership, an exceedingly rare event. Research shows numerous violations of professional standards (Nano, 2009; Levine, 2010).

What, then, do these strikingly different legal regimes tell us about the ethical orientation of each society with regard to AR? Assisted reproduction poses challenges to many of the most profound questions humans can face. Both societies recognize that human reproduction implicates the deepest aspects of ourselves, of defining who we are, who our most important connections will be, whether we will live our lives as parents, what kinds of connections our children will have to others. They implicate fundamental constitutional rights in the USA and essential human rights in the UK (Glennon, 2009). AR thus brings into question major principles of bioethics, including autonomy, non-malevolence, beneficence and justice (Beauchamp and Childress, 2008). It includes concern for human dignity as rapidly changing technological frontiers challenge our basic assumptions about human reproduction and family.

The striking differences between the UK and US regulation of AR highlight societal views regarding autonomy. The UK has developed what I will call a communitarian approach to defining the realm of human autonomy in the context of AR, while the USA demonstrates reliance on a market-based, individual approach to defining autonomy.

A communitarian approach calls upon society's members to collectively develop a structure to describe, define and regulate autonomy in AR. It is based on the belief that the interests of those involved in AR as providers, patients, surrogates, donors and donor-conceived children inevitably conflict and that their actions affect the larger society as well. Thus, the communitarian approach to defining autonomy takes a highly centralized approach to regulating AR based on an open and democratic process of evaluating societal values.

An individualistic, market-based approach to autonomy rejects the view that society best defines autonomy rights. All involved individuals, including treatment providers, should be free to define which approaches to reproduction express their values and finance their desired approach. Other concerns, including the interests of resulting children, are left to the judgement of those individuals, not society as a whole. Government's primary job is to enforce private agreements that express individual autonomy.

The UK communitarian autonomy approach has resulted in strong, mandatory, informed consent rules, clear parentage rules and access to donor identity. It strictly limits payment to donors and surrogates to reimbursement of 'reasonable expenses' to protect society's view of human dignity. Finally, it limits private ordering regarding the disposition of embryos and parentage. The US individualistic autonomy approach has few informed consent requirements, minimal regulation of the market in gametes and surrogacy, and allows the market to determine donor payment and whether donors will be anonymous or identified. In many cases parentage and use of stored embryos is left up to private ordering at the outset, while lack of legislation often leaves the status of such agreements uncertain. Each of these approaches needs to be interrogated to determine whether it has found the appropriate balance between respect for autonomy and protection of all those involved in the process.

The protection of autonomy through informed consent

Informed consent is a key ethical requirement in all medical treatment contexts. It prevents deception and coercion and provides a basis for the protection of human autonomy and dignity (Beauchamp and Childress, 2008). Given what psychological research informs us about the limits of human cognition and emotional forecasting, however, informed consent may not be enough to help participants appreciate the implications of their actions without thorough counselling (Glennon, 2010). The UK has adopted detailed requirements concerning informed consent in the broader context of AR and the specific context of gamete donation. The USA has no such requirements, nor have states adopted context-specific informed consent rules.

In the UK, the HFEA Code of Practice, 8th edition (HFEA, 2009a) sets forth a three-stage process to ensure protection for informed consent: provision of information; opportunity for counselling; and detailed written consent requirements. All clinics licensed to provide fertility treatments must comply with these requirements. Individuals considering egg or sperm donation or receipt, the contribution of their gametes to the creation, storage or use of an embryo, and non-genetically related legal parenthood must receive specified information prior to providing consent. These detailed informational requirements protect the autonomy of participants in fertility treatment.

Fertility clinics must also offer participants in fertility treatment counselling prior to obtaining informed consent. The counselling should include parentage implications, health effects and risks of treatment options. Fertility centres must offer either individual or partner counselling by an accredited, qualified counsellor, not the treating physician. Centres that violate these HFEA requirements could lose their licence or face tort litigation (HFEA, 2009a).

In the USA, informed consent requirements for AR are the same as for other medical treatment. They may be enforced through a professional licensing association and tort liability where violations lead to patient injury or unwanted treatment (Kindregan and McBrien, 2006). The tort system is only designed to deal with the failure to inform patients of medical risks involved in treatment decisions. Many of the most difficult decisions for patients, their partners and potential donors involve the legal risks, such as the disposition of stored embryos following death or divorce and the parentage implications of their actions. Physicians and many other actors involved in AR, such as sperm banks and egg donation services, are not required to provide information about these important aspects of the use of AR, nor are they knowledgeable enough to do so. Given the failure by most US states to adequately legislate on these issues, even lawyers are unable to provide authoritative counselling on these important matters (Vukadinovich, 2000). Parentage contests in the context of gamete donation and litigation over the use of stored embryos demonstrate that this 'back-end' regulation may be inadequate to protect the autonomy interests of all those involved.

Informed consent requirements are an important aspect of ensuring participant autonomy. They may also increase participants' awareness of the interests of any children they conceive through donation or surrogacy. The presence or absence of strong informed consent also forms an important backdrop to the analysis of differences in the legal status of gametes, payment for gametes, parentage issues and donor anonymity.

The legal status of donated gametes

US and UK courts have struggled to define the legal status of stored eggs, sperm and embryos. Courts take varied positions on whether gametes or embryos are property subject to contract or estate rules or whether they are so closely related to the autonomy rights of individuals that they cannot be treated as property.

In cases involving claims by individuals against providers that failed to properly preserve stored gametes, courts in both the USA and UK have considered the status of gametes under tort and other relevant law. In *Yearworth* v. *North Bristol NHS Trust* (2009) and *Kurchner* v. *State Farm Fire and Casualty Co.* (2003), plaintiffs who had stored their sperm prior to obtaining cancer treatment sought compensation for the negligent destruction of their sperm. The UK and Florida courts both found that the plaintiffs had an ownership interest in the stored sperm. The UK Court of Appeal rejected the argument that the stored sperm was not property because the men could not direct that their sperm be used, but could only request its use under the HFE Act. Instead, the Court considered the Act's stringent consent provisions 'as a powerful confirmation of their ownership' (Quigley, 2009).

US courts have gone further in their treatment of stored sperm as property. In two California cases, widows sought to use stored vials of sperm from their deceased husbands. In *Hecht* v. *Superior Court* (1993), the court found that recognition of 'an interest, in the nature of ownership' is not inconsistent with the determination that 'the value of sperm lies in its potential to create a child after fertilization, growth, and birth'. Both courts found that the deceased could control the disposition of his sperm through either a clear statement of intent in the agreement he had signed with the clinic that stored his sperm or through his will (*Hecht* v. *Superior Court*, 1993; *Johnson* v. *Superior Court*, 2000).

One state statute treats stored embryos as property alienable by agreement. Florida requires a couple and the treating physician to enter into an agreement regarding control over the disposition of eggs, sperm and pre-embryos, and provides that the agreement will govern in the event of a future dispute (F.S.A. s742.17). No provision is made for later unilateral changes once an agreement is entered, similar to the approach to other types of 'property'. Only one state, Louisiana, has legislation defining 'an in vitro fertilized human ovum' as a 'juridical person', meaning that it is not the property of the man or woman whose gametes created it. A court may appoint a curator to protect the rights of the in vitro fertilized human ovum (La. Rev. Stat. Ann. ss9: 123–126).

US courts have divided on the status of stored embryos where the gamete contributors disagree about their future use. Most influential has been *Davis* v. *Davis*, a 1992 decision by the Tennessee Supreme Court, which found that embryos 'occupy an interim category that entitles them to special respect because of their potential for human life' and recognized that the gamete providers have an 'interest in the nature of ownership'. The *Davis* Court ruled that a binding agreement between the individuals commissioning the embryo through donation of their sperm and eggs should govern embryo disposition. The *Davis* case itself lacked a binding agreement, and the Court determined that the ex-husband's interest in not procreating outweighed the ex-wife's interest in ensuring that the embryos were adopted and used by another woman.

Several other US state courts view disposition by agreement as binding, including in the context of divorce where the woman is unable to produce any other eggs to have a genetically related child (*Roman* v. *Roman*, 2006). This controversial approach has been rejected by other courts that consider embryos distinct from other types of property. They focus on the right of individuals to contemporaneously direct the use of embryos created by their gametes. One court identified 'an emerging majority view that written embryo agreements between embryo donors and fertility clinics to which all parties have consented are valid and enforceable so long as the parties have the opportunity to withdraw their consent to the terms of the agreement' (*Roman* v. *Roman*, 2006).

UK law does not regard stored embryos as property alienable by any contractual agreement at the time of donation or IVF. The use of frozen eggs, sperm or embryos requires contemporaneous agreement. Earlier agreements are never binding unless the individual is now deceased and had given written consent to post-mortem donation. Otherwise, any gamete donor or contributor to an embryo may withdraw his or her consent at any time prior to use in treatment or the implantation of the embryo (HFE Act (as amended), Schedule 3). One contributor's withdrawal of consent to embryo implantation trumps the other contributor's interest in conceiving a child even if that decision deprives the other contributor of her only opportunity to bear genetic children. This rule was upheld by the Court of Appeal and found permissible under the European Convention on Human Rights (*Evans* v. *UK*, 2008).

Preventing gamete providers from being bound by earlier agreements distinguishes gametes from property, which is alienable without later recourse. This preserves the reproductive autonomy of an egg or sperm provider to control later use. In the context of embryos, however, the right to withdraw consent until use may severely impair the autonomy and reproductive interests of the other contributor to the embryo, often the woman, who may be unable to produce genetic offspring, and for whom egg donation is significantly more physically demanding (Waldman, 2004). At minimum, laws regarding the outcomes of such conflicts must be clear and communicated to all parties prior to undertaking the creation of embryos. Each gamete contributor should be separately counselled to encourage open consideration of the consequences of the other contributor changing his or her mind.

Recruitment and payment of gamete donors

The UK currently faces a severe shortage of both sperm and egg donors. Extremely limited compensation, removal of donor anonymity and limits on the use of sperm from any one donor have created lengthy waiting lists for donated gametes in the UK. UK citizens travel to other countries to escape these shortages, and US and UK citizens both cross borders to obtain gamete donation and surrogacy services at lower cost (Audi and Chang, 2010; see Pennings and B. Gürtin, Chapter 8).

The UK and USA differ markedly in their approach to recruitment of donors and payment for gametes. The UK limits payment to reasonable expenses for donors, providing a fixed sum of £35 for each visit for sperm donors and a fixed sum of £750 per cycle of donation for egg donors (HFEA Press Release, 2011a; HFEA General Direction 0001, 2010a). The HFEA's financial limit may not be enough to reimburse donors for missed wages due to the many appointments required for both types of donation, and in particular for egg donation, which involves more extensive medical procedures and discomfort.

This policy accords with the UK's obligations as a member of the European Union, which requires that donations of tissues, including gametes, are 'voluntary and unpaid' and that compensation is limited to 'making good the expenses and inconveniences related to the donation' (European Tissues and Cells Directive, 2004/23/EC). An evaluation of British clinic practices in 2009 found that not all centres complied fully with reimbursement requirements. (HFEA Paper – Sperm Egg and Embryo Donation, 2009b). The HFEA reviewed the policy through a process that included public comment (HFEA, 2011b). This policy review resulted in increases to reimbursement payments for sperm and egg donation (HFEA Press Release, 2011a).

A second form of 'payment' involves egg-sharing. Under this approach, a woman may provide her extra eggs to other women who need eggs in exchange for treatment services. The UK regulates this procedure, and women undergoing fertility treatment are not permitted to undergo additional stimulated treatment cycles in order to give eggs to another patient (HFEA General Direction 0001, 2010a). If monetized, the value of egg-sharing arrangements is far greater than that permitted for other egg or sperm donors, and there is no clear rationale provided for this distinction (Jackson, 2007).

Finally, the UK limits payment to surrogates who carry donated sperm and/or eggs for an individual or couple to 'reasonable expenses'. UK couples who have employed surrogacy services abroad have struggled to persuade courts to approve payments in excess of permissible medical expenses, missed wages and other reimbursements for expenses. Courts asked to approve parental orders for the intended parents' cases face the difficult choice of either approving payments that exceed the law's intent or leaving children born to the surrogate parentless and stateless (*Re: X and Y*, 2008). In another international surrogacy arrangement, the judiciary recognized that recent regulatory changes require the court to make the child's welfare its 'paramount consideration', overriding other public policy concerns such as limitations on excessive payments (*In re L*, 2010). These situations highlight the difficulty of enforcing payment restrictions in the context of global fertility tourism and provide a different perspective from which to evaluate the UK's restrictions on payment.

The UK considers altruism the only acceptable basis for gamete donation, fearing that commodification could increase health risks for donors, discourage donors from raising health concerns that could affect recipients or donor-conceived children, eliminate society's moral value on the 'gift' relationship between donor and recipient and undermine social and cultural attitudes towards the body and human reproduction (Pennings, Vayena and Ahuja, Chapter 9). While some of these issues are open to empirical study, others reflect value choices that should be debated in light of the broader context, including the actual fees charged to patients for gametes by for-profit gamete banks, fertility clinics and fertility tourism.

The US approach differs markedly, and it has an abundant supply of sperm and eggs. The US government has no laws or regulations regarding payment to sperm and egg donors or egg-sharing. Prices are set by the market, and they are generally higher than in the UK. In practice, gamete banks and fertility clinics pay what they consider to be market rates to donors, and the fees offered may vary by personal characteristics or willingness to be identified to donor-conceived children. There are no federal regulations concerning what fees these entities may actually charge patients for gametes.

Few states regulate payment for gametes. Virginia explicitly exempts eggs and 'self-replicating body fluids' from its prohibition on the sale of body parts, but does not state what compensation is appropriate. Florida permits 'reasonable compensation' for egg and sperm donation, but fails to define 'reasonable'. In the absence of legal regulation, the American Society for Reproductive Medicine (ASRM) Ethics Committee issued a report supporting payment for sperm and egg donation, finding that the risks of commercialization are justified by expanded access to insemination and IVF. It found that financial or in-kind benefits can co-exist with altruistic motivations. While the report did not address what amounts are reasonable for sperm donation, it specifies that payments to egg donors in excess of $5,000 require justification and that payments exceeding $10,000 are inappropriate. It also finds that under no circumstances should payment be conditioned on the successful retrieval of eggs or the donor's personal characteristics (Ethics Committee of ASRM, 2007). Recent research shows that not all members of the ASRM follow these guidelines (Levine, 2010). The ABA Model Act 2008 also addresses payment for donated gametes and gestational carriers. It provides for payment that is 'reasonable', negotiated in good faith between the parties and not based on the characteristics of the donor or quality or genome-related traits of the gametes or embryos.

The US sperm donation business is dominated by several large sperm bank companies, all of which ship internationally. Sperm banks advertise different charges for various donor categories, and in addition many charge for 'add-ons', such as photos of donors or additional information.

Egg donation may be arranged directly through fertility clinics, but more commonly by unlicensed brokers who have 'out-hustled' clinics in developing long lists of potential donors – sometimes, it is feared, through deceptive adverts that lure potential donors on the pretence of having a recipient family ready to pay high fees for the right donor (Mundy, 2007; Advisory Group on Assisted Reproductive Technology, 2010). Egg donor agencies tend to charge a separate fee for their 'services' in matching providers and recipients, while egg donors enter into separate agreements with recipients, which may mean that prices vary from those posted on programme websites.

Commentators have noted significant gender differences in the rhetoric and payment structure that surrounds sperm and egg donation. While sperm donation banks highlight both altruism and compensation as the rewards of donation, egg donation programmes emphasize altruism, and in fact they have been known to screen out those who appear to be solely motivated by the money. Their rhetoric focuses on egg donation as a 'gift' exchange (Almeling, 2007). When defined by the time and discomfort associated with each type of donation, egg donors may be paid less than sperm donors, although good data on these fees is difficult to obtain (Krawiec, 2009; Levine, 2010).

Egg-sharing is also active in the USA, and a number of fertility clinics offer egg-sharing options to reduce fertility treatment fees for women who choose that option. The ASRM Ethics Committee expressed approval of egg-sharing programmes but cautioned that programmes should carefully address the difficult issues through counselling and informed consent procedures and ensure that donation does not interfere with the patient's own fertility needs. Once again, the Committee cautions that any fee reduction should not be conditioned on retrieval of a certain number of eggs.

An incident in March 2010 highlights the differing cultural and ethical views regarding gamete donation in the UK and USA. An American IVF clinic based in Virginia held a seminar in London designed to encourage British women to obtain donor eggs at its clinic. In order to motivate women to attend, it promised to raffle off one free cycle of IVF using the eggs of a Washington DC area donor. The HFEA condemned the raffle as 'trivialis[ing] altruistic donation' and contrary to safeguarding the status of gametes and 'the dignity of donors and recipients' (HFEA Press Release, 2010b). The ASRM, however, praised the raffle for increasing access to treatment (Stein, 2010).

Because each society weighs the incommensurable interests related to payment for gamete contribution differently, the ethical issue is difficult to resolve. Where the arguments involve measurable behaviour, such as lying about health concerns to obtain payment or whether market prices restrict access, resolution may be possible through further research. UK arguments that payments for sperm and egg donation undermine human dignity and US arguments that they are needed to ensure patient autonomy regarding fertility treatment can only be resolved with reference to each society's values. Governments must recognize, however, that their citizens are not bound by each country's values and weigh the ethics of their approaches in light of fertility tourism to less wealthy countries where concerns about safety and donor and surrogate coercion are much stronger (Pennings, 2004; Barnett and Smith, 2006; Audi and Chang, 2010). Neither country has come to grips with the costs of fertility treatment, including gamete donation, that deprive many in both countries of access to treatment and weigh other families down with significant debt.

Parentage of donor-conceived children

In the UK, the rules regarding legal parentage of donor-conceived children are clear, with one important exception. The legal status of a woman who gives birth is the most clear: any woman who gives birth to a child is the legal mother, whether or not the child was conceived with donated eggs. This means that a woman who is carrying a child as a surrogate for other intended parents is always the legal mother at birth, whether or not she is genetically related to the child. The intended parents must follow an established legal process with strict requirements to obtain a parental order to transform the intended mother into the legal mother (HFE Act (as amended)).

Legal fatherhood or parenthood by the non-birth mother in a same-sex relationship may be more complicated. The simplest situation involves those who are married or have a partner in same-sex civil unions ('partner' refers to partner in a civil union). In that situation, the husband or partner of the birth mother is the legal father or parent *unless* it is shown that the husband or partner did not consent to the conception. A husband or partner who denies parentage bears the burden of proving lack of consent to the treatment. These rules apply whether or not the treatment was conducted by an HFEA-licensed provider (HFE Act (as amended), s. 42).

The situation is treated differently if a child is born to couples who are not married or in a civil union. A man who is not married to a woman carrying a child conceived through IVF or intrauterine insemination is the legal father if, prior to the conception, he and the mother provided notice of consent to his parentage to an HFEA-licensed treatment provider who performed the insemination or IVF. Consent by both members of the couple establishes his paternity even if he is not the genetic father of the child (HFE Act (as amended), s. 37). For lesbian couples who are not in a civil partnership, a second woman may become a legal parent of a child conceived through IVF or insemination if both women consent to the parentage, the treatment is performed by an HFEA-licensed treatment provider, and the birth mother is not married to a man who consented to the treatment (HFE Act (as amended), s. 43).

Those who are not married or in a civil partnership and choose informal insemination face different rules than those who proceed through an HFEA-licensed fertility treatment provider. Where the mother is not married or in a civil partnership and undergoes an informal insemination, the biological father is the legal father, even if the man had agreed to be only the sperm donor (*Re: B (Parentage)*, 1996). He is responsible for financial maintenance and entitled to petition the court for contact time. The legal consequences of informal insemination may surprise men who believe they are informal sperm donors, not fathers. In a case that garnered widespread publicity, a British firefighter who claimed to be a sperm donor was held financially responsible for two children conceived for a lesbian couple using his sperm (Williams, 2007). The law ignores private arrangements regarding parentage. The difficulty of assessing parties' intentions in informal sperm donation was highlighted when the children's legal mother responded that the firefighter developed a relationship with the first child, but withdrew after a second child was born with disabilities. She stated that she was required to name the children's father to receive the full amount of governmental income support she needed to care for the children (Truescott and Williams, 2007).

The rules concerning informal insemination to single women or couples who are not in a marriage or civil union are clear if not well understood by the public. However, the rules regarding legal fatherhood are uncertain in one important situation: if a couple has fertility treatments, creates more embryos than needed and wishes to donate the additional embryos to a woman who is not married or in a civil union, the man's legal status regarding the child is unclear (HFEA Code of Practice 5.20, 2009a). This makes embryo donation to women who are not married or in a civil union a risky venture for the genetic father, and presumably this legal uncertainty would pose an obstacle to such donations.

The USA has far greater uncertainty about legal parentage in the context of egg and sperm donation. In many instances, conflicts regarding parentage do not have a clear legal resolution. State laws vary widely, and many states have only addressed legislation to sperm donation to married couples. The UPA 2000, ABA Model Act and most state laws provide that the husbands of married women, not the sperm donors, are the fathers of children resulting from AR. Husbands may deny paternity only when they can prove they did not consent (*Wells* v. *Wells*, 2010). The same rule applies to spouse or partners in states that have adopted same-sex marriage or civil unions.

The parentage effects of sperm donation to opposite-sex and same-sex couples not in legally recognized relationships and single women are not established in most state legislation. Sperm banks carefully protect anonymity to avoid unwanted paternity rights, and courts have not imposed paternity rights on anonymous donors. The consequences of donation by a known sperm donor are much less clear. Courts struggle with cases in which a known male's sperm was used either through a licensed physician or informally by an unmarried birth mother. The broad trend recognizes that gamete donation does not create parental status in the sperm donor where the participants agree that there will be no parental status and adjust their actions to this expectation, particularly where a licensed physician performed the insemination. One state statute that relieves a man of legal parentage when donation is through a licensed physician did not relieve a man of parentage when he donated sperm without going through a physician, asserting that it was favouring the interpretation that provided two parents for the child (*Mintz* v. *Zoernig*, 2008). In contrast, the Kansas Supreme Court recently upheld a statute that excluded the donor from paternity rights absent a written agreement providing for such rights, even in the absence of evidence that the donor had been informed of and consented to exclusion from paternity rights (*In re K.M.H.*, 2007).

State statutes must be sufficiently protective of a man's right to procreate and parent. Two state courts have struck down statutes that absolutely barred sperm donors from having any parental rights. These statutes violated the US Constitution's due process protections for the sperm donor's parental rights, which are regarded as of fundamental importance (*McIntyre* v. *Crouch*, 1989; *In the Interest of R.C.*, 1989).

Where there is no relevant statute or the statute does not clearly govern the situation at hand, courts struggle to determine parental rights.

Often, courts look to 'facts on the ground' to evaluate the parties' alleged agreements or children's welfare. For example, in one New York case, a sperm donor who had been promised no financial responsibility was found to be a legal parent where he agreed to be listed on the birth certificate and maintained some contact with the resulting child. The court did not credit the biological mother's promise to relieve the donor of financial responsibility or impose responsibility on her lesbian partner, who had participated in the creation of the child and shared parenting of the child (*P.D.* v. *S.K.*, 2007). A Pennsylvania man, however, avoided parental responsibility for twins born through sperm donation based on the parties' oral agreement where, for five years, they had acted in accordance with their agreement that he would not visit the children or have financial responsibility for them (*Ferguson* v. *McKiernan*, 2007).

Where facts support a known sperm donor's belief that, despite the use of assisted reproduction, he would be the legal father of the resulting child, courts seem reluctant to deny him parental status and permit the alleged father to try to prove his version of the facts (*Browne* v. *D'Alleva*, 2007; *Janssen* v. *Alicea*, 2010). Cases are especially challenging for courts where evidence from written documents, oral agreements and party conduct conflict, and these cases have resulted in varied outcomes (*Leckie* v. *Voorhies*, 1994; *Browne* v. *D'Alleva*, 2007). In a parentage conflict case involving one member of a lesbian couple who provided an egg to the other member of the couple, a California court, faced with a conflict between the written documentation and state law on the one hand, and the parties' shared parenting on the other, ruled in favour of the egg donor's parentage rights (*K.M.* v. *E.G.*, 2005).

The UPA 2000 distinguishes between donors and intended parents in the context of unmarried individuals. An individual who donates eggs or sperm is not a parent unless he or she is an 'intended parent'. An intended parent may become so through a written consent by the intended mother and father or where the mother, child and purported father reside together for two years following the child's birth and openly hold the child out as their own. The ABA Model Act 2008 contains the written consent and 'holding out' provisions, except it does so in a gender-neutral way equally applicable to same-sex couples. Thus, a man who donates sperm intending to be a parent but who does not have a written record signed by both him and the mother to that effect is effectively precluded from parentage under both the UPA 2000 and the ABA Model Act 2008 unless he then lives with the child and holds the child out as his own for two years following the child's birth.

At present, most states lack clear legal guidelines regarding sperm donation to women who are not in a traditional heterosexual marriage. Physicians performing egg and sperm donation do not have any legal obligation to advise participants of their rights, nor, in many instances, would they be able to do so. This lack of clarity means that individuals entering into many types of donor arrangements do so without knowing what their resulting parental rights or responsibilities will be if their informal agreements break down.

The UK's clear rules for parentage outside of the context of embryo donation to unmarried women allow the parties to be very clear about the consequences of their decisions, an important aspect of autonomy that is not currently protected in the USA because of the lack of clarity about parentage in many AR situations. However, by failing to recognize agreements regarding parentage in the situations of informal sperm donation or embryo donation to unmarried women, the UK may also limit patient autonomy.

Do donor-conceived offspring have a right to know their progenitors?

Sperm and egg donation often remains shrouded by secrecy, as families may seek to look like a biologically related family in order to avoid difficult issues concerning family relationships (Murray and Golombok, 2003; Waldman, 2006). Until recently, it was rare for gamete donors to identify themselves. This secrecy has come under attack, however, as a violation of the child's right to know his or her genetic identity, viewed by many as a human right and important to the child's health and welfare.

Vardit Ravitsky (2010) has identified four separate aspects to the broad claim in favour of 'the right to know one's genetic origins'. The first claim involves the right to know one's full medical history and relevant genetic information about the donor. The second involves the right to know personal information relevant to offsprings' development of their identity. The relational interest concerns the right to know the donor's full identity and make contact with him or her. Finally, the parental disclosure aspect concerns the child's right to know that he or she has been conceived via gamete donation.

The UK assures donor-conceived offspring of the first three aspects of the right to know, and makes the final aspect available to those who seek that information. Individuals who have reached age 18 may contact a national registry to obtain medical and identifying information about their donor, including contact information. Beginning at age 16, individuals who wish to have an intimate relationship, marry or enter into a civil union may check with the registry to see if they are genetically related due to gamete donation. The HFEA strongly advises, but does not require, parents to inform their children that they are donor-conceived. A mandate that offspring be given this information could be viewed as intruding into a protected realm of parental decision-making (HFEA, 2009a). While the UK does not require parental disclosure, registry access allows curious adults to check on their genetic status. These legal changes may have also affected the behaviour of the parents of donor-conceived children. Research shows that an increasing number of parents in the UK choose to provide this information to their donor-conceived children (Appleby, Blake and Freeman, Chapter 13).

In the USA access to information about donation and donor identity is entrusted to the market (Waldman, 2006). Most gamete donations are made anonymously, although the market for donors willing to be identified is growing. Single women and lesbian couples may prefer identifiable donors and heterosexual couples are choosing that option more often. Those who select the identifiable donor option pay a premium for that 'service', which includes obtaining permission from the donor and maintaining records over a long period of time. Without a national registry to which donor-conceived children can turn, record-keeping is a major problem, and donor information may be lost or unobtainable (Cahn, 2009).

In the absence of a legal right to donor identity generally, some donor-conceived children have sought medical information to assist them in dealing with certain medical conditions, the first aspect of donor identity claims described by Professor Ravitsky. Two state courts have rejected petitioners' efforts to obtain personally identifying information about sperm donors, but they have permitted access to certain medical information. In one case where the petitioners sued a sperm bank for failing to adequately prevent a donor from passing on a serious kidney disease, the court granted access to testimony from the donor with safeguards to protect his identity (*Johnson* v. *Superior Court*, 2000; *Doe* v. *XYZ Co.*, 2009). The limited case law makes it difficult to determine whether all states will protect donor anonymity and restrict access to medical information. However, if courts look to case law concerning adoption, they will uphold anonymity agreements and make limited exceptions for urgent medical reasons only.

No US state currently requires that donor identity be disclosed to children. Some resulting children who have been informed of the circumstances of their conception have, however, employed the Internet to locate half-siblings, identifying their donor by clinic and number

(Mundy, 2007; Appleby, Blake and Freeman, Chapter 13). Thus, access to this information is dependent on parental purchase of the right to the information at the outset and accurate record-keeping by private companies engaged in gamete donation, companies' willingness to contact an anonymous donor to see if he or she wishes to be contacted, or internet serendipity.

The US approach privileges the autonomy interests of the parents, and leaves the resulting children without any right to knowledge of their origins. At the very least the USA should maintain a national registry of medical and other important information regarding donors and recipients so donors and donor-conceived children may choose to locate each other, and donor-conceived children can avoid incestuous relationships and obtain medical information. It should also inform intended parents about the benefits of using identifiable donors and how to share information with their children. Law is not, of course, the only agent of change. Popular culture, which in 2010 featured two popular movies about known sperm donors, *The Kids are All Right* and *The Switch*, may help to create a societal context in which such information becomes the norm, as has happened in the context of adoption.

Conclusion

The UK and USA take strikingly different positions on many issues important to gamete donation. The communitarian, centrally regulated approach and the individualistic, market-based approach to autonomy in AR both hold promise and concern. This chapter identifies some important ethical concerns with each approach and argues that we should carefully consider each policy to determine whether it honours the rights and interests of all participants in the process – intended parents, gamete providers, donor-conceived children and the larger society. This review should carefully consider whether policies facilitate access to gamete donation to help people pursue their fundamental interest in family life, the extent to which they protect autonomous decision-making by all participants, including donor-conceived children, and whether the policies balance well the interests of both contributors to embryo creation. It should evaluate whether parentage rules protect child welfare and fundamental rights to be a parent. We must recognize that some variations in policy must be expected in light of the incommensurable concerns at stake. All policies, however, should be evaluated in light of the opportunities available to UK and US residents to seek gamete donation or surrogacy services in other countries, as our ethical concerns extend well beyond our own borders.

BIBLIOGRAPHY

Advisory Group on Assisted Reproductive Technology, New York State Task Force on Life and the Law, 'Thinking of becoming an egg donor: get the facts before you decide'. Available at the New York State Department of Health website: www.nyhealth.gov/publications/1127.pdf (accessed 10 August 2010).

Almeling, R. (2007). 'Selling genes, selling gender: egg agencies, sperm banks, and the medical market in genetic material'. *American Sociological Review*, 72, 319–40.

Audi, T. and Chang, A. (2010). 'Assembling the global baby'. *The Wall Street Journal*, 10 December. Available at The Wall Street Journal website: www. wsj.com.

Barnett, A. and Smith, H. (2006). 'Cruel cost of the human egg trade'. *The Observer*, 30 April, retrieved from The Observer website: observer.guardian.co.uk.

Beauchamp, T. and Childress, J. F. (2008). *Principles of Biomedical Ethics*. Cambridge University Press.

Blyth, E. *et al.* (2003). 'Assisted Human Reproduction: Contemporary Policy and Practice in the UK', in Singer, D. and Hunter, M. (eds.), *Assisted Human Reproduction: Psychological and Ethical Dilemmas*. London and Philadelphia: Whurr.

Cahn, N. R. (2009). *Test Tube Families: Why the Fertility Market Needs Legal Regulation*. New York University Press.

Connolly, M. P., Hoorens, S. and Chambers, G. M. (2010). 'The costs and consequences of assisted reproductive technology: an economic perspective'. *Human Reproduction Update*, 16, 603–13.

Ethics Committee of American Society for Reproductive Medicine (2007). 'Financial compensation of oocyte donors'. *Fertility and Sterility*, 88, 305–9.

Glennon, T. (2009). 'Regulation of Reproductive Decision-Making,' in S. Day-Sclater, F. Ebtehaj, E. Jackson and M. Richards (eds.), *Regulating Autonomy: Sex, Reproduction and Family*. Oxford: Hart Publishing.

(2010). 'Choosing one: resolving the epidemic of multiples in assisted reproduction'. *Villanova Law Review*, 55, 147–204.

Human Fertilisation and Embryology Authority (HFEA) (2004). Disclosure of Donor Information Regulations.

(2009a). Code of Practice, 8th edn.

(2009b). 'Sperm egg and embryo donation'. Available at the HFEA website: www.hfea.gov.uk.

(2010a). Directions given under the Human Fertilisation and Embryology Act 1990 as amended. Gamete and Embryo Donation Ref: 0001, version 2. Available from the HFEA website: www.hfea.gov.uk/docs/2009-06-03_GENERAL_DIRECTIONS_0001_Gamete_and_Embryo_donation_-_approved.pdf.

(2010b). Press Release: 'Statement regarding raffles and fertility treatment'. Available at the HFEA website: www.hfea.gov.uk/5679.html (accessed 16 March 2010).

(2011a). Press Release: 'HFEA agrees new policies to improve sperm and egg donation services'. 19 October 2011. Available at the HFEA website: www. hfea.gov.uk/6700.html (accessed 31 January 2012).

(2011b). 'Donating sperm and eggs: have your say ... A review of the HFEA's sperm and egg donation policies – 2011'. Available at the HFEA website: www.hfea.gov.uk/docs/2011-01-13_Donation_review_background.pdf (accessed 31 January 2012).

Jackson, E. (2007). *Medical Law: Text, Cases, and Material.* Oxford University Press.

Kindregan, C. P. and McBrien, M. (2006). *Assisted Reproductive Technology: A Lawyer's Guide to Emerging Law and Science.* American Bar Association.

Krawiec, K. (2009). 'Sunny Samaritans and egomaniacs: price-fixing in the gamete market'. *Law and Contemporary Problems,* 72, 59–90.

Levine, A. D. (2010). 'Self-regulation, compensation, and the ethical recruitment of oocyte donors'. *Hastings Center Report,* 40, 25–36.

Mundy, L. (2007). *Everything Conceivable: How Assisted Reproduction is Changing Men, Women and the World.* New York: Alfred A. Knopf.

Murray, C. and Golombok, S. (2003). 'To tell or not to tell: the decision-making process of egg donation parents'. *Human Fertility* 6, 89–95.

Nano, S. (2009). 'Most fertility clinics break the rules'. The Associated Press, 20 February 2009. Available at the Genetics and Society website: www.geneticsandsociety.org.

Pennings, G. (2004). 'Legal harmonization and reproductive tourism in Europe'. *Human Reproduction,* 19, 2689–94.

Quigley, M. (2009). 'Property: the future of human tissue?' *Medical Law Review,* 17, 457–66.

Ravitsky, V. (2010). 'Knowing where you come from: the rights of donor-conceived individuals and the meaning of genetic relatedness'. *Minnesota Journal of Law, Science and Technology,* 11, 655–84.

Spar, D. (2006). *The Baby Business.* Boston: Harvard Business School Press.

Stein, R. (2010). 'London seminar offering free IVF from Virginia clinic sparks controversy'. *Washington Post,* 18 March, A01.

Truescott, C. and Williams, R. (2007). 'Lesbian mother hits back in row over donor's support payments'. *The Observer,* 4 December, retrieved from The Observer website: observer.guardian.co.uk.

Vukadinovich, D. (2000). 'Assisted reproductive technology law obtaining informed consent for the commercial cryopreservation of embryos'. *Journal of Legal Medicine,* 21, 67–78.

Waldman, E. (2004). 'The parent trap: uncovering the myth of "coerced parenthood" in frozen embryo disputes'. *American University Law Review,* 53, 1021–62.

(2006). 'What do we tell the children?' *Capital University Law Review,* 35, 517–61.

Williams, R. (2007). 'Sperm donor to lesbian couple forced to pay child support'. *The Observer,* 4 December, retrieved from The Observer website: observer.guardian.co.uk.

CASES

Browne v. *D'Alleva*, 44 Conn. L. Reptr. 734 (Conn. Super. 2007)
Davis v. *Davis*, 842 S.W.2d 588 (Tenn. 1992)
Doe v. *Blue Cross Blue Shield of Massachusetts*, Inc., 2010 WL 1541567 (S.D.N.Y. 2010)
Doe v. *XYZ Co.*, 914 N.E.2d 117 (Mass. App. Ct. 2009)
Evans v. *United Kingdom* (2008) 46 E.H.R.R. 34
Ferguson v. *McKiernan*, 940 A.2d 1236 (Pa. 2007)
Hecht v. *Superior Court*, 20 Cal. Rptr. 275 (1993)
In the Interest of R.C., 775 P.2d 27 (Colo. 1989)
Janssen v. *Alicea*, 30 So.3d 680 (Fla App. 3 Dist. 2010)
Johnson v. *Superior Court*, 95 Cal. Rptr.2d 864 (Cal. App. 4th 2000)
In re K.M.H., 169 P.3d 1025 (Kan. 2007)
In re L (a minor) [2010] EWHC 3146 (Fam)
K.M. v. *E.G.*, 117 P.3d 673 (Cal. 2005)
Kurchner v. *State Farm Fire and Casualty Co.*, 858 So.2d 1220 (Fla. Ct. App. 2003)
Leckie v. *Voorhies*, 875 P.2d 521 (Or. Ct. App. 1994)
McIntyre v. *Crouch*, 780 P.2d 239 (Or. App. 1989)
Mintz v. *Zoernig*, 198 P.3d 861 (N.M. Ct. App. 2008)
P.D. v. *S.K.*, 17 Misc.3d 1133(A) (N.Y. Fam. Ct. 2007)
Re: B (Parentage) [1996] FLR 15
Re: X and Y (Foreign Surrogacy) [2008] EWHC 3030 (Fam)
Roman v. *Roman*, 193 S.W.3d 40 (Tex. Ct. App. 2006)
Wells v. *Wells*, 35 So.2d 1250 (Miss. App. 2010)
Yearworth v. *North Bristol NHS Trust* [2009] EWCA Civ 37

LEGISLATION

USA

American Bar Association, Model Act Governing Assisted Reproductive Technology (Approved by the ABA House of Delegates, February, 2008).
Fertility Clinic Success Rate and Certificate Act of 1992, 42 U.S.C. s263a-1 (2006)
Louisiana. Revised Statutes Annotated ss9: 123–126

UK

Human Fertilisation and Embryology Act 1990, as amended 2008

EUROPE

Directive on Setting Standards of Quality and Safety for the Donation, Procurement, Testing, Processing, Preservation, Storage and Distribution of Human Tissues and Cells (Directive 2004/23/EC)

7   Gamete and embryo donation: a legal view from Spain

Yolanda García-Ruiz and Diana Guerra-Diaz

Introduction

Spain has a strong culture of family life. Family relationships are often close and people grow up aspiring to have their own children. So, if a couple find that they are infertile and may need the assistance of a gamete donor to have children, this can be deeply disturbing. Their hopes and expectations of having 'their own' children may crumble and their feelings of esteem and personal worth can be jeopardized. Many feel deeply frustrated and find this one of the most challenging situations they have had to face in life. In Spain there is little understanding of what conception by assisted reproduction techniques (ARTs) is and no knowledge of gamete donation, and this can make the experience even more difficult for prospective parents.

It is estimated that at least three million children have been conceived in fertility clinics, according to the statistics collected by the European Society for Human Reproduction and Embryology (De Mouzon *et al.*, 2010). This figure is an underestimate, since the report only collects data from fifty-two countries and about two thirds of the global activity of ARTs. ARTs have brought a revolution with medical, social and legal implications for Spanish society. Since the birth of Spain's first IVF baby, Anna Victoria, at the Dexeus Clinic in Barcelona in 1984, Spain has experienced many changes in the development of ARTs. Expectations – and controversies – have grown with the development of egg donation and more recently with the possibility of freezing and storing eggs. Since the late 1980s, many countries have enacted laws designed to regulate these practices. However, far from achieving a consensus, legislation has been characterized by diversity, especially in the most controversial areas, such as the involvement of donors in the reproductive process. Maintaining donor anonymity, payment for donation, the risks to the health of the donor (in the case of egg donation), the relevance for children's welfare of knowing their biological origins, the importance of limiting the total number of donations by a

donor and recording donations in a donor registry have all been regulated differently in jurisdictions around the world. Currently, these
issues are raising new legal challenges that are leading to significant
legislative changes in some countries.

Several main legal controversies will be presented in this chapter and
will be discussed in the context of important ethical, economic and
psychosocial issues. These issues and legal controversies will also be
explained in relation to donors, recipients and the children who are
created using ARTs.

The evolution of legislation

In 1988 Spain was one of the first countries to enact a law on assisted
reproduction: the Spanish Act about Assisted Human Reproduction
Techniques (35/1988). This was only four years after the first regulatory legislation: the Swedish Act of Artificial Insemination 1985, n.
1140/1984. The Spanish legislators wanted to regulate the use of ARTs
and, especially, egg and sperm donation. The use of donors in ARTs
presented an important challenge to traditional family law and the 1988
Spanish Act regulating ARTs was particularly cautious in this respect.
Before 1985 artificial insemination by donor (AID) was used in many
countries without legal regulation and typically the donor was unknown
to the recipients and/or child (Lalos et al., 2003). Over the years there
have been changes in legislation concerning the anonymity of donors,
with an international trend towards revealing the identity of donors to
offspring in the belief that children are entitled to know about their
origins and their biological parents (Brewaeys et al., 2005).

The first country to introduce legislation in this regard was Sweden
in 1985 with a law giving children the right to know the identity of
their donor when they came of age (Lalos et al., 2003; Daniels et al.,
2005). Since April 2005, a change in UK law has meant that any child
born as a result of a donation of semen, eggs or embryos can access
their donor's name after they reach the age of 18 (Paul et al., 2006).
Thus, the United Kingdom has joined a small but growing number of countries with similar regulation, including Sweden, Austria,
Switzerland, Norway, Netherlands, New Zealand and some Australian
states (Daniels, 2007). Some other countries, such as Germany, have a
professional guidance that provides for access to the identity of donors
(Thorn et al., 2008).

However, matters are rather different in Spain. According to Law
14/2006 Art. 5.5, 'The donation will be anonymous and the identity of
the donor will be confidential in gamete banks, and, where appropriate,

in donor records and in the activities of the clinic.' This applies to sperm, egg and embryo donation.

AID and IVF with semen donation has been widely used in the Spanish clinics for Spanish couples and those travelling from other parts of Europe who have difficulty having children because of male sterility. In addition, in recent decades it is also being used with other patients whose problem is social rather than medical; these are women without partners or with a female partner. However, using sperm donation seems not to have caused as many moral and religious problems in Europe as has egg donation.

Before the possibility of marriage for same-sex partners, lesbian women requiring sperm donation had to misrepresent their situation to a clinic. Today, after discussions at the National Commission on Assisted Human Reproduction (the ARTs advisory body of the Ministry of Health), lesbian couples can exchange gametes with their partners, provided they are legally married. Thus, there is now equal treatment of heterosexual and homosexual people. Some assisted reproduction clinics and some governments do not accept the use of the AID by this group of patients because they believe there needs to be a medical problem of sterility to justify the use of this treatment (Englert, 1994). There have been various arguments made against the treatment of lesbian couples and single women on the grounds of supposed risks to the welfare of children (Strong and Schinfeld, 1984; Baetens *et al.*, 2000; see also Graham and Braverman, Chapter 11; Appleby, Jennings and Statham, Chapter 12), and the matter remains controversial for some (Englert, 1994).

In most European countries AID or IVF is not permitted for single women, so many of them travel to Spain for donor treatment. The fact that in Spain the donor is anonymous also leads some women or couples from countries where anonymity is not possible to come to Spain (for example, from the UK, Germany and Italy) (see Pennings and B. Gürtin, Chapter 8).

The first birth resulting from IVF with donated eggs occurred in 1984 in the USA (Lutjen *et al.*, 1984). Since then the demand for donor eggs has increased rapidly as the practice has been expanded and has been established in many ART clinics (Kan *et al.*, 1998).

There are several reasons why egg donation has been more controversial than sperm donation in Spain. Egg donation is a more difficult practice and egg donors face higher risks to their health. It also appears that women are more 'attached' to their eggs than men to their sperm. It might be said that throughout history men have 'donated' sperm, resulting in them not recognizing children, or not even being aware of their conception.

In Spain, unlike most of Europe, donors receive some financial compensation. Law 14/2006 of 26 May 2006 makes gamete and embryo donation a free contract, formal and confidential between the donor and the clinic: 'The donation will always be non-profit and not commercial. The financial compensation can be set to only compensate strictly physical discomfort, travel and loss of earnings that may arise from the donation and must not involve economic incentives.' The amount of this compensation may vary from clinic to clinic. But the guidance given by the National Commission on Assisted Human Reproduction is that the overall figure for compensation should be about 900 Euros (£775). While in a few other European countries (e.g. Cyprus and the Czech Republic) similar levels of compensation are paid, this is a much higher figure than in most countries. In the UK, for example, donors may receive out-of-pocket expenses (e.g. travel) and a compensation for loss of earnings of £61.28 (€71.25) per day up to a maximum of £250 (€290) for each course of egg or sperm donation.[1] That said, some egg donors can receive much higher payments in kind through participation in 'egg-sharing' schemes. In these procedures, women who are having IVF agree to donate some of their eggs in return for free or reduced price treatment (the clinic is paid the difference from the usual price by the recipients). In the UK IVF costs about £5,000 (€5,815) per cycle.

In Spain the number of children conceived by a donor is limited to 6. This is toward the lower range of limits set elsewhere – for example France (5), Sweden (6), Switzerland (8), New Zealand (10) and Netherlands (25). Other countries regulate in terms of numbers of families (recipients may prefer to use the same donor for all their children). These range from 3 (Austria) through 5 (Finland and New South Wales and Western Australia) to 10 in the UK and Victoria, Australia. Enforcing this limit in Spain is the responsibility of the clinics. Donors are asked about previous donations and where they have donated. Clinics are responsible for verifying the identity of the donor and checking information to ensure the limit is not exceeded. However, there is no central donor registry. Law 14/2006 of 26 May 2006 on ARTs sets out the framework for a National Donor Registry under the Ministry of Health and Consumer Affairs in which all gamete and embryo donors must be registered. Despite this and earlier legislation that enabled registration, and pressure from the National Commission on Assisted Human Reproduction, there has been a lack of political will on this matter and no national registry or activity register has been set up. Without such a facility, clinics

---

[1] In 2011 those rates were increased to a fixed sum of £35 for a visit for sperm donors and a fixed sum of £750 per cycle of donation for egg donors.

face an almost impossible task in verifying the previous donation history of donors. Indeed, it is generally assumed that the set limits of numbers of children per donor are widely breached.

Anonymity of donors

As mentioned already, Spain chose to protect the anonymity of donors in the Spanish Act about Assisted Human Reproduction Techniques 1988, and maintains this policy in the current legislation (Assisted Human Reproduction Act 2006). France, which legislated for the first time on this subject in 1994, took a similar position. This is maintained in the current French Law on Bioethics 2004, which had the intention of unifying and updating French legislation in this area. In France the law embodies a provision for review every five years. The first review report has recently been published (Law n. 94–653, 29 July 1994, relative au respect du corps humain). In this law there is an extensive section devoted to the anonymity of donors and the discussion illustrates the tensions that this issue generated within the Commission. The overwhelming preference was ultimately conservative and opted for anonymity under the law. However, the President of the Commission and many of its members accept the need to keep this issue under review and study (Assemblée Nationale, 2010).

In addition, we should note that anonymity is also protected by law in Denmark (1997), Greece (2002 and 2005), Portugal (2006), Czech Republic (2006) and Bulgaria (2007). Other states have tried to avoid the issue, in general or in some cases, by prohibiting the use of donors in ARTs (Italy, 2004) or the use of egg donors (Germany, 1990). Some states, in an attempt to reflect both the right of children to know their biological parentage and the privacy of donors, have proposed a mixed system, known as the 'double track' (Pennings, 1997, 2007). In this system, used in Iceland (1997), Canada (2004) and Belgium (2007) donors can decide whether or not to be anonymous. Obviously, this system has advantages for parents who can choose between identifiable and anonymous donors and for donors who can decide on their own anonymity. Thus, this system can preserve the privacy of donors and the private and family life of parents. However, it does not take into account the interests or rights of children to know their donor origin.

The decisions of the Spanish legislators in relation to anonymity was probably influenced by the decline in donations that occurred in Sweden (see Pennings, Vayena and Ahuja, Chapter 9, for a more general discussion of donor recruitment), after their law recognized the right of the children born following donor insemination to know their donor origin

(Art. 4, Swedish Act of Artificial Insemination (1140: 1984). Another reason that seemed obvious at the time of that decision was the lack of a culture of ARTs or widespread practice, and legislators did not want to create social and psychological difficulties for the recipients of donation and their children.

This factor was very significant in the first Spanish ARTs legislation and in the current legislation (2006). Article 5 of this Act establishes the rules for donors and the donation contract and provides that the donation will be a free, formal and *confidential* contract between the donor and the authorized clinic.

While the 1988 Spanish Act established that donation is a secret contract between the donor and the authorized clinic, the current Act (2006) has changed this concept and now donation is considered a confidential contract, but not secret. The difference is important because it is possible to acquire confidential information, if that is necessary – in this case, about the donor – whereas if the contract is secret, the application of the culture of secrecy is likely to be enforced in law (Petersen, 2006). If we have regard for the rights of children, the culture of secrecy is not a good option in legislation. However, secrecy is normal when children are born following donor insemination. In this situation, secrecy may be important for many different reasons: social and family pressure; shame because of the need for a donor in relation to infertility or sexual dysfunctions; or fear that the children might feel less love for their parents if they know that they are born following donor insemination (Golombok, 2009; this issue is further discussed by Appleby, Blake and Freeman, Chapter 13).

Donor recipients and their children

Regarding the information that children can access, the law states that '[t]he children are entitled themselves, or through their legal representatives, to obtain general information about donors which does not include identity. This same right applies to recipients of gametes and embryos' (Art. 5.5). Thus, as in some other jurisdictions where anonymity prevails, access to the fact of donation is possible, at least in principle, even though anonymity is protected.

The most recent Spanish Act uses the concept of confidentiality and establishes the anonymity of the donor but allows the children and parents the possibility of knowing general information about the donor (for example medical information), either through their legal representatives or, in special circumstances, directly. Thus, children have the possibility to know some information about the donor but the name of the donor will only be revealed in two exceptional circumstances: when there are risks to the child's life and health, or in a criminal trial in a court. In those situations it would be possible to reveal the identity of the donor but with certain restrictions, for example revelation only to clinicians or judges but not to the wider public (Art. 5.5, Spanish Act about Assisted Human Reproduction (14/2006)).

Another important aspect of donor anonymity in Spanish legislation is that the donation contract is made between the donor and an authorized clinic, not between the donor and the legal parents of the child. Article 5 of the Spanish Act (2006) establishes this rule to ensure anonymity of donors in ARTs. If the contract is made between the donor and the clinic, it is possible to apply the rules about confidentiality and about anonymity of the donor. These rules about donor anonymity could not be applied if the contract were between the donor and the couple who want a child or between the donor and a single woman. The Spanish Act about Assisted Human Reproduction (14/2006) recognizes, in Article 6, that a single woman can use assisted human reproduction techniques. If there were a private contract between her and the donor, the donor would not be protected by the rules of anonymity. The law would consider the woman who gave birth to the child as the legal mother, and the donor may be considered the legal father under Article 39.2 of the Spanish Constitution. Such a situation does arise in other jurisdictions (e.g. UK) where parenthood is only transferred from donors to the social parent if insemination takes place in a licensed clinic. And in Spain if private arrangements are made with a donor, the usual rules regulating sexual relationships outside marriage will apply.

Spanish law, working in the best interests of children, has made it possible to investigate the paternity of a child, as established in the Spanish Constitution, Article 39.2. The anonymity of donors in the legislation about ARTs is an exception to this general rule. At least hypothetically, where there is a private contract between a couple and the donor, the donor could be considered the legal father of the child by the court, because donation is considered a special circumstance. Of course, the problem is that usually children do not know that they were conceived by donation and so it is not possible for them to assert their rights in court. But there is a trend elsewhere of moving away from the protection of the anonymity of donors (Blyth and Frith, 2009). Under the UK Human Fertilisation and Embryology Act 1990, Article 31, it is open to any adult donor child to apply to a regulating authority and they will be told if they had been conceived by the same donor as a potential spouse or partner. However, in 2004 anonymity was ended. The Disclosure of Donor Information Regulations 2004 allows adult children of donation to apply to have the name and some other details of the donor. Other states have done the same: Austria (1992), Switzerland (1998), the Netherlands (2002), Norway (2003), New Zealand (2004), Western Australia (2004), Finland (2006) and New South Wales in Australia (2007).

There is a clear diversity of law on this issue. While some countries protect the right of children to know their biological parentage, others prevent this. Therefore, depending on their country of origin, children conceived by donation have the right to know their biological parents, or not (Blyth, 2006). So, there is a certain relativity of the principles underlying the legislation on reproductive donation. Perhaps the trend should be the opposite: to encourage the development of universal bio-ethical principles and 'BioLaw' rights, at least in Western jurisdictions. In any case, if the law does not protect the rights of the children born following ARTs, sooner or later they will probably demand those rights (García-Ruiz, 2004). This is a reality that cannot be ignored. For this, however, parents need to tell their children that a donor was involved in their conception and, for many reasons, this is not what usually happens, particularly in heterosexual couples (Freeman *et al.*, 2009; Appleby, Blake and Freeman, Chapter 13). Disclosure happens more generally in the case of single mothers and lesbian couples.

In Spain the law does not say anything about the obligation of the parents to tell children born from donated gametes of their origin. Although many couples before having children do say that they intend to tell their child the truth about the conception, studies have shown that most couples do not do so (Golombok *et al.*, 2002, Golombok, 2009).

In countries which retain anonymity and in which a traditional concept of family prevails, as in Spain, there is another argument for the rights of both donors and potential recipients and children born through these techniques (García-Ruiz, 2008). Since in these cultures there is still little knowledge of ARTs, and there is a belief that 'blood ties' (genetic links) are important, they try to protect children from the possible stigmatization in society in general and in particular in the situation that would arise if others knew of their donor conception. Moreover, they also believe that the donor should be protected by keeping the donation secret both now and in the future.

In addition, the contract between the donor and the authorized clinic provides an important way of controlling the number of children who are born from the same donor. In private contracts the same donor could be used many times. Failing to control the use of a donor could lead to problems in the future as it would increase the probability of marriage between half-siblings. In fact, if the clinic uses the gametes of a donor without respecting the limit that the Law has established on the number of children who are born from the same donor, the clinic would be in breach of Article 26.2 (b) 8° of Law 14/2006 of May 26.

Donor registry in Spanish legislation

As we have mentioned already, Spain has no public donor registry despite legislation for its creation.

This lack of registry is unsustainable and poses many problems. For instance, if there is no real control of the donor and there is a risk that donors will not be identified correctly, this puts in jeopardy the medical data that could be vital to the health of children in the future. Clinics may ask for identification, but if there is none forthcoming, they may 'close their eyes' and accept the donor because they need donors. The lack of control of the number of donations made by donors may increase the chances of unwitting co-sanguinity for donor couples in the future. While the current Spanish legislation fixes the maximum number of children by one donor at six, without a donor registry it is not possible to enforce this. In addition, Spain is in breach of Directive 2006/17/CE of the European Commission containing the application of the Directive 2004/23/CE from the European Parliament and Commission, concerning certain technical requirements related to donation, procurement and control of the tissues and cells of human origin and Directive 2006/86/CE from the Commission containing application of the Directive 2004/23/CE from the European Parliament and Commission, concerning the technical requirements of traceability and notification of the reactions and side-effects and certain technical requirements related to the processing, preservation, storage and distribution of human tissues and cells.

In particular, the absence of a donor registry could affect the 'traceability' that is set out in the Directives, and which applies to gamete donation in ARTs. Directive 2006/86/CE defines 'traceability' as 'the ability to locate and identify the tissue/cell during any step from procurement, through processing, testing and storage, to distribution to the recipient or disposal, which also implies the ability to identify the donor.' It is important to note that traceability implies the ability to identify the donor and without a registry this is very difficult. What is needed is to design a network of donor registers at different levels. In Spain it would be appropriate to establish registers in the Autonomous Communities that could send donor data to a national registry and the national registry could be connected with a European registry.

The creation of a network of donor registries would be a first step in meeting EU requirements for traceability in relation to the identification of donors in reproductive medicine. The authorized clinics have this data, at least in theory, and should be able to ascertain the number of donations by donor in all other centres, but what happens if the data are not correct? Has the state any responsibility here?

Donor selection

The donor selection process requires the work of a multidisciplinary team. The Spanish Law states that 'donors should be more than 18 years old, psychologically and physically healthy and with a full capacity to consent'. Their psycho-physical state must satisfy the requirements of a mandatory protocol for donors including phenotypic and psychological characteristics. The laboratory tests need to demonstrate, 'according to the state of knowledge in science and the existing technology at the time of its making, that donors do not suffer from genetic, hereditary or infectious diseases that can affect the offspring'. As for physical health tests, clinics are required to do all the assessments required by the Autonomous Community.

The donors will not get any information about the reproductive outcomes of their donations. So they will not know if their donation has produced any pregnancies or not.

The need for a psychological evaluation of potential donors is increasingly suggested to minimize the transmission of psychopathology to the offspring and ensure the successful development and completion of the donation protocol (Martin *et al.*, 2007).

A psychological evaluation protocol has been developed by the Psychology Interest Group of the Sociedad Española de Fertilidad (SEF) and this can be found in their guidelines (Grupo de Interés de Psicología Sociedad Española de Fertilidad 2010). This consists of a semi-structured interview that aims to eliminate any suspicion of psychological problems that may affect the proper outcome of the donation process.

Most sperm donors are Spanish, young, single and have upper-middle education. In a study in the Valencia Infertility Institute (IVI) (Dolz del Castellar, 2008) 87% of male donors were Spanish, which is consistent with the pattern in other studies in which donors were generally from the home country (Cook and Golombok, 1995, Thorn *et al.*, 2008). The Spanish study showed an average age of 27 years (Dolz del Castellar, 2008) which is similar to British studies carried out before donor anonymity ended in Britain (Cook and Golombok, 1995; Paul *et al.*, 2006). However, in countries where no financial reward is offered (Daniels *et al.*, 1996) or in countries where the law has ended anonymity, the average age of donors was in their 30s (Lalos *et al.*, 2003; Daniels *et al.*, 2005). Most donors were single or co-habiting, and only a small proportion were married (Cook and Golombok, 1995; Fielding *et al.*, 1998; Dolz del Castellar, 2008; Thorn *et al.*, 2008). In a study conducted by Daniels, Curson and Lewis (1996), which compares the characteristics of samples of donors who did or did not receive compensation, 76% of the no-compensation groups were married versus 9% in the compensation group. The percentage of donors with children is higher in studies where access to the donor's identity is open and where they do not receive compensation (Daniels *et al.*, 1996; Daniels *et al.*, 2005). In the Spanish study, only 10% of donors already had children (Dolz del Castellar, 2008). So in terms of demographic characteristics, we see that in countries with laws guaranteeing anonymity, donors are young, mostly single and childless, and college students. This profile is related to the method used by the clinics to attract potential donors, as it is often done through posters at universities or university magazines (Cook and Golombok, 1995; Paul *et al.*, 2006; Vives *et al.*, 2006).

Anonymity is also a major factor in the motivation of sperm donors, so in countries like Sweden where anonymity is not guaranteed we see that the motivation is primarily altruistic (Daniels *et al.*, 2005), whereas in English studies conducted before the change of the law donors were more likely to cite economic motives (Cook and Golombok, 1995). In this respect Spain differs from other countries since 27% of donors claim an economic motive (Dolz del Castellar, 2008). In countries like Germany where the status of the donor's identity is more ambiguous, there is a similar mixture of economic and altruistic reasons (Thorn *et al.*, 2008). In a study conducted in several IVF clinics in Spain, the average age of donors was around 25 years (Guerra *et al.*, 2007), similar to that found in American studies (Braverman and Corson, 2002). In other European countries the average age is slightly higher at around 30 years (Baetens *et al.*, 2000). In Spain egg donors must be less than 35 years because mature age increases the risk of Down's syndrome and reduces the quality of the eggs (Marina *et al.*, 1999).

Spanish egg donors are predominantly single (Guerra *et al.*, 2007). This is not so in other European studies, where donors are slightly older and include more married women (Baetens *et al.*, 2000; Martin *et al.*, 2007). This finding might be related to compensation payments because in countries like Spain and the United States, where compensation is permitted, the average donor age is lower and they are mostly single (Braverman and Corson, 2002; Martin *et al.*, 2007), whereas in the UK or Belgium, where there is limited compensation, the profile of age and marital status is different. In Spain single and childless women dominate (Martin *et al.*, 2007) and in a multicentre study, even with the predominance of single women, almost half of them had a child (Guerra *et al.*, 2007). It is not uncommon that they have experienced abortions before the donation (Lindheim *et al.*, 1998; Guerra *et al.*, 2007). As regards to occupation, most of them are employed (Fielding *et al.*, 1998; Kan *et al.*, 1998; Lindheim *et al.*, 1998; Guerra *et al.*, 2007; Martin *et al.*, 2007) and have a medium educational level (Guerra *et al.*, 2007) or university degree (Fielding *et al.*, 1998; Lindheim *et al.*, 1998; Martin *et al.*, 2007). Most donors cite both altruistic and financial motives. One factor that influences the pattern is anonymity. Known donors generally express a desire to help, especially when the recipients are relatives or friends (Fielding *et al.*, 1998; Baetens *et al.*, 2000). The results of studies where donors are anonymous, including Spain, show that the economic factor is a primary motivation together with some altruistic reasons, but the percentage of women who made donations for a purely altruistic motivation is lower (Guerra *et al.*, 2007; Martin *et al.*, 2007).

The Spanish samples show a profile of occasional alcohol consumption (Guerra *et al.*, 2007) that is consistent with the general culture. Regarding the consumption of other drugs, about 10% use cocaine (Dolz del Castellar, 2008), and about 5% cannabis (Lindheim, *et al.*, 1998). It is difficult to draw conclusions about psychological disorders because different studies measure different aspects (personality, psychopathology) and with different instruments. With regard to previous psychiatric problems, Klock *et al.* (1999) found that 10% of the candidates had a history of medication and 34% had received psychotherapy. Schover *et al.* (1990) reported that 64% of their sample had suffered minor depression or anxiety symptoms and Guerra *et al.* (2007) found 16% of donors had a past history of psychological disorder. Regarding the presence of psychological distress at the time of donation, Lindheim *et al.* (1998) rejected 8% of donors because of psychopathology, Guerra *et al.* (2007) 2% and Martin *et al.* (2007) 2% for personality disorder.

Conclusions

The donation of gametes is an important issue in infertility treatments because many pregnancies are achieved through the donation. The most controversial topics currently in ARTs in Spain relate to the anonymity and payment of the donors, the creation of a national donor registry with relevant information and the welfare of the donor-conceived children. Spanish legislation is not restrictive and effectively promotes the practice of ARTs, but this approach creates problems for the rights of the children to know their biological origins and for the protection of the health of women, especially those who act as egg donors.

In this area there is a need for greater knowledge about the demographic and psychological characteristics of people who come to the clinics to donate because this is important information for the recipients, as well as for the clinics.

When comparing the outcomes, there are several factors that determine the differences in the characteristics of donors that must be taken into account, such as the regulatory regime in force in the respective countries, the existence of fees or payments for the donation and the method of donor recruitment.

Spain has more liberal law compared with other jurisdictions around the world. This helps to make the country a popular destination for reproductive tourists from elsewhere in Europe. Spain's popularity may also stem from the fact that donor gametes, especially eggs, are generally available there without the long waiting lists seen in some other countries, and because of competitive pricing of ARTs treatments.

REFERENCES

Assemblée Nationale, n° 2235, *Rapport d'information fait au nom de la Mission d'information sur la revision des Lois de Bioéthique*, 20 January 2010. Available at: www.assemblee-nationale.fr/13/rap-info/i2235-t1.asp.

Baetens, P., Devroey, P., Camus, M., Van Steirteghem, A. C., *et al.* (2000). 'Counselling couples and donors for oocyte donation: the decision to use either known or anonymous oocyte'. *Human Reproduction*, 15, 476–84.

Blyth, E. (2006). 'Donor anonymity and secrecy versus openness concerning the genetic origins of the offspring: international perspectives'. *Jewish Medical Ethics*, 5, 2, 4–13.

Blyth, E. and Frith, L. (2009). 'Donor-conceived people's access to genetic and biographical history: an analysis of provisions in different jurisdictions permitting disclosure of donor identity'. *International Journal of Law, Policy and the Family*, 23, 174–91.

Braverman, A. M. and Corson, S. L. (2002). 'A comparison of oocyte donors' and gestational carriers/surrogates' attitudes towards third party reproduction'. *Journal of Assisted Reproduction and Genetics*, 19, 462–69.

Brewaeys, A., de Bruyn, J. K., Louwe, L. A. and Helmerhorst, F. M. (2005). 'Anonymous or identity-registered sperm donors? A study of Dutch recipients' choices'. *Human Reproduction*, 20, 820–4.

Cook, R. and Golombok, S. (1995). 'A survey of semen donation: phase 2 – the view of the donors'. *Human Reproduction*, 10, 951–9.

Daniels, K. (2007). 'Anonymity and openness and the recruitment of gamete donors. Part I: semen donors'. *Human Fertility*, 10, 151–8.

Daniels, K. R., Curson, R. and Lewis, G. M. (1996). 'Semen donor recruitment: a study of donors in two clinics'. *Human Reproduction*, 11, 746–51.

Daniels, K., Lalos, A., Gottlieb, C. and Lalos, O. (2005). 'Semen providers and their three families'. *Journal of Psychosomatic Obstetrics and Gynecology*, 26, 15–22.

De Mouzon, J., Goossens, V., Battacharya, S., Ferraretti, A. P., *et al.* (2010). 'European IVF-monitoring (EIM) Consortium, for the European Society of Human Reproduction and Embryology (ESHRE): Assisted reproductive technology and intrauterine inseminations in Europe, 2006: results generated from European registers by ESHRE, 2010'. *Human Reproduction*, 25, 1851–62.

Dolz del Castellar, P. (2008). 'Perfil del/la donante de gametos'. Comunicación presentada en el XXVII Congreso Nacional de la Sociedad Española de Fertilidad, Oviedo.

Englert, Y. (1994). 'Artificial insemination with donor semen: particular request'. *Human Reproduction*, 9, 1969–71.

Fielding, D., Handley, S., Duqueno, L., Weaver, S. and Lui, S. (1998). 'Motivation, attitudes and experience of donation: a follow-up of women donating eggs in assisted conception treatment'. *Journal of Community and Applied Social Psychology*, 8, 273–87.

Freeman, T., Jadva, V., Kramer, W. and Golombok, S. (2009). 'Gamete donation: parents' experiences of searching for their child's donor sibling and donor'. *Human Reproduction*, 24, 505–16.

García-Ruiz, Y. (2004). *Reproducción humana asistida: derecho, conciencia y libertad*. Granada: Comares, 1–318.

(2008). 'Incidencia de la religión y la cultura en la genética'. *Investigación, genética y derecho*. Tirant Lo Blanch, 11–35.

Golombok, S. (2009). 'Anonymity – or not – in the Donation of Gametes and Embryos', in S. Day Sclater, F. Ebtehaj, E. Jackson and M. Richards (eds.), *Regulating Autonomy. Sex, Reproduction and Family*. Oxford: Hart Publishing.

Golombok, S., Brewaeys, A., Giavazzi, M. T., Guerra, D., *et al.* (2002). 'The European study of assisted reproduction families: the transition to adolescence'. *Human Reproduction*, 17, 830–40.

Grupo de Interés de Psicología Sociedad Española de Fertilidad (2010). *Manual de intervención psicológica en Reproducción Asistida* (Guidelines). Barcelona: Edikamed.

Guerra, D., Tirado, M., Fernández, M., Dolz del Cautelar, P., *et al.* (2007). 'Psychological evaluation of egg donors at IVI centres in Spain'. Poster presented at II Congreso Internacional IVI & Simposio de Enfermería y Psicología sobre Reproducción Asistida, Barcelona.

Kan, A. K. S., Abadía, H. I., Ogunyemi, B. O., Korea, L. *et al.* (1998). 'A survey of anonymous oocyte donors: demographics'. *Human Reproduction*, 13, 2762–6.

Klock, S. C., Scout, J. E. and Davidson, M. (1999). 'Analysis of Minnesota Multiphasic Personality Inventory-2 profiles of prospective anonymous oocyte donors in relation to the outcome of the donor selection process'. *Fertility and Sterility*, 72, 1066–72.

Lalos, A., Daniels, K., Gottlieb, C. and Lalos, O. (2003). 'Recruitment and motivation of semen providers in Sweden'. *Human Reproduction*, 18, 212–16.

Lindheim, S. R., Frumovitz, M. and Saber, M. V. (1998). 'Recruitment and screening policies and procedures used to establish a paid donor oocyte registry'. *Human Reproduction*, 13, 2020–4.

Lutjen, P. J., Trounson, A., Leeton, J., Findlay, J., et al. (1984). 'The establishment and maintenance of pregnancy using in vitro fertilisation and embryo donation in a patient with primary ovarian failure'. *Nature*, 307, 174–5.

Marina, S., Expósito, R., Marina, F., Nadal, J., et al. (1999). 'Oocyte donor selection from 554 candidates'. *Human Reproduction*, 14, 2770–6.

Martin, S., Pérez, C., Salinas, A., Giménez, V., et al. (2007). 'Protocolo de actuación y perfil psicológico de donantes de ovocitos de la unidad de reproducción asistida de Quirón Bilbao'. *Revista Iberoamericana de Fertilidad y Reproducción Humana*, 24, 389–98.

Paul, S., Harbottle, S. and Stewart, J. A., 2006. 'Recruitment of sperm donors: the Newcastle-Upon-Tyne experience 1994–2003'. *Human Reproduction*, 21, 150–8.

Pennings, G. (1997). 'The "double track" policy for donor anonymity'. *Human Reproduction*, 12, 2839–44.

(2007). 'Belgian law on medically assisted reproduction and the disposition of supernumerary embryos and gametes'. *European Journal of Health Law*, 3, 251–60.

Petersen, K. (2006). 'The right of donor-conceived children to know the identity of their donor', in B. Bennet and G. F. Tomossy (eds.), *Globalization and Health*. Dordrecht: SpringerLink.

Schover, L. R., Reis, J., Collins, R. L. and Blankstein, J. (1990). 'The psychological evaluation of oocyte donors'. *Journal of Psychosomatic Obstetrics and Gynecology*, 11, 299–309.

Strong, C. and Schinfeld, J. S. (1984). 'The single woman and artificial insemination by donor'. *The Journal of Reproductive Medicine*, 29, 293–9.

Thorn, P., Katzorke, T. and Daniels, K. (2008). 'Semen donors in Germany: a study exploring motivations and attitudes'. *Human Reproduction*, 23, 2415–20.

Vives, A., Marina, D., Alcolea, R., Latre, L., et al. (2006). 'Estudio de mil donantes de semen: aceptados y no aceptados'. Comunicación presentada en el XXVI Congreso Nacional de la Sociedad Española de Fertilidad, Zaragoza.

LEGISLATION

AUSTRALIA

New South Wales
Assisted Reproductive Technology Act 2007

Victoria
Infertility Treatment Act 1995

Western Australia
Human Reproductive Technology Amendment Act 2004

AUSTRIA

Reproductive Medicine Act, 4 June 1992

BELGIUM

Loi relative à la procréation médicalement assistée et à la destination des embryons surnuméraires et des gamètes, 6 July 2007, Moniteur Belge, n° 214, 17 July 2007

BULGARIA

Health Law, Effective 1 January 2005, amended SG No. 13/8 February 2008
Regulation 28 of 20 June 2007 for assisted reproduction activities. Issued by the Ministry of Health, promulgated SG No. 55, 6 July 2007

CANADA

Assisted Human Reproduction Act, 29 March 2004, laws-lois.justice.gc.ca

CZECH REPUBLIC

Act on Research on Human Embryonic Stem Cells and Related Activities and on Amendment to some Related Acts, 26 April 2006. Amendment to Act No. 20/1966 Coll

DENMARK

Lov nr. 460 af 10. juni 1997 om kunstig befrugtning i forbindelse med lægelig behandling, diagnostik og forskning m.v.

EUROPE

Directive 2006/17/CE of the European Commission containing the application of the Directive 2004/23/CE from the European Parliament and Commission, concerning certain technical requirements related to donation, procurement and control of the tissues and cells of human origin
Directive 2006/86/CE from the Commission containing application of the Directive 2004/23/CE from the European Parliament and Commission, concerning the technical requirements of traceability and notification of the reactions and side-effects and certain technical requirements related to the processing, preservation, storage and distribution of human tissues and cells

FINLAND

Acts on Assisted Fertility Treatments (1237/2006)

FRANCE

Loi n°2004–800 du 6 août 2004, relative à la bioéthique
Amended: Loi No2011-814 du 7 juillet 2011 relative à la bioethique

GERMANY

The Embryo Protection Act, Bundesgesetzblatt, edition I, 1990

GREECE

Law 3089, 23 December 2002, Medically Assisted Human Reproduction
Law 3305/2005, Medical Assisted Reproduction

ICELAND

Regulation No. 568/1997 on Artificial Fertilization

ITALY

Legge 19 febbraio 2004, n. 40 Norme in materia di procreazione medicalmente assistita. Gaceta Ufficiale n. 45, 24 February 2004

NETHERLANDS

Conservation, Management and Provision of Data of Donors in Artificial
Insemination Act, 2002. Official Gazette of the Netherlands, n. 240, 25
April 2002

NEW ZEALAND

Human Assisted Reproductive Technology Act 2004

NORWAY

Act of 5 December 2003 No. 100 relating to the application of biotechnology
in human medicine

PORTUGAL

Law 32/2006 de Procriação medicamente assistida, Diário da República, 1.a
série No. 143–26 de Julho de 2006

SPAIN

Act about Assisted Human Reproduction Techniques (35/1988)
Ley 14/2006, de 26 de mayo, sobre técnicas de reproducción humana asistida,
B.O.E. núm. 126, 27 May 2006

SWEDEN

Act of Artificial Insemination 1985, n. 1140/1984
Replaced by the Genetic Integrity Act (2006: 351)

SWITZERLAND

Legge federale concernente la procreazione con assistenza medica (Legge sulla medicina della procreazione, LPAM), 1998

UNITED KINGDOM

Human Fertilisation and Embryology Act 1990, as amended 2008
The Human Fertilisation and Embryology Authority (Disclosure of Donor Information) Regulations 2004

8 The legal and ethical regulation of transnational donation

Guido Pennings and Zeynep B. Gürtin

Introduction

This chapter provides an overview and analysis of the phenomenon of transnational donation, an aspect of donation practices which has grown both in prevalence and significance over the past decade. After defining what we mean by 'transnational donation', we interrogate this phenomenon from different perspectives in three different sections. The first section surveys the empirical evidence and available data on transnational donation and cross-border reproductive care (CBRC), first with regard to the movements of patients and second with regard to the movements of gametes across borders. The second section analyses the potential regulatory approaches that may be developed as a response to transnational reproduction, investigating in turn the pros and cons of coerced conformity, international harmonization and moral pluralism. The final section evaluates the three main 'dangers' of CBRC – to safety, to autonomy and to justice – and analyses the ethical force, accuracy and strength of each of these arguments.

What is 'transnational donation'?

Transnational donation is one aspect of the newly emerging, and rapidly developing, phenomenon of CBRC. CBRC refers to movements across national borders to seek or facilitate infertility treatments. Within this broader phenomenon the term 'transnational donation' is reserved specifically for the pursuit of treatments involving the use of donor gametes. Although CBRC covers a wide range of assisted reproductive technologies (ARTs) – for example, pre-implantation genetic diagnosis (PGD) – infertility treatments involving donation make up a large subset of the CBRC market. This is because ARTs involving donor gametes are subject to great diversity between jurisdictions with regard both to the level and nature of regulatory control and to the availability of necessary resources (see Chapter 5, Chapter 6, and Chapter 7). It is the prevalence of such diversity, even among countries in close geographical proximity to one another, that drives transnational donation and makes it a very significant aspect of the broader CBRC phenomenon.

While the terms 'reproductive tourism' or 'fertility tourism', heavily used by the media in the coverage of CBRC, conjure up images of intended parents travelling in their quests for conception, it is also possible for providers (egg and sperm donors and surrogates) and for ex vivo reproductive cells to move across borders. In some instances, more than one of these entities may travel from or to a particular destination, as may be the case when a single woman from France travels to Belgium for treatment with sperm that has been imported from Denmark.

The different causes of CBRC may be divided into the two broad categories of legal restrictions and/or limitations of availability (Pennings et al., 2008), though each of these categories may cover a range of different circumstances. Pennings (2002) has outlined the following six causes of CBRC: (1) a type of treatment is forbidden by law for moral reasons; (2) a treatment is not available because of lack of expertise or equipment; (3) a treatment is not available because it is not considered safe enough; (4) certain categories of patients are not eligible for infertility treatment; (5) scarcity of resources leads to long waiting lists in one's home country; and (6) the out-of-pocket costs for the patients are too high. Inhorn and Patrizio (2009) have added a seventh potential reason for engaging in CBRC, namely the wish to preserve privacy. Finally, a European Society for Human Reproduction and Embryology (ESHRE) study revealed that in some countries, such as the Netherlands and the United Kingdom, people go abroad to seek a better quality of care (Shenfield et al., 2010). Each of these reasons (perhaps with the exception of (3)) could be cited by individuals pursuing CBRC specifically for treatments involving donor gametes. However, as we will discuss with reference to the empirical data available, the actual reasons why different people travel will be determined (to a very great extent) by the conditions in their home country (for example whether the country bans the treatment they require, or whether there are resource limitations) and will in turn determine their chosen destinations.

Empirical evidence on transnational donation

A major problem for a discussion of transnational donation, and CBRC more generally, remains the lack of empirical data. Although CBRC is now recognized by ART practitioners and their professional organizations, regulators, patient support groups and academics from a variety of disciplines as an area in need of rigorous and sustained attention, so far the picture remains highly fragmented. However, data have started coming in from several investigations and many studies are currently ongoing, so it will be possible to form a better-informed analyses in the not too distant future. In this section we reflect on the evidence gathered to date about transnational donation, first involving the travel of intending parents, and second involving the movements of gametes and reproductive cells across borders. While it is also possible for providers to contribute to transnational reproduction by travelling to donate sperm and eggs in other jurisdictions (see for example Carbone and Gottheim (2006) for a discussion of Canadian sperm donors being recruited by Australian clinics), there is such little evidence regarding this that we leave this possibility aside for the moment.

Intending parents in motion

To date, one of the major initiatives to plug the data gap on CBRC has been made by ESHRE. The Europe-based ESHRE study, co-ordinated by Françoise Shenfield, examines the numbers, reasons and national-ities of cross-border ART patients in six European countries (Belgium, Czech Republic, Denmark, Slovenia, Spain and Switzerland), show-ing that the broad label of CBRC covers vast heterogeneity and that important differences exist in the types of patients and types of treat-ments sought, based not only on the country of origin but also on the country of destination (Shenfield *et al.*, 2010). This study collected data from forty-six infertility centres from six European countries, selected because they were known to be popular destinations for 'reproductive tourists', and estimated that there are between 11,000 to 14,000 CBRC patients per year in Europe (Shenfield *et al.*, 2010). The patients orig-inated mainly from four countries: Italy (31.8%), Germany (14.4%), the Netherlands (12.1%) and France (8.7%). The two main reasons for travelling to another country were legal restrictions and expectations of better-quality treatment. There were, however, large differences between the countries: for German, Italian and Norwegian patients, legal restrictions were cited by more than 70% of patients, while among British citizens only 9.4% mentioned this as a reason for pursuing CBRC. The main concern (34.0%) for British patients was difficulty of access, which was mentioned far more among this group than by patients from other countries. The explanation of these differences clearly lies in the specific circumstances of infertility treatment in the home nation. For example, the United Kingdom has liberal legislation that excludes very few groups from accessing treatment, but has limited availability of funded treatment under the National Health Service, leading to expensive treatments in the private sector.

The ESHRE study, although the most complete at the moment, also has some limitations, primarily due to the inclusion of only six recipient countries, and to the participation of only a limited number of fertility centres from some of these countries, such as Spain. This may have had an effect on the nationalities of the cross-border patients recorded and on the types of treatments they were recorded as seeking. However, there is some additional information with which we can fill some of these gaps. For example, de la Fuente (2010) reports 1,919 cycles in Spain in 2008 for foreign patients. These are subdivided as 42.02% for egg donation, 31.2% for IVF/ICSI, 25.1% for cryotransfer and 1.5% for PGD. The author assumes that these numbers cover 55% of the total of cycles performed in Spain and concludes that the true number of cycles for non-residents is between 5,000 and 10,000. Additionally, Hernandez and de la Fuente (2010) indicate that 7,985 oocyte donation cycles were performed in Spain in 2007, out of a total of 13,028 cycles reported in Europe. If these numbers are accurate, they show that currently Spain conducts 61.3% of all Europe's oocyte donations, earning its reputation as Europe's 'hub' of egg donation.

We also know that Belgium received more than two thousand foreign patients for fertility treatment in 2007 (Pennings *et al.*, 2009). Although there was a considerable increase in the number of foreign patients between 2003 and 2006, numbers seem to have stabilized more recently. CBRC patients coming to Belgium originate primarily from four countries: France (38%), the Netherlands (29%), Italy (12%) and Germany (10%). Apart from Italy, these are all countries bordering Belgium. This study also demonstrated that many patients cross borders because of specific legal restrictions in their home country, and treatments sought differed markedly according to the nationality of the patient. The overwhelming majority of French patients were lesbian couples and single women looking for donor sperm treatments, since it is only heterosexual couples who have access to ARTs in France. On the other hand, many patients from the Netherlands requested intracytoplasmic sperm injection (ICSI) with non-ejaculated sperm, because the use of non-ejaculated sperm was prohibited there until 2007. The study also showed a direct influence between legislation changes and the increase of patients seeking CBRC from specific countries. For example, when the famous Law 40 was adopted in Italy in 2004, imposing all kinds of restrictions on the practice of assisted reproduction, it lead to a tremendous increase in the number of patients from Italy, also for ICSI and IVF. A second illustration is the Dutch law of 2004 on donor data that abolished gamete donor anonymity and that lead to double the number of Dutch patients seeking donor insemination in Belgium in one year.

However, in contrast to the data from Belgium and to the ESHRE study discussed above, both of which highlight legal restrictions as a major driver for CBRC, newly emerging findings from a qualitative UK-based study suggest that 'legal restrictions on forms of treatment or restrictions on categories of people who may access treatment are not major motivating factors for [UK] patients seeking treatment overseas' (Culley *et al.*, 2010). Instead the data from this study, investigating the motivations, understandings and experiences of forty-one patients who had engaged in CBRC and seven who were contemplating it, suggest that it is the shortage of egg donors, the perceived waiting times for treatment and the issues of high treatment costs that are the reasons for UK patients to resort to CBRC. These findings are clearly related to the liberal regulatory framework in the UK (which minimizes the need for patients to avoid strict legal restrictions) and, as the authors advise, they emphasize the need to keep in mind the highly variable national differences in the social and legal context of fertility treatment. In sum, although incomplete, these studies provide some sense of CBRC in Europe.

Our knowledge of CBRC in the rest of the world is even less developed. A recent study by the International Committee Monitoring Assisted Reproductive Technologies (ICMART) provides some estimates of incoming patients from 15 and outgoing patients from 11 of the 49 countries contacted – including Egypt, India and Japan in addition to several European countries and countries from Latin America (Nygren *et al.*, 2010). While this study highlights the global prevalence of CBRC, it also underlines the extreme difficulties of collecting retrospective data about this phenomenon and the need for further investigation. With regard to North America, we can refer to a survey study reporting responses from 28 Canadian clinics and 125 clinics registered by the Society of Assisted Reproductive Technologies (SART), a subsociety of the American Society for Reproductive Medicine (ASRM) (Hughes and DeJean, 2010). According to this study, the great majority of Canadians accessing ART services outside of Canada were seeking anonymous donor eggs in the USA, whereas the majority of US residents going abroad were seeking standard IVF (presumably at a lower cost) in India/Asia, Europe or Latin America. Although very little is known about the experiences of patients and providers of CBRC in other contexts at the present time, we are hopeful that various ongoing studies of CBRC by anthropologists and social scientists from a variety of global locations, such as Inhorn's investigation of transnational reproduction in the United Arab Emirates, will provide important and informative data in the near future (Inhorn and Shrivastav, 2010).

Gametes in motion

As mentioned earlier, transnational donation and CBRC need not always imply the movement of patients; it is also possible to transport eggs, sperm and embryos across national borders. In fact, of all types of transnational reproductive movements, the import and export of sperm is currently the most prolific and important (Pennings, 2010). Cryos, the world's largest sperm bank, has been instrumental in over 14,000 full-term pregnancies since 1991, and reportedly exports 85% of its 15,000–20,000 sperm donations to more than 400 clinics in 60 countries across the globe (Anonymous, 2009). The destinations of Cryos sperm include locations as culturally and geographically distant as Paraguay, Canada, Kenya and Hong Kong (Norden Report, 2006). Moreover, since 2009 Cryos has enabled international 'private customers' to purchase sperm directly from its website. Here, customers can find a choice of anonymous and non-anonymous donors, and browse profiles detailing the donor's appearance, educational achievements, interests, family history and personality, as well as baby photographs and 'staff impressions'. In addition to the original offices in Denmark, Cryos has recently opened franchises in New York and Bombay, and plans to open further franchises across Europe, Asia, Africa and Australia over the next five years. Their goal is not only to attract a greater diversity of donors, but also thereby to expand their share of the international donor sperm market.

The international transport of gametes can also be used by clinics to attract customers in a highly competitive market, with the promise of a 'simpler' cycle, with less effort required from intending parents. An example of this can be found in the activities of an Irish clinic, which is solving the shortage of donor eggs by appealing to donors from Ukraine and making use of international gamete transportation (Walsh et al., 2010). The programme is quite straightforward: frozen sperm from the male partner is shipped to Ukraine, the donor eggs are fertilized there and the embryos are returned to the Irish clinic to be transferred to the intentional mother. Thus, while their gametes traverse the globe, both the donor and the intending parents have been saved the stress, hassle and cost of international travel. This could be seen as a direct alternative to programmes that entice patients to travel to Ukraine in order to receive donor eggs, and moreover it could be argued that this method has several advantages.

First, it is a more patient-friendly procedure. Second, donor gamete screening is carried out according to the EU Tissues and Cells Directive and is thus similar to screening within Europe. Third, the data provided by this clinic generates a certain degree of confidence in the screening process, since it shows that of the 5,524 women who expressed an interest in becoming an egg donor, only 289 entered the programme after counselling (5.2% accession rate), and neither adverse effects nor complications were reported for any donors. In this instance then, moving gametes may be preferable to the travel of intending parents; yet some may argue that the international import/export of gametes also facilitates a degree of commercialism and convenience that seems to be at odds with the underlying quest to become a parent. The Indian Rotunda IVF clinic's 'CryoShip TM Global Service' for the embryos and gametes of 'intending surrogacy parents who are not keen on a long trip [to India] required for surrogacy' may be seen as an example of the latter (Rotunda, 2010).

The standards and protocols of gamete procurement, transport and use outlined in the European Union Tissues and Cells Directive (2004) have, to a certain extent, simplified the import and export of gametes across national borders, since the same standards apply to all countries within the European Economic Area. However, specific conditions for gamete donation clearly vary between nations and this may cause complexities and dilemmas regarding the movement of gametes, particularly with regard to the remuneration and anonymity of donors. The important question to bear in mind is whether clinics that import gametes donated in other countries are colluding in practices of donor recruitment that are considered unethical and prohibited in their own jurisdictions. Countries wishing to avoid such accusations may choose to define certain parameters regarding which kinds of gametes may be imported by enacting additional national laws and regulations. For example, the UK, the Netherlands and Austria have all banned the import of anonymous sperm, thus ensuring that donor sperm contravening domestic rules of donation (i.e. identifiable donors) cannot be used within their jurisdictions (Pennings, 2010).

Moreover, in addition to rules on import, some countries also state provisions for the use of gametes that are exported. For example, the UK's Human Fertilisation and Embryology Authority advises that '[t]he sperm, eggs or embryos must not be transferred if they could not lawfully be used in licensed treatment services in the UK in the manner or circumstances in which it is proposed that the sperm, eggs or embryos be used by the receiving centre' (Human Fertilisation Embryology Act 1990 as amended 2008, Section 24, items 3–4), thus requiring that any gametes or embryos exported out of the country must nevertheless be used in ways that are commensurate with UK regulation (HFEA, 2010). Such export restrictions could also generate multiple hurdles for the growing business of moving gametes across international borders.

The regulation of CBRC

The existence and growth of CBRC is often regarded as 'a problem' which poses a range of regulatory dilemmas for states. Although as discussed with reference to the available empirical data, CBRC is not always motivated by restrictive legislation, circumstances pertaining directly or indirectly to the regulation of ARTs in the home country play a large role in feeding the traffic for transnational donation. Thus, in addition to the practical questions surrounding CBRC, such as how many patients are going abroad, where they are going and what effect this extra-territorial treatment will have on the national health system (e.g. McKelvey et al., 2009), states (or at least those that consider CBRC a problem) are also required to engage with the ethical and regulatory implications of transnational reproduction. Concerns voiced might include the extent to which it is fair for some citizens to be able to 'buy their way out' of the moral choices given legislative force in their states (Hervey, 1998), the extent to which CBRC will result in the exploitation of 'foreign women's reproductive capacities as a service' (Taylor, 2009) and the appropriate balance to strike between the moral views of the majority and the rights and freedoms of the individual (Blyth and Farrand, 2005). While responses to such deliberations will likely determine the manner in which particular states respond to CBRC, here we will discuss three possible options: coercing conformity from their citizens; seeking international harmonization; and exercising moral pluralism (Pennings, 2002).

Coerced conformity

In the absence of international harmonization, states that are particularly troubled by CBRC and the possibilities it affords may choose to adopt policies that seek to coerce their citizens into conforming to their ART legislation. There are several ways in which they might do this: they could attempt to restrict the freedom of movement of their citizens; they could introduce control and criminal charges for patients engaging in CBRC, or for practitioners and organizations that facilitate such movements; or they could request the collaboration and assistance of potential CBRC destinations. However, there are serious – ethical and practical – problems with each of these potential approaches.

First, without even getting into the moral problematic, it should be stated that it would be practically unfeasible to restrict the movement of citizens travelling for CBRC, since in a globalized world where many people engage in international travel on an annual basis, it would be impossible to know for certain who is planning to have infertility treatment. Not only are such motivations private, but they are also easily hidden. This is already the case when patients leave jurisdictions in which donor gametes are forbidden and highly stigmatized in order to secretly access such treatments (Inhorn and Shrivastav, 2010). Unlike the cases pertaining to restricting the travel of women wanting to access abortion services (Pennings, 2002), infertile couples or women wanting to access ARTs do not (necessarily) have physiologically determinable characteristics (i.e. pregnancy) that would 'give away' their reasons for wanting to travel. Moreover, within Europe the free movement of services is guaranteed by Articles 59 and 60 of the European Community treaty and it would be an infringement of the rights of persons to deny them the ability to travel to receive the services they desire (Pennings, 2002).

Turkey recently became the first country to regulate against CBRC for donor gametes as it made several significant amendments to its ART regulation. According to Articles 18.6 and 18.7 in the new regulation, it is forbidden to refer patients abroad for donor treatments, and in the event of a discovery, at any point, of such prohibited activities, 'the person who has conducted this procedure, the persons who have referred patients or acted as an intermediary, the impregnated person, and the donor' will be reported to the state prosecutor. Turkish clinics engaged in providing or facilitating CBRC with donor gametes will be closed down for three months in the first instance, and indefinitely on subsequent instances, with all involved professionals having their practice certificates nullified. These strict prohibitions against CBRC involving donor gametes have been justified with reference to (the existing) item 231 of the Turkish Penal Code, according to which it is illegal to 'change or obscure a child's ancestry', with a punishment of one to three years' imprisonment. According to Irfan Şencan, the director of the Ministry of Health's Treatment Services department, the new ban on reproductive travel was added in response to the growth of this phenomenon in recent years: 'It is a way of breaking Turkish law abroad', he argued (Gürtin-Broadbent, 2010). However, it can be proposed that, rather than eliminating transnational donation, this legislation will only result in exacerbating the difficulties faced by infertile couples and women wishing to access donor treatments, by forcing them to partake in reproductive travel without the collaboration of their practitioners.

Trying to enlist the help of potential CBRC destinations is also a difficult proposal. Although such nations could be asked to enforce a citizenship or permanent residency requirement in order to treat patients (simply to curtail reproductive travellers), this places a considerable regulatory burden on them. It is not up to a CRBC destination to impose moral rules that differ from its own, simply in order to assist another jurisdiction to regulate its citizens. Moreover, there are significant financial advantages to being a CBRC-provider nation, so potential destinations are unlikely – on an economic basis – to deter their international 'customers'.

International harmonization

Harmonization in this context refers to the effort to gain international consensus among different jurisdictions on the regulation of ART practices, including what treatments are practised; to whom and under what conditions they are available; and the financial costs of infertility treatments.

There is some reason to believe that harmonization can be successfully achieved within a limited geographical location, an example of which may be the situation in Nordic countries. Cohen writes:

Ten years ago, oocyte freezing was allowed in Denmark and Sweden but not in Norway. Oocyte donation was forbidden in Norway and Sweden but allowed in Denmark. Norwegian couples were seeking microinsemination in Denmark and Sweden because of a ban on the method in their country. There is now harmonization of the laws: since 2003 sperm donation in connection with IVF and oocyte donation are permitted in all three countries. Reproductive tourism seems to have stopped (Cohen, 2006: 146).

This case represents a small victory for harmonization over reproductive travel (if you wish to characterize it as this), but it was effective over a small, and culturally similar, area in which each country decided to permit those ARTs that were available in their neighbours. Nevertheless, other differences remain. Denmark, contrary to the two other countries, still maintains donor anonymity.

Harmonization on a larger scale does not seem to be possible, precisely because even within Europe there are great differences between the moral codes and regulatory frameworks that govern the practice of assisted reproduction (see Gürtin and Vayena, Chapter 5). Thus far, rather than regulatory harmonization, what has been pursued within Europe is agreement on certain basic principles that can act as a 'lowest common denominator'. Once broad principles are agreed upon, Member States have remained largely free to interpret and translate them into application. For example, even though the EU Tissues and Cells Directive (2004), Article 12(1) provides that 'Donors may receive compensation which is strictly limited to making good the expenses and inconveniences related to the donation', those countries that have ratified the Directive can nevertheless define for themselves the conditions and amount of such compensation. As a result, compensation or reimbursement for a cycle of egg donation is €1000 (about £890) in Spain, and £250 (about €300) in the United Kingdom.

The main problem associated with aiming for harmonization is that each country regards its own legislation as correct and would therefore like others to follow its example without changing its own structures. Furthermore, it is unclear whether harmonization should be attempted in the direction of greater permissiveness (i.e. anything that is allowed by one country will be allowed by all) or in the direction of greater prohibition (i.e. anything that is prohibited by one country will be prohibited by all). While the former has been characterized as a 'slippery slope' scenario towards complete deregulation (Millns, 2002), the latter has the risk of becoming entirely draconian. Moreover, unless it is universally agreed, harmonization towards greater prohibition may in fact do little other than incite travel to even further locations (outside the zone of harmonization). In short, it can be argued that harmonization, even within Europe, is an impractical and unfeasible option.

Moral pluralism

The final regulatory option that states might consider is to enact moral pluralism regarding citizens that seek locally prohibited ART services in other jurisdictions. This requires states to accept CBRC as the result of a (reasonable) difference of opinions and perhaps even to view it as a pragmatic solution: 'a safety valve that reduces moral conflict and expresses minimal recognition of the others' moral autonomy' (Pennings, 2004: 2689). States could adopt the stance that although they prohibit certain ARTs, they recognize it as the right of those who have a different moral assessment to pursue such treatments in other locations, and display tolerance to enactments of 'moral pluralism in motion' (Pennings, 2002). Such an approach will not only enable intending parents – or moral dissenters – to pursue the treatments they desire without undue coercion, but also reduce internal pressure for regulatory change or confrontations that can arise as a result of such moral differences. Instead of spending energy trying to minimize or put a stop to 'reproductive tourism' – a case of either locking the stable door after the horse has bolted or a demonstration of draconian intolerance – states may fare a great deal better by concentrating their efforts on defining procedural and practical steps to enable their citizens to engage in CBRC in the safest and most ethical way possible.

Of course, if CBRC is assessed to be unduly dangerous or unethical, states may wish as far as possible to regulate their citizens' involvement in such activities, rather than tolerating moral pluralism or reproductive travellers. In the next section we analyse the arguments that have been put forward regarding the potential dangers of CBRC to safety, autonomy and justice, and assess the extent to which these perceived risks are accurate and whether they could be a justification to curtail reproductive travel.

The dangers of CBRC

Since the start of the discussion on CBRC, there have been many warnings regarding the potential dangers of such practices for health care systems, clinics and especially for patients and donors. Such concerns were not without reason. For example, in 2005 serious shortcomings were demonstrated in Romanian clinics, in which oocyte donors had not given their informed consent; had inadequate information regarding the possible health risks of the procedure; and had not received follow-up care when complications resulted (Magureanu, 2005). Such practices are undoubtedly related to increased commercialization and the desire by some in the field of ARTs to make a lot of money. However, although exacerbated by the potential of an international market, such dangers for the welfare of donors are the result of poor national regulations or surveillance services, rather than of CBRC per se.

Several societies have also issued statements to warn patients against the dangers of infertility treatment outside their home countries. Among these are the ESHRE Ethics and Law Task Force, the Human Fertilisation and Embryology Authority (HFEA), the Donor Conception Network, the International Federation of Gynecology and Obstetrics (FIGO) and Infertility Consumer Support for Infertility (iCSi). Analysis of these statements shows that the main concerns regard the violation of safety and quality standards; financial implications; confidentiality of patient information; the lack or insufficiency of counselling; legal conflicts; professional responsibilities;

donor anonymity; and justice. Some propose that patients should be provided with a list of questions or items to raise when approaching or screening foreign clinics. However, a major shortcoming of these patient checklists is that they only contain questions, rather than answers. Besides the obvious problem that clinics may give false or incomplete answers, there is also the problem that patients may not have the resources necessary to collate sufficient information, or will not always know how to evaluate or interpret the information they have gathered.

Safety

The main medical dangers associated with bad practice in ARTs is ovarian hyperstimulation syndrome (OHSS) and multiple pregnancies. Both are frequently mentioned as having increased in the context of CBRC. There is some evidence that higher numbers of embryos are replaced in foreign patients, for example in Belgium (Pennings *et al.*, 2009). However, this finding has to be interpreted with caution since it may be partially explained by the fact that a larger proportion of foreign patients have already undergone several cycles of unsuccessful treatment at home and are on average older than the Belgian patients. Another study suggested that overseas treatments were responsible for a large proportion of high order multiple pregnancies encountered in the UK (McKelvey *et al.*, 2009). However, it is again of note that this study only showed that patients receiving treatment overseas were significantly less likely to have embryo reduction, and not that more embryos were transferred to them.

Arguments against CBRC based on fears to safety are a double-edged sword, since if examined rationally, they suggest not that patients should not travel, but only that they should not travel from more safe to less safe nations in order to receive infertility treatments. For countries that still have (very) high multiple pregnancy rates (such as Russia, Ukraine and the United Kingdom), an argument based on safety should actually encourage them to travel to destinations (such as Sweden and Belgium) that have much lower levels of multiple pregnancies and associated risks in ARTs (de Mouzon *et al.*, 2010). If we base arguments solely on safety concerns, then we would need to promote the travel of patients whose care abroad would be safer than in their own countries. Thus, safety concerns, although clearly relevant to the assessment of potential CBRC destinations, does not in itself provide a sound argument against infertility treatment across national borders.

Autonomy

There is an important concern regarding the impact of CBRC on the patient's autonomy. Autonomy refers to the right of the patient to decide about their own medical treatment on the basis of their own life plans and values. Threats to autonomy may be related to whether there is provision of counselling: the ability of smooth communication between providers and patients; the uses of the Internet; and the procedures of referral.

Adequate counselling is key to ensuring the informed consent and autonomy of patients receiving ARTs. Within the context of medically assisted reproduction, information and counselling should be provided on potential complications, multiple pregnancies, success rates and future consequences of the treatment. Specifically for treatment involving donor gametes, it is essential to provide counselling about the potential ethical, psychological and legal implications.

Why would there be less or less good counselling for foreign patients? The two most likely reasons would be communication problems (language but also general cultural aspects) and commercialization. Counselling patients in another language than one's mother tongue always adds new difficulties. One may appeal to the services of an interpreter, but most psychologists are not particularly happy with this solution. Interpreters can function as an additional step causing loss of meaning (lost in translation), particularly when discussing highly personal and sensitive topics related to self-esteem, family-building, sexuality and emotions. There may also be culturally sensitive issues that are unknown to the counsellor in the foreign clinic.

Regarding commercialization, the concern is that clinics with a clear for-profit motive will skip aspects of infertility treatment that they consider as secondary and non-essential (i.e. non-medical and non-technical aspects without a direct bearing on success rates) as a means to reduce costs, and thus counselling services would suffer. However, although one may expect some differences between private and public clinics, all clinics – and private clinics even more so – have an interest in offering a good service in a highly competitive market (Castilla *et al.*, 2009). Thus, money and the desire to attract customers may also be a good motivator to abide by the rules of good patient care. Indeed, many clinics advertise their conformity to clinical guidelines and the European Tissues and Cells Directive, as well as stringent donor recruitment procedures, prominently on their websites to gain the trust of potential customers. Moreover, since different countries and clinics within Europe have different standards for counselling, it is once again possible for some patients to receive a much better service outside their home countries.

Another potential cause for concern regarding autonomy is the fact that most patients choose their clinic through the Internet. There are very few studies on the quality and reliability of information on clinic websites and on the influence of the Internet on the ART market. However, these are clearly very important intermediary structures that connect consumers and providers, especially across national borders. Frequently raised issues are that success rates are exaggerated; potential risks are downplayed; and subtle commercial strategies are used to entice potential patients. Although to date there have been no scientific studies specifically on the use of such websites in CBRC, we know that the majority of ART patients use the Internet as their main source of information (Blyth, 2010). The ESHRE study also demonstrated that there are large international differences in source selection, with Swedish, German and British patients using the Internet most, while Italian patients relied most often on their local doctors, using the Internet in only 25 per cent of cases (Shenfield *et al.*, 2010). Although it has never been proven, the underlying assumption seems to be that the Internet is the least reliable source of information. At first sight, the solution is relatively easy: doctors and patient organizations (which are almost invisible in the total picture at the moment) should play a greater role. However, this solution is riddled with all kinds of problems (Pennings *et al.*, 2008). For example, there may be legal restrictions that do not allow doctors to refer patients for treatments forbidden in their home country (Gürtin-Broadbent, 2010) or local doctors may simply not be familiar with the international situation, or they may be ignorant about the quality of foreign clinics. The responsibility of the referring physician would depend on the type of referral. If (s)he refers to a specific clinic, (s)he should be aware of the general quality of the treatment provided in that clinic. The actual treatment of the patient, however, remains the responsibility of the treating doctor. When the doctor refers to another country, simply on his or her knowledge of the legality of the treatment, (s)he cannot be held accountable when things go wrong.

CBRC enables patients in restrictive countries to realize their life plans abroad. To that extent, it can only be seen as positive. Also regarding the practical conditions to guarantee patient autonomy when they decide to go abroad, the concerns that are raised seem to be largely unfounded. Obviously, more empirical data on patients' experiences are needed, but, at least for the moment, there is no hard evidence that counselling, information provision and referral are insufficient.

Justice

Since the start of the discussion, issues around justice have been used to argue against CBRC, on the grounds that only the rich can afford to travel. There are several reasons that support this view: first, travelling brings extra costs (such as hotels, fees and plane tickets); second, patients leaving their country normally also forsake the chance of reimbursement from the social security system; and third, treatment to foreign patients is almost always provided by profit-based private clinics. However, although these factors might be true, it is also paradoxically the case that some patients resort to CBRC for financial reasons, and are able to access treatment at a cheaper price abroad than they can in their home countries. In assessing arguments regarding justice, such patients travelling for cheaper treatments should be distinguished from patients with other types of motivations (such as law evasion or avoiding waiting lists).

It is also important to bear in mind that justice has two dimensions: access and equality. Just access to treatment dictates that no one should be denied access without a good reason. If reproduction is considered as a basic need, we can argue that financial means (or lack thereof) should not determine a person's ability to access infertility treatment. This suggests that if people who live in a country with little reimbursement from either public or private health insurance cannot afford to pay for treatment in their own country, they should then be able to travel freely to other locations where they may be able to afford treatment. Such a scenario clearly applies to many American CBRC patients (de Brito and Kaycoff, 2010). In these cases, it can be argued that CBRC improves access, and consequently leads to greater justice.

However, those pursuing a justice argument tend to focus more on equality than on access. Equality can be improved in two ways: either by making sure that no one has access or that everyone has access to treatment. The remarkable point about this argument, and also its greatest weakness, is that in a situation of inequality where full coverage is not possible, justice can only be obtained by denying treatment to everyone. However, if infertility is recognized as a disease, as it was by the World Health Organization and the ICMART glossary on assisted reproduction (Zegers-Hochschild *et al.*, 2009), then its treatment should be considered a basic need, and thus such a position becomes untenable.

When one considers the second group of patients who leave the country for other reasons than finances, we get a completely different situation. Some people feel that these patients are 'buying their way out' of the regulations in force in their home countries, because by paying to travel they circumvent laws while poorer people are denied such choices (Hervey, 1998). Two points should be made here. First, this argument gives a strong impression of 'blaming the victim': patients who are excluded from receiving treatment at home (either because of personal characteristics such as age or sexual orientation, or because the treatment in question is prohibited) are forced to travel in search of treatment as 'reproductive exiles' (Inhorn and Patrizio, 2009). If one gives priority to personal autonomy above societal rights, they do nothing wrong. If they have been unjustly excluded from treatment, their movement to access treatment elsewhere simply corrects the situation. Second, one should avoid a morality of envy, which dictates that 'if I cannot have it, then nobody should'. Even though poor people might not have the means to escape their domestic restrictions, that does not make it wrong for more fortunate individuals to make the most of their resources.

Conclusion

Many misunderstandings are generated by the fact that CBRC is still considered as a monolith, organized by the same rules, triggered by the same causes and resulting in the same outcomes. Empirical evidence to date has demolished this picture, revealing instead many trajectories of CBRC with different reasons and under diverse conditions. Travelling across borders does not necessarily (or even frequently) lead to lower safety standards, nor does it automatically correspond to worse counselling or insufficient patient information, to higher multiple pregnancy rates or to the exploitation of unethically recruited donors. CBRC defines not one phenomenon, but a range of heterogeneous activities, the practical and ethical details of which depend to a great extent on the origin, destination and reasons for travelling of the various components. Here we have conceptualized 'transnational donation' as a subset of CBRC practices, have evaluated the available empirical data on the movements of intending parents and gametes, considered the regulatory options of jurisdictions and assessed the potential dangers associated with such reproductive travel. Since it is unrealistic to aim for its elimination, or to ignore its existence, we believe that the best response to transnational donation would be better international recognition; greater attention to practical and ethical considerations to improve the conditions of its practice; and improved provision of information for potential patients.

REFERENCES

Anonymous (2009). 'Business booms at world's biggest sperm bank'. Available at: www.google.com/hostednews/afp/article/ALeqM5hBNU1WQrNjmPogMWhQc1XYQly65Q.

Blyth, E. (2010). 'Fertility patients' experiences of cross-border reproductive care'. *Fertility and Sterility*, 94, 11–5.

Blyth, E. and Farrand, A. (2005). 'Reproductive tourism – a price worth paying for reproductive autonomy?' *Critical Social Policy*, 25, 91–114.

Carbone, J. and Gottheim, P. (2006). 'Markets, subsidies, regulation, and trust: building ethical understandings into the market for infertility services'. *Journal of Gender, Race and Justice*, 9, 509–47.

Castilla, J. A., Hernandez, E., Caballo, Y., Navarro, J. L., *et al.* (2009). 'Assisted reproductive technologies in public and private clinics'. *Reproductive BioMedicine Online*, 19, 872–8.

Cohen, J. (2006). 'Procreative tourism and reproductive freedom'. *Reproductive BioMedicine Online*, 13, 145–6.

Culley, L., Hudson, N., Blyth, E., Norton, W., *et al.* (2010). 'Travelling abroad for fertility treatment: an exploratory study of UK residents seeking cross-border care'. *Human Reproduction*, 25 suppl. 1: i78.

de Brito, L. and Kaycoff, K. K. (2010). 'Decision-making factors that influence U.S. patients in selecting overseas egg donor programs and how clinics can appeal to those potential patients'. *Human Reproduction*, 25, suppl. 1: i153–4.

de Mouzon, J., Goossens, V., Battacharya, S., Castilla, J. A., Ferraretti, A. P., Korsak, V., Kupka, M., Nygren, K. G., Nyboe Andersen, A. and The European IVF-monitoring Consortium, for the European Society of Human Reproduction and Embryology (2010). 'Assisted reproductive technology in Europe, 2006: results generated from European registers by ESHRE'. *Human Reproduction*, 25(8): 1851–62.

de la Fuente, L. A. (2010). 'Cross border reproductive care in Spain'. Presentation at the ESHRE meeting 'Cross border reproductive care', 14 May 2010, Paris.

Gürtin-Broadbent, Z. (2010). 'Problems with legislating against "reproductive tourism"'. *BioNews*, 550.

Hernandez, J. and de la Fuente, L. A (2010). 'Spanish views: facts/concerns'. Presentation at the ESHRE meeting 'Cross border reproductive care', 14 May 2010, Paris.

Hervey, T. K. (1998). 'Buy baby: the European Union and regulation of human reproduction'. *Oxford Journal of Legal Studies*, 8, 207–33.

Hughes, E. J. and DeJean, D. (2010). 'Cross-border fertility services in North America: a survey of Canadian and American providers'. *Fertility and Sterility*, 94, e16–9.

Human Fertilisation and Embryology Authority (HFEA) (2010). 'FAQs about transferring, importing and exporting from abroad'. Available at: www.hfea.gov.uk/patient-questions-importing.html (accessed July 2010).

Inhorn, M. C. and Patrizio, P. (2009). 'Rethinking reproductive "tourism" as reproductive "exile"'. *Fertility and Sterility*, 92, 904–6.

Inhorn, M. C. and Shrivastav, P. (2010). 'Globalization and reproductive tourism in the United Arab Emirates'. *Asia-Pacific Journal of Public Health*, 22, suppl., 68S–74S.

Magureanu, G. (2005). 'Egg donation and conflict within the Romanian legal framework'. Paper presented at CORE European seminar: Human egg trading and the exploitation of women. Brussels, European Parliament, 30 June 2005. Available at: www.handsoffourovaries.com/pdfs/appendixg. pdf.

McKelvey, A., David, A. L., Shenfield, F. and Jauniaux, E. R. (2009). 'The impact of cross-border reproductive care or fertility tourism on NHS maternity services'. *British Journal of Obstetrics and Gynaecology*, 116, 1520–3.

Millns, S. (2002). 'Reproducing inequalities: assisted conception and the challenge of legal pluralism'. *Journal of Social Welfare and Family Law*, 24, 19–36.

Norden Report (2006). *Assisted Reproduction in the Nordic Countries. A Comparative Study of Policies and Regulation*. Available at: www.norden. org/en/publications/publications/2006–505 (accessed July 2010).

Nygren, K., Adamson, D., Zegers-Hochschild, F. and de Mouzon, J. (2010). 'Cross-border fertility care—International Committee Monitoring Assisted Reproductive Technologies global survey: 2006 data and estimates'. *Fertility and Sterility*, 94, e4–e10.

Pennings, G. (2002). 'Reproductive tourism as moral pluralism in motion'. *Journal of Medical Ethics*, 28, 337–41.

   (2004). 'Legal harmonization and reproductive tourism in Europe'. *Human Reproduction*, 19, 2689–94.

   (2010). 'The rough guide to insemination: cross-border travelling for donor semen due to different regulations'. *Facts, Views and Vision in OBGYN*. Monograph, 55–60.

Pennings, G., de Wert, G., Shenfield, F., Cohen, J., et al. (2008). 'ESHRE Task Force on Ethics and Law 15: Cross-border reproductive care'. *Human Reproduction*, 23, 2182–4.

Pennings, G., Autin, C., Decleer, W., Delbaere, A., et al. (2009). 'Cross-border reproductive care in Belgium'. *Human Reproduction*, 24, 3108–18.

Rotunda – The Centre for Human Reproduction website – www.iwannaget-pregnant.com/ (accessed July 2010).

Shenfield, F., De Mouzon, J., Pennings, G., Ferraretti, A-P., et al. (2010). 'ESHRE Taskforce on Cross Border Reproductive Care, Cross border reproductive care in six European countries'. *Human Reproduction*, 25, 1361–8.

Taylor, A. (2009). 'Experts attack "fertility tourism" industry'. *Bionews*, 526.

Walsh, A. P. H., Shkrobot, L. V., Omar, A. B., Walsh, D. J., et al. (2010). 'EU screening applied to anonymous oocyte donors from Ukraine: logistics, results and reproductive outcomes from an Irish IVF programme'. *Human Reproduction*, 25, suppl. 1, i154.

Zegers-Hochschild, F., Adamson, G. D., de Mouzon, J., Isihara, O. et al.(2009). 'The International Committee for Monitoring Assisted Reproductive

Technology (ICMART) and the World Health Organization (WHO) Revised Glossary on ART Terminology'. *Human Reproduction*, 24, 2683–7.

LEGISLATION

EUROPE

Directive 2004/23/EC of the European Parliament and of the Council of 31 March 2004 on setting standards of quality and safety for the donation, procurement, testing, processing, preservation, storage and distribution of human tissues and cells. *Official Journal of the European Union* L 102: 48–58

UK

Human Fertilisation Embryology Act 1990, as amended 2008

9   Balancing ethical criteria for the recruitment of gamete donors

Guido Pennings, Effy Vayena and Kamal Ahuja

Introduction

Patients and clinics are constantly searching for donors. The increasing gap between supply and demand in most countries shows beyond doubt that the current systems are unable to attract a sufficient number of donors. The first suggestion for a solution is always the same: let's pay. However, payment for body material is, at least in Europe, generally rejected on ethical grounds. Several alternative modes of compensation are currently applied. Still, the efforts made by clinics and/or governments to increase the donor pool are fairly limited. In order to curb commercialization, a number of countries do not allow clinics to take their own initiatives to attract donors. This entails that the task lies completely with the government. However, compared to the campaigns for blood and organs, governments show very little interest in organizing widespread awareness campaigns for gamete donation. Moreover, the rare campaigns that are set up are so little advertised that they might as well not be done. Only seldom are special organizations (such as the National Gamete Donation Trust in the UK) set up to alleviate the shortage of gamete donors. The most likely explanation for this reticence is that most governments and responsible institutions are not convinced of the moral status of the procedure and as a consequence do not want to associate themselves with this topic.

The practice of gamete donation is a complex system in which multiple ethical rules, legal restrictions and medical facts intermingle. Things are further complicated by the fact that there are many different types of donors. The different categories are based on dimensions with ethical, social and psychological consequences: gamete type (oocyte and sperm donors), anonymity (known, identifiable and anonymous donors) and remuneration (volunteer, commercial and patient donors) (Purewal and van den Akker, 2009). Given space restrictions, we will focus on the major findings and trends.

150

Anonymity

In the last decade, several European countries have adopted legislation to impose gamete donor identifiability (Blyth and Frith, 2009). Many people in countries where identifiability is the legal rule blame the abolishment of anonymity for the current shortage of gamete donors. Anonymity as a rule plays a different role in donor recruitment than payment: it does not attract donors but facilitates their recruitment. Many practitioners believe that the abundance of sperm donors in Denmark and egg donors in Spain is only possible because of the anonymity there. In countries where anonymity was abandoned (e.g. Sweden, the United Kingdom, the Netherlands), there has been a sharp drop in the number of donors (at least initially). It would have been surprising if this had not been the case. A certain type of donor is recruited through the rules, mainly regarding payment and anonymity. When these rules change, the donor population will also change (Pennings, 2005a). It was perfectly predictable that when existing donors were asked whether they would still donate if the anonymity rule were abandoned, the majority (but notably less in Australia and New Zealand) said they would cease to donate (Daniels, 2007). A new rule means that a new population should be addressed in the campaigns so that new donors who agree with these rules can be attracted.

Many people have a rather simplistic view of the gamete donation practice. They believe that one can alter one rule and leave the rest as they are. The rules, however, can best be compared with Mikado pick-up sticks: peripheral rules can be changed relatively easily, but central rules, such as anonymity and payment, will almost inevitably bring about and require other additional changes (Pennings, 2010). So, in summary, the abolishment of anonymity has had the expected negative effect on the number of donors in the countries that originally respected anonymity. But newly adapted (and most likely expensive) campaigns are able to regain the same level of donation that existed during the pre-identifiability period, as was demonstrated in the UK (Blyth and Frith, 2008; Pacey, 2010). Still, reaching the pre-identifiability level may not be sufficient to cover the demand since a peripheral rule connected to the altered anonymity rule may have a highly limiting effect on the use of the donor gametes. This peripheral rule is the possibility for the donor to set upper limits on the number of children born from their donation, an option that does not exist in systems that work with anonymous donors.

Anonymity in essence regulates the interaction between donor and recipients. Its most important consequence is that it closes the relationship completely: after the donation, no party can contact another party. This is an aspect that can be very highly appreciated both by the donor and by the recipients. Anonymity prevents all kinds of possible complications and conflicts regarding rights, duties and so on in the future. If this closure is a precondition for a candidate donor to donate, then abolishing this rule will reduce the number of donors. This cannot be the end of the argument, though, since donors may request all kinds of things. Society's attitude towards donation of body material is not solely focused on attracting the highest number of donors: society wants to recruit the highest number of donors while respecting a number of ethical rules. Every rule excludes a number of donors but that in itself is not a sufficient reason to abandon the rule. A country that believes that a child has a right to know its genetic origin, cannot reintroduce anonymity. Countries such as France that put more emphasis on social parenthood can, on the contrary, impose anonymity. Given the fact that both sides in the debate have strong arguments for their position, it seems reasonable for governments not to take sides and allow the participants to decide how they want to organize their family and what kind of relationship they want with the other persons involved. This can be done by adopting a 'double track' system (Pennings, 1997). In this system, both the donor and the recipients decide whether they want to be identifiable or anonymous. Beside the fact that this is a liberal structure that allows competent participants to decide for themselves, it does not exclude potential donors and thus promotes recruitment. In Belgium, for instance, the general rule is anonymity, but this rule can be broken when both donor and recipient(s) agree to be known to each other. Research has shown that, when given the choice, the decision on known or anonymous donation is a matter of negotiation between the parties and depends on aspects such as a genetic link with the donor and the importance of knowing the donor as a person. At the same time, both donor and recipients may feel uncomfortable with the close presence of the other (and all the possible complication this entails) and opt for the anonymous exchange (Baetens *et al.*, 2000). The double track policy represents the best attempt to balance the rights of donors and recipients. The decision about the best interests of the offspring is, like in many other instances, left to the future parents.

Payment

The question of payment for body material has been around for decades (Titmuss, 1970). Whether gamete donors should receive financial remuneration for their donation still is a major controversy in medically assisted reproduction. In the general perception, *to donate* means *to give a gift*. A great part of the controversy stems from the different views of what the 'gift' is and whether it remains a 'gift' even if a price tag is attached to it. An interesting twist in the debate is the role that remuneration can or should play in recruiting donors. Some data have shown a decrease in the number of donors when payment ceases (Anonymous, 2010). The evidence from countries (like France) that forbid all payment clearly shows, however, that people still come forward to donate even if no remuneration is offered (Guerin, 1998). Other studies have concluded that a recruitment strategy that targets the right kind of donor can successfully bypass the compensation issue (Daniels *et al.*, 2006). The core questions are whether gamete donation should be a purely altruistic act and to what extent or under what conditions financial compensation is morally acceptable. Lack of consensus on whether a donor should receive any money at all and, if yes, what this should be for (i.e. payment for a service, compensation for lost earnings or simply minimal reimbursement of costs incurred by the donor through the act of donation such as travel costs to the donation site, etc.) is evident in the variety of laws and guidelines. The differences in practice are vast. In the USA donor payment is not regulated and clinics operate on a free market model. Egg donors in particular may receive huge amounts of money. A recent study of recruitment advertisements for oocyte donors in US college newspapers reported fees up to US$50,000 (Levine, 2010).

The American Society for Reproductive Medicine's (ASRM) guidelines on the issue of oocyte donation recommend financial compensation but propose that up to US$5,000 is a reasonable compensation and set a maximum upper limit of US$10,000 (Ethics Committee of the American Society for Reproductive Medicine, 2007). This sum is based on a calculation of estimated hours spent for oocyte donation multiplied by US$60–70 which is the hourly compensation for sperm donation. A survey of American clinics in 2007 showed that the average payment for oocyte donors (in clinics which are members of the Society for Assisted Reproductive Technology) did not exceed US$5,000. Semen donors are also compensated, but in most places payment is based on sample acceptability (quality and sperm count) and the amount varies between US$50 and US$100 (Almeling, 2007). The situation is distinctly different in neighbouring Canada, which forbids payment to gamete donors according to legislation passed in 2004. The law allows reimbursement of expenses for receipted expenditures, which includes for sperm donors travel expenses (such as transportation, meals and accommodation), child care costs (for attending clinic appointment), counselling services, health care services (provided and prescribed by health care providers); compensation for egg donors includes all the above and, in addition, the costs for medication.

In Europe the situation is highly variable. In contrast to the ASRM, the professional organization of European fertility specialists, the European Society for Human Reproduction and Embryology (ESHRE) views the 'direct payment for reproductive material as unethical'. It does, however, accept 'reasonable compensation for the effort of the donor' (ESHRE Task Force on Ethics and Law, 2002). A survey of European states conducted by the EU's Health and Consumer Protection Directorate General found that most states regulate non-remuneration by law in the context of preventing organ trading and trafficking as dictated by the EU Tissues and Cells Directive 2004/23/EC. However, even within these states, some allow reimbursement of expenses and others of inconveniences. The remaining states have no regulation or operate on non-binding national and international guidelines (EU Health and Consumer Protection, Directorate General, 2006). Specific amounts of payment are not commonly mentioned in the guidelines and most tend to use vague language. Nevertheless, there is general acceptance that costs incurred due to donation (i.e. travel costs and medication) should be reimbursed. However, there exists considerable disagreement on whether people should be paid for the risk they take, the inconvenience they experience and the service they provide.

These different approaches and practices have been justified by the use of arguments based either on moral principles or pragmatism and they evolve around the issue of protection of the donor, the offspring or society as a whole. In the following sections we summarize the arguments for and against payment of gamete donors.

Donors should not be paid

Article 21 of the Council of Europe's Convention for the Protection of Human Rights and Dignity of the Human Being with regard to the Application of Biology and Medicine: Convention on Human Rights and Biomedicine (1997) clearly states that 'the human body and its parts as such should not give rise to financial gain'. This is a widely accepted position and the same point appears in other regulatory documents and guidelines (Nuffield Council, 1995; Directive 2004/23/EC). The rejection of payment is based on the argument that the body and its parts should not be treated as commodities because this denies their dignity and sacred worth (Holland, 2001). Moreover, gametes with the potential to become embryos and possibly persons come even closer to the notion of selling and buying humans. The 'human dignity' argument is particularly appealing to regulators and it is widely used in ethical debates about regulating biomedicine and biotechnology (Caulfield and Brownsword, 2006). However, it remains a vague argument because there is no clear definition of human dignity and it is therefore hard to show which aspects of dignity are violated in the case of paid donors.

The argument goes on to raise the concern of exploitation. If a monetary gain can be made, people in financial need will be more tempted to sell their gametes. Depending on the price they are offered, those individuals may end up underestimating the physical and psychological risks of gamete donation (Steinbock, 2004). This argument is stronger in the case of oocyte donation as the risks associated with ovarian stimulation and oocyte retrieval are much higher than for semen donation. Financially disadvantaged individuals, such as young women, are more vulnerable and therefore more at risk of exploitation. Vulnerability, however, is a complex concept and it is difficult to define precisely all its nuances. Is an athletic, beautiful, Ivy League university student with very high SAT scores a vulnerable individual when she is offered over US$35,000 for her oocytes? Is a young, beautiful, educated Indian woman vulnerable if she is offered US$1,000 for her oocytes? It could be argued that when there is financial remuneration, the risk of exploitation increases. Whether there actually is exploitation can be determined on a case-by-case basis. Still, prohibition of payment is a relatively easy way to protect vulnerable individuals (Rao, 2006).

Payment, especially when the amount is high, may also jeopardize informed consent, which is frequently seen as a safeguard against exploitation (Nuffield Council on Bioethics, 1995). The donor in need may underestimate the risks of donation and, if operating under undue inducement, the consent is not free and voluntary as it ought to be.

Beyond the arguments that address the need to protect donors, a second set of arguments focuses on the welfare of the child. One pragmatic argument against payment raises the concern that prospective donors who donate just for money might not disclose important information about their medical history and might put potential offspring at risk (Yee, 2009). Psychological issues or abusive behaviour have been quoted as examples (Schover et al., 1992). However, standard medical and psychological screening of donors would normally suffice to avoid this problem. Another argument in this context states that children who find out that they were conceived as a result of a financial transaction might be psychologically adversely affected (Johnson, 1997). There is limited evidence to support or refute this argument but there is evidence suggesting that, in case of disclosure to the offspring, the 'gift nature' of the donation is important (Thorn, 2007).

A broader argument against payment is that it may exacerbate inequities. Those who can afford to pay for gametes will be more likely to receive treatment and to have children. This point is linked to a eugenics argument. In a free market for gametes, human traits and characteristics will be valued selectively. The price will not be compensation for the risk or the inconvenience of the donor but for the trait itself (i.e. being blond, tall or athletic) (Schonfeld, 2003). Furthermore, if people can pay more for certain genetic traits, well-off couples will be able to buy 'better' eggs and sperm, while poorer couples will be unable to select and will be consigned to fate. This argument has been fuelled by the payments that have been made for specific traits to egg donors in the USA. However, this argument does not hold for European countries where a maximum limit is imposed on the amount that can be offered to the donor. As a consequence, many poor, uneducated women present themselves as candidate donors. Moreover, most European clinics do not allow the recipients to choose their donor.

The altruism argument is further extended to the societal level. The Nuffield Council report argues for the need to encourage the 'altruistic culture' in our societies. If individuals with purely altruistic motives can be recruited for donation through recruitment strategies, there will be less need for commercial donors (Nuffield Council on Bioethics, 1995). Gamete donation should not be perceived as business. On the contrary, it should be an act of altruism within a culture that rewards altruism. This raises an interesting point that is rarely discussed, namely the amount of money that the clinic should be allowed to ask from the recipients of the donor gametes. According to the non-commercialization rule, the clinic should not charge more than the expenses they made to recruit the donors and to obtain and store the gametes. There is surprisingly little interest from regulators in this point. Furthermore, there is also the issue of how fertility treatment and reproductive medicine is perceived by the broader public. The argument here points to the 'bad image' if such services are perceived to be just big business. This reputation would erode public trust in science and medicine.

Donors should be paid

People who argue for payment of gamete donors do not necessarily argue in favour of a free market approach. On the contrary, even the proponents of payment heavily criticize the phenomena observed in the USA with special egg donors receiving large sums of money for their donations (Levine, 2010). Most people arguing in favour of paying donors call for reasonable amounts. The difficulty, however, is to determine what constitutes 'reasonable' payment and how this should be calculated.

The main argument for payment is fairness. Donors should be compensated for the risk they take, the burden of the procedures, the inconvenience, the discomfort they experience and the time they spend for the donation. This also happens for other services in our societies (Macklin, 1996). In fact, a parallel has been drawn between gamete donors and clinical trial volunteers. Payment to health volunteers in clinical trials for the temporary donation of their bodies to medical research is widely accepted (although the prices vary dramatically). If people are compensated for taking a risk and bearing the burden in that case, why not for donating their gametes? Paying reasonable fees for the service of donation would also prevent unfair differences in the compensation, such as the ones observed today where donors with certain traits end up receiving more money. The money will be paid for the service and not for the product. The American Society for Reproductive Medicine guidelines for compensation of egg donors explicitly state that 'compensation should not vary according to the planned use of the oocytes (e.g. research or clinical care), the number or quality of oocytes retrieved, the outcome of prior donation cycles, or the donor's ethnic or other personal characteristics' (Ethics Committee of the American Society for Reproductive Medicine, 2007).

Another popular and pragmatic argument for payment relates to the impact of payment on recruitment. There is a shortage of gamete donors worldwide and financial incentives will most likely increase the number of donors. Conversely, lack of financial incentives will discourage donors. Several studies have been undertaken to establish what motivates people to donate gametes and consequently what the best strategies to recruit them should look like. While it is not easy to draw a clear conclusion (even systematic reviews of such studies cite serious limitations), it is evident that there is a wide spectrum of motives (Purewal and van den Akker, 2009). Gamete donors are donating for purely altruistic reasons, for altruistic and financial or just financial reasons. Undoubtedly, financial incentives are important. Some recent studies from Canada where payment for gamete donation has been abolished pointed to a dramatic reduction in sperm donation. Of the forty sperm banks that existed in Canada, only one is still in operation (Anonymous, 2010).

In the broader context of payment for donation, an alternative approach has been proposed: the so-called 'all inclusive' model (Craft and Thornhill, 2005). In this model, payment for specific expenses, inconvenience and so on is replaced by a predetermined sum of money that covers everything. As a consequence, payment is legitimate but mixed with expenses. No exact figure is proposed and obviously, if such a model were to be adopted, it would have to be calculated based on local indexes. In theory, this transparent arrangement will deter illegal transactions and exploitation. In addition, it will reduce the administrative load that clinics face when processing receipts for reimbursement of expenses. If the sum is reasonable (to avoid the concerns raised earlier about undue inducement), this presents a middle ground approach (Pennings, 2005a).

Summarizing the different practices and arguments for and against donor payment, three major models emerge: the market model (unlimited sums paid to donors) based on the rule of supply and demand; the reimbursement model (reimbursement of expenses incurred by the donor) based on the belief that altruism is the only morally acceptable motive for donation; and the reimbursement/compensation model (reimbursement of expenses and compensation but too low to constitute undue inducement) based on the idea that services are compensated for and that it is fair for gamete donors to be compensated as well. In the discussion on payment of healthy volunteers for clinical trials, Dickert and Grady discussed three very similar models: the market model (unlimited payment), the reimbursement model (only expenses paid) and the 'wage model'. The wage model is based on the notion that clinical research requires little skill but time, effort and inconvenience. Therefore, research subjects should be paid hourly wages similar to those for unskilled labour (Dickert and Grady, 1999). They rightly argued that with the wage approach, the risk of undue inducement is significantly reduced, as subjects would have alternative options for the same financial gain; the principle of fairness would not be violated as similar people would be treated similarly; and standardization among clinical research centres in terms of subject payment could be achieved.

In our view, a compensation scheme based on the 'wage model' for clinical trial subjects can be applied to gamete donors. Such an approach would address the major concern of undue inducement since the gain cannot be that high and donors must have preferred to donate rather than to do something else for the same money. It would also address the concern of unfairness since donors would receive something for the service they provide and would avoid the issue of valuing certain genetic traits more than others. Finally, donors would not be compensated for the gametes themselves (seen as a commodity) but for the time they spend and the inconveniences they encounter.

Egg-sharing

Egg sharers are fertility patients who have been diagnosed as subfertile and who are considering IVF. The concept of egg-sharing was first raised in the UK in 1992 by three women patients from the northeast of England who proposed sharing their oocytes with women looking for treatment with donor eggs. Against a national background of too few egg donors and a more local background of too few funds for any further treatment, they asked if they could exchange their eggs in return for another cycle of IVF treatment. The Human Fertilisation and Embryology Authority (HFEA) reviewed the concept extensively and, after many debates and public consultations, in 2000 incorporated egg-sharing into the Code of Practice.

The ethical claims of egg-sharing have been the subject of a long and exhaustive debate over the past twenty years. The detractors argued that subsidized treatment is remuneration in all but name, that treatment outcome favours the recipient (who pays) and that the sharer is giving up half of her eggs before she has even become pregnant (thereby reducing her chances). The first concerns arose from an interpretation of the 1990 Human Fertilisation and Embryology Act and its accompanying Code of Practice for fertility clinics, which specifically declared 'that no money or other benefit shall be given or received in respect of any supply of gametes or embryos'. The authorities and other clinics were concerned that subsidized IVF treatment in return for donating a random portion of eggs could be seen as 'payment'. However, subsequent studies of the motivation of egg sharers indicate that financial reward is not their main incentive; a survey found egg sharers in the UK to be 'well informed women who carefully consider the issues involved' (Ahuja et al., 1998) and disapproved of cash rewards. They were also well educated, middle class and, as judged by their moving accounts and goodwill messages to the future children of their recipients, totally committed to the underlying theme of mutual help (Ahuja et al., 1998). However, despite such repeated findings, the controversies were not resolved until 2004 when a review for the HFEA concluded that egg-sharing was morally acceptable (Human Fertilisation and Embryology Authority, 2005).

The main problem with egg-sharing as an intermediate system is that it falls between two paradigms: altruistic donation and commercial transaction. One has to decide, through analogical reasoning, whether the intermediate positions (reimbursement, payment in kind etc.) link best with one rather than the other paradigm. The underlying idea is that once we have decided this point, we know whether or not it is acceptable. We are confronted with the conviction that the donation of body material is only acceptable if it is purely altruistically moti-vated. The argument against payment has overshot itself and has been extended to any kind of benefit that the donor might receive. Any bene-fit is sufficient to disqualify the system. However, it is one thing to ban payment to prevent commodification of the human body. It is quite another to forbid other types of benefits that do not have this effect. Two counterarguments are worth mentioning here. First, to forbid any benefit is a very strict position. One could adopt the alternative position that an act is morally praiseworthy to the extent that it is motivated by the need of the other(s). The latter would fit better with the empirical fact that most (if not all) actions are done for more than one reason. Second, some people seem to mix up moral praiseworthiness and moral acceptability. These are different standards and, from a moral point of view, it is more important to be able to decide acceptability. Our start-ing point is that benefits can be offered (i.e. it is morally acceptable) as incentives for people to donate as long as these incentives do not lead to the commercialization and commodification of the human body.

It is this pragmatic altruism that defines the place of egg-sharing in ART today, for the simple fact is that egg-sharing simultaneously solves the principal problems of the sharer and the recipient: the former receives the IVF treatment she needs but cannot afford and the lat-ter obtains the eggs which she can no longer produce. Many patients perceive the system as a win–win procedure (Blyth, 2004). Moreover, neither has a treatment which she otherwise need not have had. The risks – such as ovarian hyperstimulation – are still there, of course. But now there is a difference in the relativity of those risks because the donor is also a patient, and not merely a donor. The former has a vested interest in the treatment that goes beyond pure altruism but, as the studies have found, egg sharers do not perceive it to be blatant commer-cialism. Finally, the benefits are conferred equally between the recipi-ent and the donor: both parties have an almost equally high chance of a successful pregnancy (Ahuja and Simons, 2005). Other studies also confirmed that egg-sharing does not reduce the chance of success of either party (Thum *et al.*, 2003).

According to one group, egg-sharing in exchange for a free cycle (or part of a cycle) of IVF is a compensation that far surpasses the amount allowed for other donors. The other group argues that a treatment cycle should not be considered as payment and thus should not be compared with the other types of compensation. The question is whether the free cycle should be recalculated in a monetary amount. Depending on the country and clinic, the amount can be several thousand euro. This is a considerable sum of money that may, according to the chairman of the British Medical Association Ethics Committee, 'constitute an inducement that may jeopardize the validity of the woman's informed consent' (Anonymous, 2005). However, the question whether something is undue inducement or whether it is payment is not the same. Even if we agree that there is a certain degree of inducement, that does not mean that it is payment. This is important because payment has other reprehensible aspects beside undue inducement such as exploitation and commodification.

There are indications that some egg sharers are reluctant to do so but that they go ahead because of their desire to have a child (Rapport, 2003). The prediction has been made that if these women could obtain their treatment without offering their oocytes, egg-sharing would be less attractive for them (Blyth, 2004). Corroborating evidence for this statement was provided by a legal experiment in Belgium. In July 2003 Belgium started to provide full reimbursement for six IVF cycles. Since that date, the number of egg sharers dropped by approximately 70 per cent (Pennings and Devroey, 2006). The conclusion that can be drawn from this reaction is that these women were mainly motivated by the cost reduction. It does not show that altruism was not part of at least some of these women's motives. The studies on the motivations of egg sharers show that they have multiple reasons for sharing. The sharp decline in egg sharers nevertheless shows that a number of these women do not part with their eggs fully voluntarily. Some might consider this to be a sufficient reason to forbid the practice. However, this is too easy an answer. When the broader picture is taken into account, one should realize that even the women who feel strong pressure are not helped or protected by forbidding the practice. The ideal solution would be to prevent a situation where people in need of infertility treatment have to donate their oocytes to receive treatment. This can be done by reducing the out-of-pocket costs of the treatment for the patients either through health insurance or through direct cost reduction.

Reciprocity

The scarcity of donor gametes stimulates the discussion on acceptable systems of recruitment. Other fields equally confronted with a shortage of donor material, such as blood and organs, may serve as an inspiration.

In fact, there already exists a large variety of systems within the practice of oocyte donation, mainly the result of attempts to alleviate the shortage. Fundamental rules like anonymity were reconsidered and in some systems abandoned because of the shortage. Direct donation, where the recipient knows the donor and vice versa, is an option both for gametes and organs. For oocytes (and organs) cross-donation is applied: a donor recruited by recipient X donates to recipient Y and vice versa. In France this system is called 'personalised anonymity' since it allows the protection of the donor's anonymity. Such systems are important because they reveal morally relevant deviations from the ideal 'pure altruism'. Cross-donation, for instance, introduces an element of exchange (i.e. something is asked in return): donor A gives to a certain recipient b in exchange for an equivalent gift by donor B recruited by recipient b to recipient a who recruited donor A. A new variant of this system has been called 'mirror exchange' and was originally invented and applied in the fertility clinic Stichting Geertgen in the Netherlands (Pennings, 2005b). Very simply put, the partner of the person who needs gametes donates in exchange for the gametes of the opposite sex. The man of a woman who needs oocytes donates sperm in exchange for the oocytes donated by the woman of a man who needs sperm. This scheme is then broadened so that the donated gametes are directed into an oocyte and sperm pool and allocated to candidate recipients on the waiting list. For practical and moral reasons, this 'indirect' system is preferable. Persons who donate are awarded bonus points that are attributed to their partners, who then move up on the waiting list. This system, like cross-donation, holds a quid pro quo element that conflicts with the idea of pure altruism. More importantly, the system is based on the principle of fairness. According to this principle, a person is obligated to contribute his or her fair share of the costs if he or she has voluntarily accepted the benefits conferred by the cooperative scheme (Simmons, 1979). In other words, a person who accepts donor gametes as part of his or her parental project as a couple, should, if he or she fulfils the medical and genetic conditions, also contribute to the system from which he or she benefits. Moreover, the system is also open to single women and lesbian couples since it does not matter who reciprocates; it can be the person who benefits herself or her female partner. However, this system cannot rely exclusively on the principle of reciprocity. Some partners will be rejected as donors because of medical and/or genetic contraindications. This will be the case, for instance, for older women. Non-contributors should, on the basis of the bonus points they receive for waiting time, medical urgency and so on, still have the possibility to receive gametes, but they may have to wait longer than those who contribute.

The mirror exchange system has a considerable number of advantages: more donors will be recruited; the benefit for the donor (less waiting time) is strictly non-commercial; the female donor is also a patient and thus undergoes the medical risks for the stimulation in part for her own benefit (like egg sharers); contributors can make good their obligation to reciprocate; the system is compatible with the identifiability of donors; infertile couples are easier to motivate; and, finally, people who need donor gametes for their own family-building are best informed about and prepared for the psychological, social and ethical ramifications involved in gamete donation (Pennings, 2007).

Most people have to get used to the underlying idea, despite the fact that reciprocity as a rule of justice is universally accepted. Three major counterarguments can be distinguished. First, there exists the chance that the recipient becomes pregnant while the donor does not, which may lead to psychological problems. Besides the fact that in most countries it is unlikely that the donor will ever know about the outcome of the treatment of the recipients, the system can easily be adapted to accommodate this objection by allowing people who find it difficult to live with this possibility to postpone their donation. This can be done by allowing them to come back only after their own pregnancy. The second argument focuses on the voluntariness of the donation. Just as for the question of altruism, one should avoid an almost absolute interpretation of the ethical criteria. Every type of reward, benefit or incentive can be interpreted as a kind of threat to voluntariness. Still, offering a reduction in waiting time can hardly be considered as 'an offer one cannot refuse'. This danger might be an additional reason for not imposing strict reciprocity (where only people who donate have access to the waiting list). However, while voluntariness refers to the donors being free from coercion, there is one form of coercion that cannot be avoided here: the fact that recipients of gametes have a moral obligation to donate. If they benefit from the system, they are morally obliged to reciprocate.

The final problem with the exchange is the asymmetry between oocyte and sperm donation. However, whether or not there is an imbalance depends on the criteria with which one measures. Although the medical efforts and risks differ between the two types of gamete donation, the psychosocial aspects are comparable. Moreover, both donors (as a couple) receive what they need in order to build a family. Again, the solution may be found in an adaptation of the procedure. The imbalance can be reduced by introducing a form of egg-sharing: the woman who donates her eggs receives a free IVF cycle instead of an intrauterine insemination with donor sperm. This reduces the waiting time (the treatment coincides with the donation) and increases her chances of success. More elaborate adaptations can be introduced if considered necessary.

Although the system was presented almost five years ago, there is very little enthusiasm for it. Only the Working Party on Sperm Donation Services in the UK has recommended that 'research on sperm sharing schemes should be facilitated to permit further evaluation of this option' (British Fertility Society, 2008). Many people seem to prefer the violation of the payment rule rather than a system that abides by a fundamental rule of justice. Moreover, there is evidence that the system works. In an Italian clinic, 80 per cent of the women whose partner needed donor sperm accepted sharing their oocytes. In 2001 this clinic introduced a system which guaranteed women who needed donor eggs that they would receive them within 8 months (without donation the mean waiting time was 2 years) if their male partner donated sperm. Approximately 60 per cent of the men accepted, and in one year they recruited 30 new semen donors from the sample of partners (Ferraretti *et al.*, 2006). The data from Stichting Geertgen in the Netherlands indicate that, between August 2006 and May 2007, 54 couples received counselling for mirror exchange. This resulted in 18 sperm donors and 22 oocyte donors of which 12 opted for the egg-sharing option (a free immediate IVF cycle instead of intrauterine insemination).

Conclusion

The recruitment of gamete donors is a complex issue. The patients, the professionals and governments have to make an effort to tackle the problem. Governments play a crucial role in this task, either by imposing regulation of gamete donation (which frequently comes down to introducing restrictions) or by adopting a laissez-faire approach. In most European countries governments want to keep control over the whole procedure and the rules governing it. They make it their responsibility through regulation. At the moment they are found wanting. Very little money and effort is spent on awareness campaigns for gamete donation. However, the practical aspects are only secondary to the real issue: in which ethical framework do we, as a society, place assisted reproduction with donor gametes? To answer that question, we need a broad societal debate. It would also require a sustained effort to change the ambiguity towards gamete donation that still lives in society and thus indirectly hampers donor recruitment. Moreover, we urgently need a more critical analysis of ethical standards that are brought forward.

Altruism and voluntariness are no absolute criteria. A detailed analysis of the precise conditions and rules of a particular system may reveal that they fall within the range of morally acceptable variants. Just as in the fields of organ and blood donation, we need creativity in designing new systems and flexibility in the application of existing systems if we want to get anywhere close to a reasonable coverage of the need for donor gametes.

REFERENCES

Ahuja, K. K. and Simons, E. G. (2005). 'Egg-sharing: an evidence based solution to donor egg shortages'. *The Obstetrician & Gynaecologist*, 7, 112–16.
Ahuja, K. K, Simons, E. G., Mostyn, B. J. and Bowen-Simpkins, P. (1998). 'An assessment of the motives and morals of egg-share donors: policy of "payments" to egg donors requires a fair review'. *Human Reproduction*, 13, 2671–8.
Almeling, R. (2007). 'Selling genes, selling gender: egg agencies, sperm banks, and the medical market in genetic material'. *American Sociological Review*, 72, 319–40.
Anonymous (2005). 'BMA response to new guidance on sperm and egg donation, UK. Medical News Today, 8 October 2005'. Available at: www.medicalnewstoday.com/releases/31744.php (accessed 5 May 2006).
Baetens, P., Devroey, P., Camus, M., Van Steirteghem, A. *et al.* (2000). 'Counselling couples and donors for oocyte donation: the decision to use either known or anonymous oocytes'. *Human Reproduction*, 15, 476–84.
Blyth, E. (2004). 'Patient experiences of an "egg sharing" programme'. *Human Fertility*, 7, 157–62.
Blyth, E. and Frith, L. (2008). 'The UK's gamete donor "crisis" – a critical analysis'. *Critical Social Policy*, 28, 74–95.
Blyth, E. (2009). 'Donor-conceived people's access to genetic and biographical history: an analysis of provisions in different jurisdictions permitting disclosure of donor identity'. *International Journal of Law, Policy and the Family*, 23, 174–91.
British Fertility Society Working Party on Sperm Donation Services in the UK (2008). 'Report and recommendations'. *Human Fertility*, 11, 147–58.
Caulfield, T. and Brownsword, R. (2006). 'Science and society: human dignity: a guide to policy making in the biotechnology era?' *Nature Reviews Genetics*, 7, 72–6.
Collier, R. (2010). 'Sperm donor pool shrivels when payments cease'. *Canadian Medical Association Journal*, 182, 233–4.
Craft, I. and Thornhill, A. (2005). 'Would "all-inclusive" compensation attract more gamete donors to balance their loss of anonymity?' *Reproductive Biomedicine Online*, 10, 301–6.
Daniels, K. (2007). 'Anonymity and openness and the recruitment of gamete donors. Part I: semen donors'. *Human Fertility*, 10, 151–8.
Daniels, K., Feyles, V., Nisker, J., Perez-y-Perez, M., *et al.* (2006). 'Sperm donation: implications of Canada's Assisted Human Reproduction Act

2004 for recipients, donors, health professionals, and institutions'. *Journal of Obstetrics and Gynaecology Canada*, 28, 608–15.

Dickert, N. and Grady, C. (1999). 'What's the price of a research subject? Approaches to payment for research participation'. *New England Journal of Medicine*, 341, 198–203.

ESHRE Task Force on Ethics and Law (2002).'Gamete and embryo donation'. *Human Reproduction*, 17, 1407–8.

Ethics Committee of the American Society for Reproductive Medicine (2007). 'Financial compensation of oocyte donors'. *Fertility and Sterility*, 88, 305–9.

EU Health and Consumer Protection, Directorate General (2006). *Report on the Regulation of Reproductive Cell Donation in the European Union*.

Ferraretti, A-P., Pennings, G., Gianarolli, L. and Magli, M. C. (2006). 'Semen donor recruitment in an oocyte donation programme'. *Human Reproduction*, 21, 2482–5.

Guerin, J-F. (1998). 'Payments to gamete donors. The donation of gametes is possible without paying donors: experience of the French CECOS Federation'. *Human Reproduction*, 13, 1129–31.

Holland, S. (2001). 'Contested commodities at both ends of life: buying and selling gametes, embryos, and body tissues'. *Kennedy Institute of Ethics Journal*, 11, 263–84.

Human Fertilisation and Embryology Authority (2005). SEED Report. Available at: www.hfea.gov.uk/534.html.

Johnson, M. H. (1997). 'The culture of unpaid and voluntary egg donation should be strengthened'. *British Medical Journal*, 314, 1401–2.

Levine, A. (2010). 'Self-regulation, compensation, and the ethical recruitment of oocyte donors'. *Hastings Center Report*, 40, 25–36.

Macklin, R. (1996) 'What is wrong with commodification?', in C. B. Cohen (ed.), *New Ways of Making Babies: the Case of Egg Donation*. Bloomington: Indiana University Press.

Nuffield Council on Bioethics (1995). *Human Tissue: Ethical and Legal Issues*.

Pacey, A. (2010). 'Sperm donor recruitment in the UK'. *The Obstetrician and Gynaecologist*, 12, 43–8.

Pennings, G. (1997). 'The "double track" policy for donor anonymity'. *Human Reproduction*, 12, 2839–44.

  (2005a). 'Commentary on Craft and Thornhill: new ethical strategies to recruit gamete donors'. *Reproductive Biomedicine Online*, 10, 307–9.

  (2005b) 'Gamete donation in a system of need-adjusted reciprocity'. *Human Reproduction*, 20, 2990–3.

  (2007). 'Mirror gametes donation'. *Journal of Psychosomatic Obstetrics & Gynecology*, 28, 187–91.

  (2010). 'The rough guide to insemination: cross-border travelling for donor semen due to different regulations'. *Facts, Views and Vision in Obstetrics and Gynaecology*, Monograph, 55–60.

Pennings, G. and Devroey, P. (2006). 'Subsidized in-vitro fertilization treatment and the effect on the number of egg sharers'. *Reproductive Biomedicine Online*, 13, 8–10.

Purewal S. and van den Akker, O. B. A. (2009). 'Systematic review of oocyte donation: investigating attitudes, motivations and experiences'. *Human Reproduction Update*, 15, 499–515.

Rao, R. (2006). 'Coercion, commercialization, and commodification: the ethics of compensation for egg donors in stem cell research'. *Berkeley Technology Law Journal*, 21, 1055–66.

Rapport, F. (2003). 'Exploring the beliefs and experiences of potential egg share donors'. *Journal of Advanced Nursing*, 43, 28–42.

Schonfeld, T. (2003). 'Smart men, beautiful women: social values and gamete commodification'. *Bulletin of Science, Technology and Society*, 23, 168–73.

Schover, L. R., Rothmann, S. A. and Collins, R. L. (1992). 'The personality and motivation of semen donors : a comparison with oocyte donors'. *Human Reproduction*, 7, 575–9.

Simmons, A. J. (1979). 'The principle of fair play'. *Philosophy and Public Affairs*, 8, 307–37.

Steinbock, B. (2004). 'Payment for egg donation and surrogacy'. *Mt Sinai Journal of Medicine*, 71, 255–65.

Thorn, P. (2007). 'Donor insemination: the needs of the children'. *Creating Families*, Spring, 8–12.

Thum, M. Y., Gafar, A., Wren, M., Faris, R., *et al.* (2003). 'Does egg-sharing compromise the chance of donors or recipients achieving a live birth?' *Human Reproduction*, 18, 2363–7.

Titmuss, R. (1970). *The Gift Relationship: From Human Blood to Social Policy.* New York: Pantheon Press.

Yee, S. (2009). '"Gift without a price tag": altruism in anonymous semen donation'. *Human Reproduction*, 24, 3–13.

LEGISLATION

EUROPEAN PARLIAMENT AND COUNCIL

Convention for the Protection of Human Rights and Dignity of the Human Being with regard to the Application of Biology and Medicine: Convention on Human Rights and Biomedicine 1997. Available at: http://conventions. coe.int/Treaty/EN/Treaties/Html/164.htm (accessed July 2010).

Directive 2004/23/EC of 31 March 2004 on setting standards of quality and safety for the donation, procurement, testing, processing, preservation, storage and distribution of human tissues and cells. *Official Journal of the European Union*, L.102/48–58

UK

Human Fertilisation and Embryology Act 1990

10   Challenges in intra-family donation

Effy Vayena and Susan Golombok

Definition and prevalence

Intra-family donation is gamete donation between family members of various degrees of blood or kin relationship. Most intra-family donation involves intra-generational donation between siblings or cousins, most commonly egg donation between sisters or sisters-in-law. Less frequently there is intergenerational donation: usually father to son, daughter to mother or niece to aunt.

There is little data on the prevalence of intra-family donation. Surveys conducted in North America report only the types of intra-family donation that are accepted in the participating centres but provide no information on the number of requests or actual procedures performed (Marshall, 2002; ASRM Ethics Committee Report, 2003). Similarly, the International Committee on Monitoring Assisted Reproductive Technologies (ICMART), which collects data from national IVF registers, does not collect data on specific types of donation. In the early days of IVF egg donors tended to be known. Some US fertility experts advocated sister-to-sister donation rather than anonymous donation (Lessor, 1993). Studies at that time reported positive attitudes towards egg donation by sisters among infertile couples (Sauer, 1988) and the broader public (Lessor, *et al.*, 1990).

Today, most donations involve unknown donors. However, there appears to have been a recent rise in the use of known donors, including family members, in the UK and elsewhere. A study from Canada of the emotional and psychological impact of altruistic donation on known egg donors reported that 39 per cent of respondents had donated to a sister or cousin (Yee *et al.*, 2007). There is also anecdotal information that UK fertility clinics have recently experienced an increase in requests to use sibling donors, possibly as a result of a shortage of donor eggs (Moorhead, 2009). The most up-to-date information comes from a survey of UK clinics conducted in April 2010 by the Human Fertilisation and Embryology Authority (HFEA, 2010). More than 40 per cent of clinics reported receiving a request at least monthly for treatment using gametes donated by a family member, and more than three-quarters of clinics received such a request at least twice a year. The most frequent requests were for sister-to-sister or brother-to-brother donation, although other types such as father-to-son, daughter-to-mother and cousin-to-cousin donations were also occasionally requested. Half of the clinics reported carrying out treatment involving intra-familial donation at least four times per year.

Some UK clinics operate a pool egg donation system, offering recipients a choice of using their relative's egg (generally sisters) or that of an unknown donor from the pool. Significantly, up to half of recipients choose a stranger's egg from the pool. It would seem that in a situation of scarcity some may turn to their family as a source of available and affordable eggs, but, given the choice, may prefer to avoid the relational complications of using an intra-familial egg donor.

Regulation and professional guidelines

Intra-familial donation is permitted and practised in many countries. In countries that have regulated ARTs there is usually no distinction made between intra-family and other forms of donation and, therefore, what applies to these cases is the same as for donation in general. Some countries with no regulation have issued guidelines. The American Society for Reproductive Medicine (ASRM) produced an ethics committee report in 2003 on family members as gamete donors and surrogates. This guidance suggested the use of family members as donors or surrogates is generally ethically acceptable with brother-to-brother and sister-to-sister as the most acceptable. It found intergenerational donation was 'especially challenging' and donation involving consanguineous relations that give a 'strong impression of incest' should be prohibited. The report calls for special attention in terms of consent and counselling for this type of donation and the need for ART centres to have clear policies. While recognizing the ethical and psychological complexities, the overall tone of the report is positive. But it recommends that if any requests for intra-familial donation raise consistent concerns about potentially problematic family relationships or undue pressure on the donor, the centre should have the right to refuse treatment.

In 2007 New Zealand's Advisory Committee on Assisted Reproductive Technology (ACART) issued 'Guidelines on Donation of Eggs or Sperm between Certain Family Members'. This document spells out the principles that should always be taken into account including the welfare of all involved, especially of the offspring. It states that the children should be made aware of their donor origins and be able to access information about the donor. It also specifies which requests will need to be reviewed by the National Ethics Committee on Assisted Reproductive Technology (ECART) when it comes to donation from family members. These include all requests other than: the donation of eggs by a sister or cousin of the recipient, when both are over the age of 20; donation of sperm by a brother or cousin of the recipient's husband, when both are 20 or older; donated eggs from the partner of the recipient woman and sperm by a brother or cousin of the recipient woman when both are over 20 – the age of majority at the time the guideline was developed (ACART, 2007).

Most recently, guidelines have been forthcoming from the European Society for Human Reproduction and Embryology's Task Force on Ethics and Law (ESHRE Task force on Ethics and Law, 2011). They found intra-family medically assisted reproduction to be a morally acceptable practice in some situations and under some conditions. They regard both combined and separate counselling of recipients and donors as crucial as it may contribute to both well-considered decision-making and risk reduction. But they argue that such treatments should be withheld in case of undue pressures on the donor or where there is a high risk of serious harm (psycho-social and/or genetic) for the possible child. While they see no a priori moral objection to intergenerational donation, they conclude that first-degree relative intergenerational donation needs special scrutiny in view of the increased risk of undermining autonomous choice. Cases involving third-degree consanguinity are found to be acceptable, in principle, while first- or second-degree consanguinity should be ruled out.

The ESHRE report also considers the issue of incest. They suggest that while most countries have laws and regulations forbidding consanguinity and incest which apply to sex, marriage and reproduction between closer than third-degree (genetic) relatives, such laws were written before the era of assisted reproduction and may therefore not explicitly rule out non-coital forms of reproduction between such relatives. However, they suggest that clinicians should conform to 'the spirit' of such regulation and rule out first- and second-degree consanguineous medically assisted reproduction. But as they point out, such cases are very unlikely to be proposed. They also consider cases where there is a semblance of incest and first- or second-degree consanguinity. One of their examples is of an adult daughter donating eggs to her mother whose new partner's sperm will be used to conceive the child.

As this involves what they term reproduction between genetically unrelated adults, there is no consanguinity. They suggest the relationship is not incestuous because the daughter has no parent–child relationship with the mother's new partner. They conclude that unless serious moral objections can be found about these cases, where there is no coitus, no mixing of gametes of close relatives and no co-parenting of the gamete producers, such arrangements are acceptable (see also Pennings, 2001).

In this context the UK is unusual as it does have specific legislation governing assisted reproduction which has extended the prohibition of incest to intra-familial donation. As in other jurisdictions, UK law prohibits both marrying and sexual intercourse between close relatives linked by blood (first- and second-degree) and affinity (adoptive parents and children)(Sexual Offences Act, 2003; Marriage (Prohibited Degrees of Relationship) Act, 2004). The same list of forbidden relatives[1] was applied in the situation of assisted reproduction where legislation (Human Fertilisation and Embryology Act, 1990, as amended) prevents those on the list from donating to each other if they plan to co-parent the children. The legislation embodies a notion of what Pennings (2001) has called 'intentional incest'. Donation to close relatives is not forbidden. So, for example, a case of a brother donating to an infertile sister who was using donor eggs would be lawful. However, a similar case treated in the USA, where again the sister used donated eggs, would have been illegal in the UK because the sister and brother who cohabited planned also to jointly parent the children.

Recently the Human Fertilisation and Embryology Authority (HFEA) has considered further extending the ban to rule out any mixing of gametes from close relatives. This and other issues concerning intra-familial donations are part of a current HFEA public consultation on donation policies.

---

[1] Lists of forbidden relatives vary across jurisdictions and the UK list has changed over time. When the prohibitions embodied in cannon law were transferred into state legislation (The Marriage Act 1835) the list included the deceased wife's sister. Biblical doctrine saw marriage as creating 'one flesh' between husband and wife so in-laws were treated as blood relations and so included in the table of forbidden kindred and affinity. After a long period of parliamentary debates this prohibition was removed under the Deceased Wife's Sister Marriage Act of 1907 (Anderson, 1982). At an earlier time cousin marriage had been included in cannon law prohibitions. Such patterns of 'close marriage' became a very common and widespread pattern among the middle strata across Europe, North America and their colonies in the late eighteenth, and through the 'long' nineteenth centuries (Davidoff, 2006).

A rather different approach to regulation has been taken in Japan. In 2003 a panel attached to the Ministry of Health's Science Council produced a set of guidelines on ART including the proposal to ban sibling donation. The arguments used to justify the ban were that such arrangements could unsettle family relationships or could lead to undue pressure for donation (Watts, 2003; Mayeda, 2006). These arguments are not particular to Japan. They have been raised by other regulators as issues of concern, but many other countries have chosen to allow a case-by-case assessment of each individual request by the health practitioner and clinic team or an ethics committee.

In New Zealand's programme for personal donors (donors found and chosen by recipients) there were some who chose brothers. All participants in the programme were united in their wish for a donor personally known to them, whose personality was familiar and who they liked as a person. But while some couples had chosen brothers as donors because the child's social father would be closer genetically to the child, others saw disadvantages in the family connection and preferred to use a friend instead. Those who preferred friends cited the possibility of feelings of obligation to donate to a family member, the 'closeness' of the situation and the complexity of relationships that would be created as reasons for their preference (Adair and Purdie, 1996).

Reasons for intra-familial donation

One of the reasons for seeking a gamete donor within the family can be the maintenance of a genetic link between both parents and the child (Adair and Purdie, 1996). Families who use an unknown (and unrelated) donor have children who are blood relatives of only one of the parents; many settle for this and such families are found to function very well (Daniels, 2005; Golombok *et al.*, 2006; Grace and Daniels, 2007). However, some would prefer a genetic link with both parents (Pennings, 2001). This may be achieved, for example, by using a sister as an egg donor. In some cases it may be family membership that is important, rather than any genetic connection between donor and recipient; an example here would be having an egg donation from a sister-in-law.

The few studies that have investigated motivations for intra-familial donation have found that the wish for a genetic link between the donor and recipient, the fear of genetic material from an unknown donor and the child's physical resemblance to the parents were of importance (Baetens *et al.*, 2000; Greenfeld and Klock, 2004; Winter and Daniluk, 2004), with the significance of the genetic link appearing to be more important for men than for women (Brewaeys *et al.*, 1997). A practical reason for seeking intra-family donation is the acceleration of treatment. Generally there is a shortage of gamete donors and waiting periods for couples who wish to undertake fertility treatment can be long. Finding a family donor can speed up the process. There is a widely held view that as many countries move towards removing donor anonymity, fewer gamete donors will come forward and couples will be forced to look for alternatives. In countries where donors are receiving remuneration, particularly egg donors, reducing this expense may also be driving the quest to find a relative as a donor.

Relatives who volunteer to donate their gametes are primarily motivated by altruism and the wish to help members of their family overcome their infertility. This is a consistent finding in studies examining donor motivation (Purewal and van den Akker, 2009). A personal relationship with the recipient appears to play the most significant role; love for the sibling, in particular, is cited as the main motive by egg donors. The perceived importance of motherhood and coming from a large family were also reported as reasons to donate (Warren and Blood, 2003). In intergenerational donation, similarly there is a strong sense of helping the parent or child, and of providing a 'gift from the heart' (Lessor, 1993; Nikolettos *et al.*, 2003; Winter and Daniluk, 2004).

Issues related to consanguinity and perceptions of incest have already been discussed, but aside from these questions, intra-family donation would still raise distinct ethical concerns more complex than using a known or unknown donor from outside the family. With intra-family donation, traditional family relations are altered to produce new patterns of blood, gestational and social relationships among family members, challenging those involved to work out some moral dilemmas and psychological uncertainties. These issues may affect the donor, the donor's own children, the parents and their offspring, as well as the wider family in a variety of ways. We will discuss the key issues arising in intra-family donation for the various parties involved and present some new data from the first longitudinal study to examine families created by intra-family donation (Jadva *et al.*, 2011).

The donor relative

Intra-family donors tend to be motivated by the need to help their relatives create a family and alleviate their suffering from infertility. In an ideal situation this is an altruistic gesture by the donor who is fully aware of the physical and psychosocial implications of donation. He or she either initiates the process or is responsive to a request from the recipients. There is often a concern that emotional pressure may be put on the relative to donate. This pressure may be external, caused by other family members or internal, driven by feelings of obligation to help the relative. This issue has been discussed in detail in the context of live organ donation and the analysis can also be applied here (Crouch and Elliott, 1999). Emotional pressure could lead to coercion and so restrict the would-be donor's autonomy. While this can occur, it is impossible to make blanket statements, and of course this can happen with any known donor, not only family members. The individual's relationship to the recipient, to other family members and his or her perception of the family as a whole, including religious views, will influence the decision-making process and subsequently the extent to which the donor can make a free decision. Some commentators have suggested that it may be impossible to make a free decision, for example when parents request a child's involvement (i.e. the son to donate sperm to his father), given the role of parental authority and possible issues of dependence, financial or otherwise (Sureau and Shenfield, 1995). On the other hand, Finch and Mason (1993) have shown that rather than being viewed as an obligation, giving assistance to family members is usually carefully negotiated and often has advantages for the donor as well as the recipient. A sister who donates her eggs, for example, may not only enhance feelings of family solidarity but also her own identity as a caring sister: an altruistic gift relationship of the kind discussed by Titmuss (1970). Finch and Mason have also shown that family members may not wish to be beholden to each other so it would not necessarily be in the best interests of those in need of gametes to put undue pressure on relatives who might donate.

The measures that are typically taken to protect the donor's autonomy are the informed consent process and counselling. Both are *sine qua non* in all donations and certainly in intra-family donation, but still there are questions to be asked. A consent process operates on the basis of personal autonomy. The individual is presumed to be capable of making a free and rational decision after having received the relevant information. The consent process cannot, however, ensure that the donor has reached a 'free' decision uninfluenced by the relationship with his or her relatives. In thinking about intra-family donation, the concept of 'relational autonomy' might be more useful. This concept acknowledges the importance of personal autonomy but also how this is influenced and shaped by various relationships and the broader social context (Mullen, 2001). Therefore, it provides a richer understanding of what a 'free choice' actually is and all of the factors that can lead an individual to consider a particular action as free (MacLeon and

Sherwin, 2000). In practical terms, recognition of relational autonomy can lead to better processes for recruitment of intra-family donors (how the options are presented) and better consent processes (how the risks and benefits are discussed) while it can further inform the counselling process. In live organ donation it is usual practice to interview the would-be donor and the recipient independently. If the donor is found to be at all reluctant to donate, 'medical reasons' are found which make the donor unsuitable.

A specific question about the counselling process is the extent to which it can prepare the donor for what the future holds. The donor (if the treatment is successful) will be the genetic parent of the offspring but within the family would have a different social role. So, for example, with sisters the donor will be aunt to the child and her own children will be half-siblings of the donor child. While the donor may see herself as a rather special aunt, her own children may remain unaware of their new half-siblings and the mother may prefer to emphasize her sisterhood with the donor and her motherhood of the child she has carried (Lessor, 1993). As these half-siblings may resemble one another, there will always be a risk that they or others may come to realise the true relationship between them, and it is not known how those who become aware that they are half-siblings rather than cousins will feel about their family circumstances. In brother-to-sister donation where the sister uses donated eggs, the social mother would be the gestational mother but without a genetic relationship to the child, and the genetic father would be the social uncle, while some cousins would be half-siblings. With daughter-to-mother donation, the genetic mother would be the child's social sibling and the social mother would be the child's genetic grandmother. It is maybe difficult to imagine at the time of a donation how one might feel in the future about the offspring with whom (unlike in unknown donation) one would have a social relationship and under circumstances that cannot be known at the time of the donation (for example, the donor might end up not having children of their own).

Furthermore, the donor will inevitably be involved in any failed attempts at conception or in conceptions of unhealthy children. Failed cycles have been reported as having a major psychological impact on donors (Purewal and van Akker, 2009). The donor can suffer through treatment failure even though he or she is not the patient. Similarly, if the child suffers from a genetic disease or disability, there is a risk that the donor might feel at least partially responsible. The potential for emotional harm for the donor should not be underestimated. In unknown donation the donor would most likely not know the outcome of his or her donation and therefore this type of harm would be avoided.

Altruistic donation usually receives social recognition, and such recognition may contribute to the donor's satisfaction and well-being. Intra-family donation, however, may completely lack this particular element or may even create an adverse reaction (Marshall, 2002). Some intra-family donations are not viewed positively as they appear to resemble incest (even if they do not) or they are kept a close secret so there is no opportunity for recognition or appreciation.

There are few studies addressing these issues and those that do tend to have relatively small samples. Findings about the post-donation experience of intra-family donors are therefore not conclusive and appear somewhat contradictory (Winter and Daniluk, 2004). In one recent follow-up study of oocyte donors who donated to known recipients including family members, most donors were satisfied with the physical and emotional implications of their donation and only a small minority reported difficulties and distress when seeing the child (Yee *et al.*, 2007).

The family

An issue that extends beyond the donor to the family network is how family relationships might be affected by the donation. The empirical data show diverse outcomes. In an older study, 75 per cent of known semen donors said that their relationship with the recipients had become closer while the remainder felt that their relationship had deteriorated (Adair and Purdie, 1996). Other studies have reported a strengthening of relationships between the donor and recipients (Winter and Daniluk, 2004). An investigation from the Netherlands of known oocyte donation reported that 88 per cent of the recipients described their relationship with the donor as close and friendly or fairly close and friendly; only a small minority seemed to have problems (Van Berkel *et al.*, 2007). However, we should note that these studies concern known donors, most of whom were not family members. The two issues that may profoundly affect family relationships are boundaries between the donor and recipients, and secrecy. Both raise ethical conundrums.

At this point we will describe some of the results from the ongoing study being carried out by one of the authors and her colleagues. As part of a longitudinal investigation of a representative sample of British families created by gamete donation (Golombok *et al.*, 2004, 2005, 2006 and 2011), 9 families were identified where the child had been conceived using the egg of a family member. Of these egg donors 6 were sisters of the mother and 3 were sisters-in-law, of whom 1 was the wife of the mother's brother, 1 was the wife of the father's brother and 1 was the female partner of the father's sister (Jadva *et al.*, 2011). Interviews about family relationships were carried out when the children were 1, 3 and 7 years old. Most of the families were middle class and half the group came from black British, Asian or other ethnic minority groups. This is a surprisingly high proportion and while the numbers are very small, it at least raises the question of whether sister/sister-in-law dona- tion may be particularly favoured in some cultures. Whereas having a donor from within the family, and the genetic or familial links that this provides, were seen as an advantage by some, for others there were more practical considerations in view of the long waiting list for an anonymous egg donor.

In most families it had been agreed that the donor would be the child's aunt and nothing more but in two families it was decided that the donor would have a special role such as a godmother. There was no evidence whatsoever of donors wishing to adopt a mothering role, a situation that parallels that of surrogate mothers who do not view the child they carry for another couple as their own (Jadva *et al.*, 2003). One mother whose egg donor was her sister commented: 'She's very, um, I don't know what the word is really, not detached, but just very much, you know, stepped back … If she sends a card she always sends it "to my nephew", you know, that kind of thing.' Another mother said: 'She's my sister, so she is my daughter's auntie, and she is very much her auntie, and that is her role.'

The mothers themselves appeared secure in their role as mother of the child and many commented that they rarely thought about the relative being the child's genetic parent. However, some mothers were concerned to ensure that the child viewed them as their mother. For one mother this was given as a reason for not telling her child about the egg donor: 'I suppose I just wouldn't want her to be confused about who she was and who her mother was.' Another mother who had been open with her child said: 'We're always very clear that she's come from mummy that she grew in mummy's tummy so she knows that that connection is there. I don't want her to think that my sister is her mummy.'

In all but one of the families the mother and child were in regular contact with the donor, although over time this reduced somewhat. At age 7, 2 (of 5 participating at that point) were in contact at least once a month, 2 less frequently and 1 was in telephone contact only. The chil- dren tended to have less frequent contact than the mother. The moth- ers continued to rate their own and the child's relationship with the donor as harmonious with the exception of one mother who reported some dissatisfaction and coldness but no major conflict or hostility. All of the mothers felt that the donor's involvement with the child was positive apart from one mother who felt ambivalent.

At the time of the child's first birthday, 6 of the mothers planned to tell the child about their donor origins, with the remaining 3 having decided against telling. However, by the time the child was 7 years old, only one set of parents had actually done so. Of the 4 remaining families who were interviewed at age 7, 3 still planned to tell, one at age 7, one at age 10 and one at age 18. These mothers had not yet disclosed this information as they felt that their child was too young to understand. Previous research on children conceived by anonymous gamete donation has shown that if parents do not tell their child about their genetic origins by early school age, they tend not to do so (Golombok *et al.*, 2002a, 2002b). Thus it seems likely that almost all of these children conceived by intra-family donation will grow up unaware that a person they know as their aunt is actually their genetic mother.

Although most mothers had not disclosed the donor conception to their child, many had told other family members including parents, their partner's parents, their siblings and their partner's siblings. They had not, however, always told the full story. Some had mentioned having fertility treatment but not the use of a donated egg, and some had been open about the donated egg but not about the identity of the donor. In some cases, the egg donor's family or the egg donor's partner's family were not aware of the egg donation, that is that a child born into the family was related to them in a way that differed from their understanding of their relationship to that child.

If family members are aware of the donation but the child is not, the child may find out by accident or inadvertently due to resemblance. One mother expressed her anxiety about the similarity in appearance between her child and the donor's children and talked about being taunted by her mother-in-law who had not been told: 'Yesterday I went to my mother-in-law's and she looked at her and said she looks like … she looks like your nephew … it's hard to swallow.' Another mother was concerned about her child and her sister's [the donor's] child working it out for themselves because they looked alike: 'As babies my sister's [donor's] daughter and my daughter looked very, very alike, you know they could have been twins … If ever a situation came up when perhaps one of them clicked onto something or just felt they looked alike we would tell them straight away … because then you've got a situation where cousins aren't really cousins, they're brothers and sisters and it gets complicated.'

The one family who had been open with their child from the start, where the donor was the mother's sister, did not have any regrets, in spite of the child informing her entire school: 'There was a lovely moment when they had an assembly where everyone was talking about how they were special and what's special about you and my daughter's hand shot up and I thought to myself what is she going to say, she's never put her hand up and she isn't usually one to volunteer, so up shoots her hand and the teacher said why are you special and she said I'm special because I come from my mummy's sister's egg and the teacher said oh did you, that does make you special!'

Although this sample is small, it was drawn from a larger, representative sample of families with a child conceived by egg donation. An advantage of the study is that the families were recruited while the children were still in infancy, thus avoiding the potential biases associated with opting in or out of the investigation once the child had formed a relationship with the donor or had acquired the capacity to understand the true nature of this relationship. Moreover, the families were followed up until the child entered middle childhood, that is beyond the age at which children develop an understanding of the meaning of biological relationships (e.g. Solomon et al., 1996; Brodzinsky and Pinderhughes, 2002; Williams and Smith, 2010).

The concern that intra-family donation would have an adverse impact on family relationships appears to be unfounded. Although the donors themselves were not interviewed so no conclusions can be drawn about their feelings or experiences, for example, about whether they felt under pressure to donate or whether they are satisfied with their level of involvement with the child, data obtained from mothers suggests that egg donation by a sister or sister-in-law did not have a detrimental effect on the relationship between the donor and either the parents or the child. Without exception, the two sets of adults clearly maintained their social roles within the family as mother and father, and aunt and uncle, respectively, and there was no evidence that either of the parties involved wanted it any other way.

But it is noteworthy that in only one family had the child been told about their genetic origins by the time they reached 7 years old. This was in spite of the greater risk that these children would find out by accident about the circumstances of their birth than children conceived by anonymous gamete donation. In addition to the usual concerns experienced by parents regarding the disclosure of donor conception to their child, such as the fear that this would distress the child or that the child would love the non-genetic parent less (Cook et al., 1995; Golombok et al., 2002a, 2002b), the reluctance of parents whose child was conceived using the egg of a relative to be open with their child stems from the desire to avoid the unknowable complications that could potentially arise within the extended family.

Tension may rise when the recipient couple and the donor do not agree on the boundaries they wish to draw. Should the donor be actively involved in the child's life? How involved should he or she be? Should he or she have a say in parenting decisions? In a traditional family, an aunt or uncle or grandparent may be significantly involved, or not, in the life of the couple and their children. Should a social uncle or aunt who is also the genetic father or mother of the child have more rights to involvement in the child's life? This question can be asked in moral, legal and psychological terms. The answers will differ. From the legal point of view the answer is straightforward. In most situations in many jurisdictions parental rights and duties are transferred from the donor to the recipient parents. Morally speaking, it is generally accepted that a donor does not have any parental obligations to the offspring nor any parental rights because he or she has made a free decision to transfer such rights to other people (Bayne, 2003; Fuscaldo, 2006) and this remains the case if the donor is a relative. However, the opposite has been argued, namely, that gamete donors have parental responsibilities because such a responsibility is by default not transferable (Weinberg, 2008). In theory, at least, a known donor could claim rights and duties; indeed, disputes may arise about the extent to which a known donor may be involved in a child's life or, in some situations in some jurisdictions, may be able to claim parental rights and duties. With intra-familial donation the donor will already have a kindred role in the child's life. A donor may bond with the child and may feel to some extent that the child is their 'own', especially if there is a resemblance. In the study by Winter and Daniluk (2004), the oocyte donors who donated to their sister reported their anxiety at first meeting their niece or nephew arising from the fear that the child would resemble them too much, or that they would experience maternal feelings. All three women in this study, however, seemed to have no boundary confusion and were able to maintain a clear line between their roles as donor and aunt. The Dutch study by Van Berkel *et al.* (2007) found that contact with the donor remained good and frequent after the birth of the child, and half of the recipients saw their donor daily or once a week. Only a minority of parents reported problems in their relationship with the donor because of too much interference by the donor in the child's life.

Gamete recipients might have difficulties accepting a very involved 'uncle' or 'aunt'. They might find it particularly difficult to deal with such an issue in the context of the gratitude they would inevitably feel to someone who gave them a 'gift from the heart'. Gratitude towards the donor and a sense of reciprocity, allowing the donor to be involved in the child's life, may, however, create tension and difficult relationships. Such tension might spill over to other family members who may or may not know about the donation depending on who has been told. Conversely, one could argue that the close involvement of the donor may actually be welcome and enhance the family network, bringing family members much closer to each other. As yet, we know very little about how such relationships play out in different families. There is a need for further longitudinal data on how such families function, the specific issues that they face and how they resolve them in both the short and long term.

Secrecy is another issue of relevance to intra-family donation. As donors are family members who may have regular contact with the recipients, it may be more difficult for families who wish to do so to keep the donation secret. The evidence here is again inconclusive. Some early studies of intra-family donation found that the majority of donors had not informed other members of the family (Purewal and van den Akker, 2009). Others have reported a tendency towards openness (Yee et al., 2007; Van Berkel et al., 2007). A complicating factor is that the donor and the recipients may have different values, views and beliefs regarding this issue. Although secrecy about genetic parentage has increasingly been viewed as undesirable, with parents who do not disclose donor conception to their children considered to be self-serving, Smart (2009) points out that secrets may be felt to be necessary for the preservation of family relationships. This may be particularly likely in the case of intra-family donation as not only are parent–child relationships perceived to be at risk but also relationships between the nuclear family and wider kin. As we described earlier, only one of those in the longitudinal study had told their child of their donor origins by age 7.

The offspring

The welfare of the child is a central theme in most debates about ARTs. This dictates that the child's best interests should always be taken into account and that treatment should not be undertaken if it is probable that the child may suffer physical or psychological harm. In intra-family donation the welfare of the potential child remains of prime concern. While the probability of physical risk is not higher than in donation in general (assuming consanguinity is avoided), concerns focus on the probability of psychological and social harm. Of particular relevance is the issue of disclosure to the child, and the impact of information about the donor conception on the child's psychological well-being. Studies have shown that in families created with the help of a donor, parent–child relationships have not been negatively affected following disclosure if the child is told by the parents early in childhood (Rumball and Adair, 1999; MacDougal, 2007; Jadva *et al.*, 2009) (see Appleby, Blake and Freeman, Chapter 13). In addition, studies investigating donor offspring's perceptions of family functioning in relation to disclosure showed that parents' disclosing together was predictive of more positive family functioning (Berger and Paul, 2008).

Despite the advice from counsellors and other health care practitioners to tell children, most parents of children conceived by donor gametes do not do so. Research conducted in the UK, for example, has found that in spite of parents' intention to be open with children about their donor conception, less than half actually disclose (Golombok *et al.*, 2002a, 2002b; Golombok *et al.*, 2011). The reasons parents give for their decision not to tell are to protect the child and maintain family relationships (Cook *et al.*, 1995; Murray and Golombok, 2003). The common argument for disclosure is the right of the child to know about their donor conception and to prevent children learning about this from someone other than the parents. With known donation, most studies have reported the reluctance of parents to disclose this information to the child. The need for secrecy in order to protect the family as a whole has been suggested as a reason for non-disclosure of intra-family donation but the studies are not conclusive regarding the role this actually plays (Purewal and van den Akker, 2009).

Disclosure in intra-family donation may have far-reaching implications and certainly has the potential to alter the dynamics of relationships in the extended family. The situation whereby family members are aware of the donor conception but the child is not is similar to that of many families with a child conceived using an anonymous donor, thus creating a risk that unintentionally the child will find out about their origins. However, intra-family donation brings additional layers of complexity. It may be more distressing to a child to discover that their donor is a family member – to discover not only that they lack a biological link with one of their parents but also that an aunt, uncle, grandmother or grandfather is not exactly who they thought they were. Also, they could inadvertently discover the truth about their origins through their resemblance to other family members. A unique aspect of secrecy about intra-family donation that does not apply to anonymous gamete donation is that the children are unaware that the donor's children, whom they will know, are their (genetic) half-siblings. In the case of sister-to-sister donation, for example, their cousins are actually their (genetic) half-brothers and half-sisters.

The question here is whether offspring are better off knowing about the involvement of a relative in their conception or not, given the unknown consequences, since so many other people will inevitably be affected. Until information can be obtained directly from the offspring of intra-family donation, predictions about their thoughts and feelings about being conceived using the gametes of a family member remain purely speculative. It might be expected that their reaction to this information would depend on the quality of their relationship with their parents, and also with the family member to whom they find themselves more closely related than previously thought. Finding out that you are the biological daughter of a much-loved aunt may provoke a rather a different response than the discovery that you are the biological daughter of a disapproving one. Good relationships with both the social mother and the new-found genetic mother may cause the child to feel more secure; bad relationships with the two 'mothers' may lead to double psychological trouble. On a more positive note, in contrast to the offspring of anonymous donors, there is no need to search for the donor and donor siblings in the quest for information about genetic relatives. Not only do children born from the gametes of a family member know who their donor relatives are but they also know what they are like.

Research on children conceived through anonymous gamete donation indicates that the earlier they are told about their conception, the more easily they accept this information and incorporate it into their sense of self. Those who find out in adolescence or in adulthood are more likely to feel shocked, distressed and deceived (Turner and Coyle, 2000; Jadva et al., 2009). It is conceivable that the additional challenges presented by intra-family donation may exacerbate the more negative feelings of those who learn of their origins later in life. They may feel deceived not just by their parents but by their family as a whole.

If we accept that truth-telling has a higher moral value and that secrecy has a deleterious effect on family functioning, then disclosure would be the recommended approach. The words of Baroness Mary Warnock about disclosure in donation hold true in intra-family donation as well: 'I cannot argue that children who are told of their origins … are necessarily happier or better off in any way that can be estimated. But I do believe that if they are not told they are being wrongly treated'

(1987: 151). What makes the issue of disclosure difficult to resolve from an ethical perspective is that it automatically involves the donor, the recipient, the partner of the recipient and the child as well as other family members. If they do not all share the same beliefs and wishes about disclosure, a conflict is created between their respective individual rights. The principles of individual autonomy, beneficence and fairness are simultaneously at stake and may be at odds. It is not clear that these principles are in any certain hierarchy and it is therefore challenging to determine how they may coexist and what compromises need to be made.

A practical arrangement that may prevent future conflict is where recipients and donors decide prior to the donation about the issue of the disclosure. In the study by Van Berkel, about 53 per cent of the recipients and donors had made an agreement before the egg donation about how to deal with disclosure to the child. The agreements included whether the parents would disclose together with the donor, and at what point (Van Berkel *et al.*, 2007). This is merely a practical arrangement that may help prevent potential conflict, but it does not necessarily guarantee the well-being of the child, nor does it resolve the ethical dilemmas that may arise.

Conclusions

Intra-family donation is a complex arrangement and there is still much uncertainty about its ethical acceptability. Although it may be an appropriate solution for some families, it may be detrimental for others. The principles of autonomy, relational autonomy and non-maleficence are at stake and may conflict. While such principles may be competing in the use of other medical interventions, at least a favourable risk/benefit ratio for the patient is the minimum required standard in order to accept a procedure. However, it is problematic to use the risk/benefit approach here as there is not only one person/patient but at least three (plus the extended family) and also because we cannot accurately estimate the risk and benefit as the psychological risks for all involved are unknown.

Further empirical data will help us make a better assessment of the risks and benefits involved and therefore form more robust arguments. It would seem to be premature to try to prohibit intra-family donation based on the speculation that it might be harmful. Given our current knowledge and in light of the ethical issues involved, a careful case-by-case analysis of each request may be the most reasonable approach.

REFERENCES

Adair, V. and Purdie, A. (1996). 'Donor insemination programmes with personal donors: issues of secrecy'. *Human Reproduction*, 11, 2558–63.

Advisory Committee on Assisted Reproductive Technology (ACART) (2007). *Guidelines on Donation of Eggs or Sperm between Certain Family Members.* New Zealand.

American Society of Reproductive Medicine (ASRM) Ethics Committee Report (2003). 'Family members as gamete donors and surrogates'. *Fertility and Sterility*, 80, 1124–30.

Anderson, N. F. (1982). 'The "marriage with a Deceased Wife's Sister Bill" controversy: incest anxiety and the defence of family purity in Victorian England'. *Journal of British Studies*, 21, 67–86.

Baetens, P., Devroey, P., Camus, M., Van Steirteghem, A., et al. (2000). 'Counselling couples and donors for oocyte donation: the decision to use either known or anonymous oocytes'. *Human Reproduction*, 15, 476–84.

Bayne, T. (2003). 'Gamete donation and parental responsibility'. *Journal of Applied Philosophy*, 20, 77–87.

Berger, R. and Paul, M. (2008). 'Family secrets and family functioning: the case of donor assistance'. *Family Process*, 47, 553–66.

Brewaeys, A., Golombok, S., Naaktgeboren, N., de Bruyn, J. K., et al. (1997). 'Donor insemination: Dutch parents' opinions about confidentiality and donor anonymity and the emotional adjustment of their children'. *Human Reproduction*, 12, 1591–7.

Brodzinsky, D. and Pinderhughes, E. (2002). 'Parenting and Child Development in Adoptive Families', in M. H. Bornstein (ed.), *Handbook of Parenting*, vol. 1. Mahwah: Lawrence Erlbaum Associates, pp. 279–312.

Cook, R., Golombok, S., Bish, A. and Murray, C. (1995). 'Keeping secrets: A study of parental attitudes toward telling about donor insemination'. *American Journal of Orthopsychiatry*, 65, 549–59.

Crouch, R. and Elliott, C. (1999). 'Moral agency and the family: the case of living related organ transplantation'. *Cambridge Quarterly of Healthcare Ethics*, 8, 275–87.

Daniels, K. (2005). 'Is blood really thicker than water? Assisted reproduction and its impact on our thinking about family'. *Journal of Psychosomatic Obstetrics and Gynaecology*, 26, 265–70.

Davidoff, L. (2006). '"Close Marriage" in the Nineteenth and Twentieth Century Middle Strata', in F. Ebtehaj, B. Lindley and M. Richards (eds.), *Kinship Matters*. Oxford: Hart Publishing.

ESHRE Task Force on Ethics and Law (2011). 'Intra-familial medically assisted reproduction'. *Human Reproduction*, 26, 504–9.

Finch, J. and Mason, J. (1993). *Negotiating Family Responsibilities*. London: Routledge.

Fuscaldo, G. (2006). 'Genetic ties: are they morally binding?' *Bioethics*, 20, 64–76.

Golombok, S., Brewaeys, A., Giavazzi, M. T., Guerra, D., et al. (2002a). 'The European study of assisted reproduction families: the transition to adolescence'. *Human Reproduction*, 17, 830–40.

Golombok, S., MacCallum, F., Goodman, E. and Rutter, M. (2002b). 'Families with children conceived by donor insemination: A follow-up at age 12'. *Child Development*, 73, 952–68.

Golombok, S., Lycett, E., MacCallum, F., Jadva, V., et al. (2004). 'Parenting infants conceived by gamete donation'. *Journal of Family Psychology*, 18, 443–52.

Golombok, S., Jadva, V., Lycett, E., Murray, C., et al. (2005). 'Families created by gamete donation: follow-up at age 2'. *Human Reproduction*, 20, 286–93.

Golombok, S., Murray, C., Jadva, V., Lycett, E., et al. (2006). 'Non-genetic and non-gestational parenthood: consequences for parent-child relationships and the psychological well-being of mothers, fathers and children at age 3'. *Human Reproduction*, 21, 1918–24.

Golombok, S., Readings, J., Blake, L., Casey, P., Mellish, L., Marks, A. and Jadva, V. (2011). 'Children conceived by gamete donation: the impact of openness about donor conception on psychological adjustment and parent–child relationships at age 7'. *Journal of Family Psychology*, 25, 230–9.

Grace, V. M. and Daniels, K. R. (2007). 'The (ir)relevance of genetics: engendering parallel worlds of procreation and reproduction'. *Sociology of Health and Illness*, 29, 692–710.

Greenfeld, D. and Klock, S. (2004). 'Disclosure decisions among known and anonymous oocyte donation recipients'. *Fertility and Sterility*, 81, 1565–71.

Human Fertilisation and Embryology Authority (HFEA) (2010). *Donation Review: Update and Early Options*. Paper number 561. London: HFEA.

Jadva, V., Murray, C., Lycett, E., MacCallum, F., et al. (2003). 'Surrogacy: the experiences of surrogate mothers'. *Human Reproduction*, 18, 2196–204.

Jadva, V., Freeman, T., Kramer, W., and Golombok, S. (2009). 'The experiences of adolescents and adults conceived by sperm donation: comparisons by age of disclosure and family type'. *Human Reproduction*, 24, 1909–19.

Jadva, V., Blake, L., Casey, P., Readings, J., Blake, L. and Golombok, S. (2011). 'A longitudinal study of recipients' views and experiences of intra-family egg donation'. *Human Reproduction*, 26, 2777–82.

Lessor, R. (1993). 'All in the family: social processes in ovarian egg donation between sisters'. *Sociology of Health and Illness*, 15, 393–413.

Lessor, R., Reitz, K., Balmaceda, J., and Asch, R. (1990). 'A survey of public attitudes towards egg donation between sisters'. *Human Reproduction*, 5, 889–92.

MacDougal, K. (2007). 'Strategies for disclosure: how parents approach telling their children that they were conceived with donor gametes'. *Fertility and Sterility*, 87, 524–33.

MacLeon, C. and Sherwin, S. (2000). 'Relational autonomy, self-trust in health care for patients who are oppressed', in C. Mackenzie and N. Stol-Jar (eds.), *Relational Autonomy: Feminist Perspectives on Autonomy, Agency and the Social Self.* New York: Oxford University Press.

Marshall, L. (2002). 'Ethical and legal issues in the use of related donors for therapeutic insemination'. *Urologic Clinics of North America*, 29, 855–61.

Mayeda, M. (2006). 'Present state of reproductive medicine in Japan – ethical issues with a focus on those seen in court cases'. *Biomed Central Medical Ethics*, 7, 1–16.

Moorhead, J. (2009). 'My sister's egg gave me a baby'. *The Guardian*. 22 August.

Mullen, M. (2001). 'What oocyte donors aren't told?' *American Journal of Bioethics*, 4, 1–2.

Murray. C. and Golombok, S. (2003). 'To tell or not to tell: the decision-making process of egg donation parents'. *Human Fertility*, 6, 89–95.

Nikolettos, N., Assimakopoulos, B. and Hatzissabas, I. (2003). 'Intrafamilial sperm donation: ethical questions and concerns'. *Human Reproduction*, 18, 933–6.

Pennings, G. (2001). 'Incest, gamete donation by siblings and the importance of the genetic link'. *Reproductive Biomedicine Online*, 4, 13–15.

Purewal, S. and van den Akker, O. (2009). 'Systematic review of oocyte donation: investigating attitudes, motivations and experiences'. *Human Reproduction Update*, 15, 499–515.

Rumball, A. and Adair, V. (1999). 'Telling the story: parents' scripts for donor offspring'. *Human Reproduction*, 14, 1392–9.

Sauer, H. (1988). 'Survey of attitudes regarding the use of siblings for gamete donation'. *Fertility and Sterility*, 49, 721–2.

Smart, C. (2009). 'Family secrets: law and understandings of openness in everyday relationships'. *Journal of Social Policy*, 38, 551–67.

Solomon, G., Johnson, S., Zaitchik, D. and Carey, S. (1996). 'Like father, like son: young children's understanding of how and why offspring resemble their parents'. *Child Development*, 67, 151–71.

Sureau, C. and Shenfield, F. (1995). 'Should gamete donation between family members be restricted?: Oocyte donation by a daughter'. *Human Reproduction*, 10, 1334.

Titmuss, R. M. (1970). *The Gift Relationship: From Human Blood to Social Policy.* Harmondsworth: Pelican.

Turner, A. J. and Coyle, A. (2000). 'What does it mean to be a donor offspring? The identity experiences of adults conceived by donor insemination and the implications for counselling and therapy'. *Human Reproduction*, 15, 2041–51.

Van Berkel, D., Candido, A. and Pijffers, W. H. (2007). 'Becoming a mother by non-anonymous egg donation: secrecy and the relationship between egg recipient, egg donor and egg donation child'. *Journal of Psychosomatic Obstetrics and Genecology*, 28, 97–104.

Warnock, M. (1987). 'The good of the child'. *Bioethics*, 2, 141–55.

Warren, N. and Blood, J. (2003). 'Who donates? Why donate? An exploration of the characteristics and motivations of known egg donors: the Victoria Australia experience'. *Journal of Fertility and Counselling*, 10, 2–24.

Watts, J. (2003). 'Panel advises against egg and sperm donations from siblings'. *The Lancet*, 361, 1532.

Weinberg, R. (2008). 'The moral responsibility of sperm donation'. *Bioethics*, 22, 166–78.

Williams, J. and Smith, L. (2010). 'Concept of kinship relations and inheritance in childhood and adolescence'. *British Journal of Developmental Psychology*, 28, 523–46.

Winter, A. and Daniluk, J. A. (2004). 'A gift from the heart: the experiences of women whose egg donations helped their sisters become mothers'. *Journal of Counseling and Development*, 82, 483–95.

Yee, S., Hitkari, J. and Greenblatt, E. (2007). 'A follow-up study of women who donated oocytes to known recipient couples for altruistic reasons'. *Human Reproduction*, 22, 2040–50.

LEGISLATION

Deceased Wife's Sister Marriage Act 1907
Human Fertilisation and Embryology Act 1990, as amended
Marriage (Prohibited Degrees of Relationship) Act 2004
Sexual Offences Act 2003
The Marriage Act 1835

11 ARTs and the single parent

Susanna Graham and Andrea Braverman

What are single parents by choice?

Single parents by choice (SPCs) are single men (single fathers by choice), or women (single mothers by choice), who actively choose to parent a child without a partner. The term single mother by choice (SMC) has been used to describe a distinct group of women who differ in a number of ways from mothers who either conceive accidently or become single after separation or divorce (Chan *et al.*, 1998; Mannis, 1999; Murray and Golombok, 2005a, 2005b). They are often older women, predominantly heterosexual, in their thirties and forties, well educated and financially independent (Murray and Golombok, 2005a, 2005b; Hertz, 2006; Jadva *et al.*, 2009a). There is currently a dearth of academic literature concerning single fathers by choice (SFCs) and little is known about such men or the children they raise.

Routes to single parenthood by choice

An SPC decides to have a child knowing that they will parent that child, at least initially, without a partner. This can be achieved via various routes and does not necessarily have to incorporate the use of Assisted Reproductive Technologies (ARTs). A woman could embark upon single motherhood by choice through sexual intercourse, donor insemination (DI) at a clinic, self-insemination with a known or anonymous donor, as well as through adoption or fostering (Bock, 2000; Hertz, 2006). Research has shown that different women choose different methods depending upon their circumstances, the options available to them and their beliefs about the morality of different methods. For example, some women may feel it is wrong to deceive a man by purposefully getting pregnant through a sexual encounter (Bock, 2000; Murray and Golombok, 2005a) while others feel that adoption is a morally superior route to single motherhood (Mannis,

1999; Morrissette, 2008). However, for many women adoption is seen as a last resort (Hertz, 2006), wanting instead to experience pregnancy and have genetically related children. Indeed, Jadva *et al.* (2009a), in their survey of 291 women using the US-based website 'choice moms', found that the most common method used to become an SMC was DI at a clinic: single motherhood by choice was most commonly pursued through the use of ARTs.

The choices available to single men wishing to embark upon parenthood alone are more limited. Unless he wishes to pursue adoption or fostering, he will also need to access ARTs. To become an SFC to his own biological child, a man requires the assistance of at least one woman to act as a surrogate and, if he wants to separate the genetics and gestation, the additional assistance of an egg donor and IVF team.

The ethical debate

This chapter will focus on the ethical debate surrounding single men and women becoming parents through the use of ARTs. This phenomenon has sparked much debate, encapsulating arguments surrounding reproductive rights (Correia and Broderick, 2009), the welfare of resulting offspring, non-discrimination against unmarried individuals and professional autonomy (Ethics Committee of the American Society for Reproductive Medicine, 2009) as well as the issues already inherent in the use of surrogacy and donated gametes (see Chapters 13 and 16). In essence, when discussing the acceptability of single parenthood by choice through ARTs, the rights of the single person to have access to care to conceive are weighed against the welfare of the resulting child.

The experience of parenthood is considered to be central to the individual identity and life-plan of most people in most societies (Boivin and Pennings, 2005). There is no reason to assume that just because a man or woman is single, they do not have an interest in having children, nor that the desire for a genetic link to one's child is weaker for single men and women than it is with married heterosexual couples. Parenthood is generally considered a liberty right (Robinson, 1997; Boivin and Pennings, 2005), indicating that other persons, or the state, should not interfere with a person's choice to have, or not have, children. Adhering to this liberty right, one should not interfere with a single person's choice to parent. Indeed, many children are coitally conceived by single persons, as they are able to have children without the assistance of ARTs.

However, if a woman chooses to be an SPC and does not have a donor for home insemination or coitus or if a man does not have an available traditional surrogate, should these individuals be able to access clinic-based ARTs for assistance in becoming a single parent? Should donor gametes and surrogacy be available to single persons who request them, not as a result of infertility, but a desire to parent their own biological child without a partner? The fact that these single men and women are making an active choice to parent alone, and doing so in a way that separates reproduction from sex, means that other individuals are involved in the creation of the SPC family. The concern in facilitating such a family form is that it might put the welfare of the child into jeopardy. Does being raised by single parents harm children? What is the effect of the knowledge that half one's genetic parentage is from an egg or sperm donor? Does a single person's wish for their own genetic child outweigh the child's right to know their genetic parentage?

By discussing such questions, this chapter will outline some of the criticisms raised against single parenthood by choice via ARTs, exploring how the phenomenon is represented in popular discourse and how this informs ethical debate. It will explore what we know about the men and women who embark upon single parenthood by choice, their motivations and experiences, and how these relate to the criticisms of their choice. This will provide insights into the issues at play for the individuals involved in these emerging family forms, going beyond ethical principles, to see what is at stake for them. Research detailing the well-being of children in these families will be presented, and its implications for our discussion of the acceptability of the use of ARTs by single persons explored. Finally, we will argue that, although there is very limited research, there is no evidence to suggest that single parenthood by choice causes harm to the children conceived, and therefore no compelling evidence to suggest that access to ARTs should not be available to single people. However, as will be shown throughout this chapter, these emerging family forms call into question our ideas regarding family, motherhood and fatherhood, and the responsibilities they entail. Perhaps the most important voice to hear is that of the child conceived into the SPC family, the child whose father is a sperm donor, or the child who has been raised by their father but conceived with the help of an egg donor and surrogate. What are their views, their experiences of their family form? Although there is currently no evidence to suggest that ARTs should not be available to single people or that there should be a 'Big Brother' approach to prohibiting single people from conceiving spontaneously, we need comprehensive research following the effects of such family forms.

Single parenthood by choice and the ideal family

Much of the concern surrounding single men and women making an active decision to become SPCs pertains to our ideals of what we think a family *should* be like. ARTs have become widespread amongst infertile heterosexual couples but their role in creating families consisting of single parents has generated a debate regarding who should have access to these technologies and what sort of families should be formed through their use. Unfamiliar or novel concepts are often evaluated in terms of divergence from the norm (Moscovici, 1984 in Correia and Broderick, 2009). Consequently, in the case of SMCs or SFCs, these family forms are compared to the 'gold standard' family: the traditional nuclear family with its mother, father and genetically related children. This traditional imagery constructs the father as the provider while the mother stays at home to raise her coitally conceived children. Of course, this idea has already been challenged and markedly redefined with the advent of high divorce and out-of-wedlock birth rates, as well as adoption, heterosexual couples using third-party ARTs, and women's rights movements. However, despite shifts in our ideas of what a family constitutes, and the reality that family forms are indeed changing, the deviances from this 'gold standard' remain prominent in the debate regarding ARTs and emerging family forms. The choice to create a family that diverges from this norm is criticized; the nuclear family is depicted as 'natural' and 'good' while families such as the single mother or father by choice or, indeed by circumstance, are deemed 'unnatural' and 'bad' (Correia and Broderick, 2009).

The welfare of the child: do children need a mother and a father?

Through focusing upon the deviances away from the nuclear family ideal, the popular discourse surrounding SPCs has emphasized the negative effects the lack of both a mother and a father could have on a resulting child. US SMC, Louise Sloan (2007), for example, was described as 'the epitome of selfishness' for 'deliberately handicapping' her future child by 'condemning him to a fatherless life' (Weathers, 2007). The importance of fathers also caused much debate when the Human Fertilisation and Embryology Act 1990, as amended 2008, removed the requirement for clinics to consider a child's 'need for a father' in decisions about whether or not to offer fertility treatment, and instead replaced it with the 'need for supportive parenting'. The Act was described by Conservative MP Iain Duncan Smith as 'the last nail in the coffin for traditional family life' (Gamble, 2009) and as another blow for fatherhood.

The need for a father

The presumption that a child needs a father draws on stereotypes about what mothering and fathering entail, as well as a vast body of literature concerning the outcomes for children raised in single-parent families. Studies comparing differences in parenting between mothers and fathers have shown that mothers spend more time interacting with their children (Yeung, 2001; Hawkins *et al.*, 2006) and that fathering involves more breadwinning, stereotypical masculine tasks and play with children (Hawkins *et al.*, 2006). The conclusion drawn is that men and women parent in different ways and these are both vital to child psychological and gender development. The importance placed on a child's need for a father has also been inferred from research comparing father present and father absent families: children raised in families headed by a married heterosexual couple have been compared with those raised in single mother families formed through divorce or separation. Such research has shown that children growing up in single mother families are more likely than children living with continuously married parents to experience a variety of cognitive, emotional and behavioural problems (Dunn *et al.*, 1998; Amato, 2005; Coleman and Glenn, 2009). Thus the 'essential father' theory has evolved: the father is a disciplinarian, problem solver, and playmate who provides crucially masculine parenting. Proponents have claimed that boys need fathers to develop appropriate masculine identity and to inhibit antisocial behaviours and girls need fathers to help deter promiscuity, teen pregnancy and substance abuse (Blankenhorn, 1995; Popenoe, 1996).

The negative outcomes for children in these single-parent families have been presumed to be applicable to SMC families and therefore the ethics of actively choosing to parent a child in the absence of an available father has been questioned. However, many of the poor outcomes detailed in this research can be attributed to socio-economic disadvantage, conflict, maternal depression and lack of social support. With SMCs found to be financially secure (Murray and Golombok, 2005a; Hertz, 2006; Jadva *et al.*, 2009a), no more likely to experience psychological difficulties than married mothers using DI (Murray and Golombok, 2005a) and well supported (Hertz, 2006; Jadva *et al.*, 2009a), as well as their children not experiencing the conflict, nor the 'father loss' that follows from a divorce or separation, these negative outcomes may not apply to children in SMC families. In addition, research has not identified any gender-exclusive parenting abilities (Biblarz and Stacey, 2010); married mothers and fathers may differ in their parenting styles within the traditional division of labour, but this does not mean that women can't or won't take on these traditionally masculine parenting traits and therefore questions the presumption that a child needs a father per se.

Gender bias

SFCs are, of course, also founding families with only one parent. At the heart of the criticisms of single fatherhood by choice, however, is the implicit bias that fathers cannot 'mother' their children and that such mothering is essential for child development. Single mother homes, if still not seen as an ideal situation, have been modelled to be successful. However, similar models for men are rare, both in reality and the media. In the 1960s the show *My Three Sons* portrayed a single widowed father with his sons, and in the 1970s *The Courtship of Eddie's Father* also depicted a single widowed father. In both cases, being a single parent was not by choice but by circumstance. By 2003 *Two and a Half Men* depicted a divorced father *choosing* to be a single parent with his son. However, in most of the television shows, the family is dependent upon a female caregiver; the men are portrayed as incapable of parenting alone.

With the rarity of single father families by circumstance in the general population, the decision to actively seek lone fatherhood, the decision to 'deprive' their child a mother, appears to spark more criticism than single motherhood by choice. As Ian Mucklejohn, a British SFC with triplets conceived through egg donation and surrogacy in the USA, stated, 'If I was a woman no-one would be interested' (Whitney, 2001). Arguments have been made from both a psychoanalytic and socio-learning theory that healthy psychological development is impossible without a father (Grill, 2005). Ironically, theories do not even address the concept of an SFC, but the converse of these arguments may be assumed to hold true. If the concern for children raised by single mothers is focused upon the lack of an appropriate male role model and disciplinarian, the reverse would be concerns that a child would not have an appropriate female role model, nor a nurturing parent. Indeed, research comparing outcomes for children raised in single father and single mother-led families has shown that more single mothers than fathers were skilled at developmental styles of parenting and actively involved with their children (Buchanan *et al.*, 1992; Hall *et al.*, 1995; Hawkins *et al.*, 2006). However, these were not single parent by choice families and the single mother and father-led families compared in these studies were formed through vastly different processes, with single fathers often widowed or gaining custody of children due to concerns about the mother's ability to parent. Therefore, men who intend to parent their children without a mother from the outset may well differ substantially. Indeed, initial studies of gay male couples who parent show that these men are highly motivated in parenting and adopt parenting practices more feminine than do typical heterosexual fathers (Johnson and O'Connor, 2002), with some gay fathers even describing themselves engaging in 'mothering' (Mallon, 2004). It may be assumed that SFCs may be similar in this respect.

Does a child need two (known) parents?

Biblarz and Stacey's (2010) extensive review examining whether the gender of parents matter, that is whether a child needs a mother and a father, did not identify any gender-exclusive parenting abilities. It therefore appears that on a practical level a child may not need a father to be present in order to provide typically masculine parenting, but does this mean that a child does not need a *father*? In the UK a child conceived to a single woman by an unknown sperm donor at a licensed clinic will have no legal father: there will not be a man named on their birth certificate. In a context where the importance of fatherhood is being emphasised and there are moves to encourage men to take on rights and responsibilities by requiring a father's name on birth certificates (Welfare Reform Act 2009), the total absence of a father, in name or person, in SMC families sets these apart from most other single parent families where there is a father but he is living apart from his children. Proponents such as Velleman have claimed that 'gamete donation purposefully severs a connection of the sort that normally informs a person's sense of identity' (2005: 363). When single men or women use anonymously donated gametes to become parents, their children are not only being brought up without a man or woman acting as their social father or mother but also without the knowledge of their genetic parent that Velleman argues is necessary for their pursuit of self-knowledge and identity formation. Do children conceived through donated gametes to single parents by choice feel the need to know about or even form a relationship with their other genetic parent? Children may not need the practical influence of both a mother and a father, but do they need to know who these genetic parents are for their own identity formation? Moreover, Biblarz and Stacey conclude that although the gender of the parents does not seem to matter, 'compared to all other family forms, families headed by (at least) two committed, compatible parents are generally best for children' (2010: 17). Rather than focusing the debate pertaining to the ethics of single parenthood by choice on the idea that a child has a specific need for a mother and a father, we should perhaps be questioning whether a child is harmed by only having one (known) parent.

Buying babies

Single parenthood by choice, as achieved through ARTs, creates single-parent families in novel ways. Rather than being formed after separation or bereavement, in the case of single parents by circumstance, single parenthood by choice is actively sought from the outset. It is this active choice that at times provokes criticism: rather than single motherhood being an unfortunate circumstance to find oneself in, and men blamed for their absenteeism, women who make the decision to become a single mother with ARTs can be seen to be actively negating men from family life. Of course this active intention to become a single mother and the fact that the women seeking it are older professional women may not be novel. Indeed, an investigation that focused upon the single-parent families in the National Child Development Study, which traces the development of 17,500 children born in the UK during one week in 1958, found that almost half of the mothers of illegitimate children were 30 years of age or over when their child was born (Ferri, 1976). We do not know the method by which these children were conceived, nor whether there was a desire for the father to be involved, but these women certainly seem to share some of the characteristics of what we now call SMCs. What is novel about single motherhood by choice, therefore, is perhaps not the social practice of an older, professional single woman deliberately becoming a single parent but the concept of this family form itself. The term 'single mother by choice', coined by Jane Mattes to describe the support group she and fellow single mothers founded in 1982, describes a collection of 'single women who *chose* to become mothers; single mothers who are mature and responsible and who feel empowered rather than victimized' (Mattes, 1997: xxi). It is the public expression of this *choice*, the phenomenon becoming more visible within society, both in terms of single women openly accessing formal ART services and the attention it is given in the media,[1] which makes single motherhood by choice a novel, emerging family form.

This active *choice* to become a single mother brings concerns not just for the welfare of the child but also the way in which this family has been formed. A *Daily Mail* article, provocatively entitled, 'Daddies be Damned' (Davies, 2009), portrayed SMCs as using men solely for their genetic contribution to the resulting child; they didn't want a father for their child, they just wanted to choose a man who could provide good genes. In the USA, with its privatized commercial fertility business, single women can literally browse hundreds of donor profiles with detailed descriptions of their medical and family history, personality traits, hobbies and baby pictures before paying vast amounts of money for the donor of their choice. One single mother described picking a 'father' from a catalogue of sperm donors as 'a strange and somewhat creepy process' with a feeling of 'sheer consumerism' as if she were 'buying a baby' (Soiseth, 2008: 103–4). Despite the highly regulated UK fertility system where there is little information available about prospective donors, single British women attending private clinics for DI still draw the criticism of consumerism. Many of the public comments to the *Daily Mail* article (Davies, 2009) described SMCs as selfish career women who wanted the latest, must-have accessory: a baby. The choice to parent alone is likened to loveless 'designer breeding ... having it all as if it was a right' and it is suggested that these women should 'spend their money on another Prada handbag ... not a person with feelings and needs' (A reader's response to Davies, 2009). Single women, even those with medically diagnosed infertility, are very unlikely to have their treatment funded by the NHS and so if they want to pursue clinic-based ARTs, will need to do so in the private sector where they can face costs of £850 for donor sperm for their treatment cycle (London Sperm Bank, 2011) and over £800 for unstimulated intra-uterine insemination (IUI) or £3,400 plus the cost of drugs for IVF (Bridge, 2011). In the UK, where over 70 per cent of IVF treatment is performed in the private sector (HFEA, 2010), it is perhaps surprising that single women draw this consumer criticism whereas their married counterparts may not. The single women are perhaps seen as 'buying' goods at the private clinic, a child who they cannot have 'naturally', whereas heterosexual couples of reproductive age are viewed more sympathetically

---

[1] In 2010 alone, two Hollywood films, 'The Back-up Plan' and 'The Switch', and the British radio soap, 'The Archers,' depicted single professional women choosing to become mothers through the use of donor sperm.

with regards pursuing private fertility treatment in the context of their infertility and the 'postcode lottery' of NHS treatment.

Single fatherhood by choice, when achieved through ARTs, involves spending considerably larger amounts of money than single women using donor sperm. One man who used an egg donor and gestational surrogate to become an SFC reported spending $300,000 in the process (Bhattacharya, 2006). With such high costs and the ability to choose desirable traits in egg donors and surrogates comes the fear that children are becoming commodified.

The social use of ARTs

Of course the use of ARTs, and more specifically the use of donated gametes, to conceive children is not a new phenomenon. Heterosexual couples have long used DI to overcome male factor infertility. More recently surrogacy and egg donation have been used when a female partner cannot conceive or carry a pregnancy to term. Who should have access to these ARTs has, however, been the focus of much debate. In the British parliamentary discussions regarding the Human Fertilisation and Embryology (HFE) Bill some feared that donor insemination would be used by single women, lesbian couples or unmarried heterosexual couples and it was therefore proposed that assisted conception should be restricted to married couples. The House of Lords rejected this amendment to the bill by only one vote. It was in this context of unresolved discussion about who fertility treatment should be available to that the duty to consider the 'welfare of the child' and in particular 'the need of that child for a father' was added to the bill (Gamble, 2009).

At stake in the discussions of the HFE Act 1990 was a discussion not just about what sort of families could be formed with the use of ARTs but under what circumstances ARTs would be indicated. With single motherhood by choice, DI is not used for male factor infertility but because of the lack of a male partner; it is not used for medical reasons but social ones. Likewise, single fatherhood by choice requires an egg donor and gestational surrogate, not because of female infertility but due to the decision to father alone. Donor gametes are used as a means to have children without a partner of the opposite sex, not as a substitute for the gametes of an infertile partner. ART use by single persons is therefore constructed as a chance to become a parent, given the lack of a reproductive partner, rather than a medical necessity brought about by a couple's infertility. With ARTs traditionally being indicated only in the presence of fertility problems, requests for ARTs by men and women without a medically defined fertility problem question how

ARTs should be used. Are ARTs a treatment for infertility or are they merely a means for an individual to have a (genetically related) child?

Using ARTs in the absence of infertility has been described as transgressing too many boundaries (Haimes and Weiner, 2000); the ideological, because of its apparent flouting of the importance of mothers or fathers; the structural, because of its advocacy of the one-parent household; and the biogenetic, because of its avoidance of sexual intercourse. Where third-party assisted reproduction has, in the past, been shrouded with secrecy, allowing the nuclear family ideal to be preserved, or at least the image of it, SPCs draw attention to the ART practice itself; there is no social father or mother to act as the genetic parent and so the question of 'where is my mother?' or 'where is my father?' becomes inevitable. The ethics of parenthood through gamete donation, the meaning of the gamete donor and/or surrogate in kinship terms and the impact of these novel family forms on the resulting child are all highlighted by single men or women being able to openly use ARTs to become single-parent families.

Single parents by choice – what do we know?

There is a small but growing body of literature concerning SMCs, their reasons for actively embarking upon single motherhood, their methods of doing so and experiences of motherhood, as well as a small number of studies examining the parent–child relationship and psychological development of children conceived to these women. There is not, as yet, a comparable body of literature regarding the single men who actively choose parenthood, nor the development of children in these families. As will be shown in the following sections, the existing literature concerning SPCs goes some way to addressing whether the welfare of the child in these family forms is at risk and therefore the ethics of single persons accessing ARTs. Indeed, many of the ethical concerns and public criticisms raised against single parenthood by choice are, in fact, concerns shared by many of the individuals who are embarking on this route to parenthood. Research indicates that these parents strive to do all they can to address and allay these concerns and protect the welfare of their own children.

The decision to become a single mother by choice

Contrary to views that the decision to become an SMC is a selfish, reckless choice (Davies, 2009), research has shown that the decision has, in fact, often been a lengthy, well-planned and purposeful one

(Mannis, 1999; Bock, 2000; Murray and Golombok, 2005a). The responsible nature of this decision-making process is often emphasized, with the women shown to make changes to their lifestyle, planning ahead to make sure they can provide both financially and emotionally for their child (Hertz and Ferguson, 1997; Bock, 2000; Hertz, 2006; Jadva *et al.*, 2009a). The women have often saved money, moved to a child-friendly neighbourhood, made changes to their career and ensured they have a good social network around them who can help with childcare (Hertz, 2006; Jadva *et al.*, 2009a). Indeed, in many of the self-help books on the market (see for example, Mattes, 1997; Sloan, 2007; Morrissette, 2008) sections are devoted to topics such as 'Am I single mother material?' and 'Can I afford it?', suggesting that one should only embark upon single motherhood if one is in a stable position to do so.

In relation to the ethical debate concerning single motherhood by choice's active divergence from the ideal nuclear family norm, it is interesting to see some SMCs actually trying to maintain inclusion in this norm. Bock, in her research detailing her participant observation in an SMC support group in California, describes a 'mother hierarchy' (2000: 83) where married, heterosexual and economically stable women who become mothers in their twenties and early thirties live within the 'charmed circle', while unmarried, lesbian, poor, or age-inappropriate mothers live in the outer limits. The SMCs in the support group tried to legitimize and normalize their positions as single mothers by aligning themselves as closely as possible with the nuclear family ideal rather than the single mothers that they felt society deemed problematic. These women argued for their place within this 'charmed circle' by virtue of the emotional maturity, financial stability and the planned nature of their conception that they believed justified them becoming mothers, even though their marital status and the lack of a partner and father for their child would generally preclude it (Bock, 2000). Whereas they believed other single mothers were chastised for being sexually promiscuous, lazy, unmotivated and dependent on welfare, by appropriating the term 'single mother by *choice*', these mid-life, middle-class, single women implicitly claimed their entitlement to motherhood (Bock, 2000).

In line with the argument that single people may have as much desire to parent as individuals in a married heterosexual relationship (Robinson, 1997; Boivin and Pennings, 2005; Correia and Broderick, 2009), the SMC literature suggests that the decision to embark upon motherhood alone seems to stem from an underlying desire to mother and nurture (Mannis, 1999; Murray and Golombok, 2005a; Jadva *et al.*,

2009a). However, despite Bock's (2000) participants appropriating the term 'single mother by *choice*' to legitimize their decision to mother alone, research suggests that this choice has only been made when these women realized that they were single and had limited prospects of finding a partner with whom to have a child in the time frame that their increasing age and decreasing fertility would allow (Hertz, 2006; Jadva *et al.*, 2009a). Many SMCs report they would have rather become mothers in the context of a relationship (Mannis, 1999; Bock, 2000; Hertz, 2006; Jadva *et al.*, 2009a; Murray and Golombok, 2005a), preferring a nuclear family arrangement to that of a single-parent family. In contrast to the view that women are purposefully denying a child a father, research therefore suggests that these single women only embark upon motherhood when they believe they are in a position to offer a child a stable family home and realize that their fertility will not let them wait any longer for the possibility of the nuclear family ideal.

Decision to become a single father by choice

With an absence of academic literature concerning single fatherhood by choice, nor a body of support groups and accompanying literature aimed at such men, little is known about the men who embark on this choice, nor their motivations and experiences. However, one pundit in the USA commented that:

the main reason why men (or straight men, anyway) want to have children through a surrogate [is] so they can be assured that they won't lose the child upon divorce or separation. A woman can have a child and know that unless the situation is exceptional or she behaves outrageously, she'll always be a regular part of her child's life. For men, being a father is a roll of the dice – if mom decides she doesn't want you around anymore, it can be hard to preserve your relationship with your child ... something the mainstream media doesn't like to talk about (Sacks, 2009).

In clinical practice, men presenting to be SPCs often cite similar reasons to those voiced by their female counterparts. Men state that they are ready to be a parent, indicating that the biological clock is one comprised of emotions about readiness to parent and concerns about being a 'too old' parent, not just biological capacity to reproduce. Ironically, examples of older fathers abound and these emotions may be dismissed or their importance diminished through the prejudice that the age of the father is not as imperative as that of the mother. However, as all single parents consider their anticipated longevity, age is just as critical a consideration as fertility for both single mothers and fathers by choice.

Experiences of single mothers by choice

In contrast to the view that single-parent families are resource-, time- and social capital-lacking, initial research suggests that this is not in fact the case. Small-scale studies in the UK and the USA, as well as a much larger web-based survey, have found that SMCs tend to be financially stable (Mannis, 1999; Murray and Golombok, 2005a; Jadva *et al.*, 2009a) and although these women have decided to parent their child without a partner, this does not mean that they are unsupported in their parenting. Women in these studies reported that they got much support from friends and family (Hertz and Ferguson, 1997; Jadva *et al.*, 2009a) and instead of relying upon a nuclear family arrangement, pulled together an ensemble of people to support them. SMCs have reported that they have no more difficulties than other mothers (Jadva *et al.*, 2009a) with some even stating they had fewer difficulties and enjoyed being able to make their own decisions about parenting techniques as well as devoting all their time and attention to the child without taking a partner's needs and wants into consideration. From this limited research, it seems that SMC families may not experience the difficulties they are assumed to face.

The role of the 'father'

Much of the ethical concern regarding single motherhood by choice has focused upon a child's need for a father. This also seems to be something that SMCs are themselves concerned about. Despite these children not having a 'father' in the traditional sense of the word, research has indicated that SMCs go out of their way to make sure their children have a balanced upbringing that includes a male influence. Of the SMCs who took part in Jadva *et al.*'s (2009a) online questionnaire about their experiences of single motherhood, 74 per cent were concerned about their child growing up without a father. The women thought it was important for their children to have male role models and a large majority stated that their child had such a role model in their life. Trying to counteract the absence of a father by making sure male role models are available to their children is also a theme prominent in other studies (see for example Hertz and Ferguson, 1997; Hertz, 2002, 2006; Murray and Golombok, 2005a).

In addition to men being involved as role models, the importance SMCs seem to place on being open and honest with their child about their conception (Murray and Golombok, 2005a; Jadva *et al.*, 2009b) has meant sperm donors also become physically or metaphorically visible within some families (Hertz, 2002; 2006). DI, when used by heterosexual couples, has traditionally been surrounded with secrecy and shame and despite advice that parents should tell their offspring about their donor conception, few disclose such information (see Appleby, Blake and Freeman, Chapter 13). This therefore raises questions regarding children's right to know their conception details and genetic heritage. SMCs, however, appear to be much more likely to disclose their use of DI than heterosexual couples (Klock *et al.*, 1996; Brewaeys, 2001; Scheib *et al.*, 2005; Murray and Golombok, 2005a, 2005b; Jadva *et al.*, 2009b) and do so at an earlier age (Jadva *et al.*, 2009b). The absence of a father in these families also makes it more likely that the child, as well as friends and family, will enquire about the child's origins. Indeed, according to Mattes (1997), SMC and author of a best selling guidebook for single women who are considering or have chosen motherhood, what to tell children about their fathers – 'the daddy question' – is the biggest concern of SMCs and a topic covered at length in other SMC self-help literature (see, for example, Sloan, 2007; Morrissette, 2008). Moreover, as mentioned earlier, when single women use donor sperm, the semen sample is no longer just a 'treatment' for a man's infertility but a means to pregnancy without a male partner. Another man does not claim the role of father and therefore the sperm donor is more likely to be publicly represented as the child's father (Kirkman, 2004). This therefore brings other issues into play; rather than the traditional secrecy surrounding sperm donation, SMC children have to construct meaning and roles for the man whose sperm their mother used to conceive them. Is a sperm donor a father? If there is no other man to take on this role, should a donor take on the rights and responsibilities fatherhood entails? What would the offspring in SMC families expect from their sperm donor if meeting them later in life? It appears that donor-conceived children from single-mother households are more likely to use the terms 'dad' or 'father' to describe their donor than children from two-parent families (Scheib *et al.*, 2005; Jadva *et al.*, 2009b). However, what 'dad' or 'father' means to these children remains unknown.

Far from men, and fathers, being rejected and invisible from SMC families, it appears that men are actively incorporated into daily life. Moreover, the single-mother household is often seen as a temporary status. Murray and Golombok (2005a) found that most of the single mothers who had used DI in their study hoped to find a partner in the future; they wanted companionship for themselves and a father for their child. The temporary nature of single motherhood by choice is also a concept discussed by Hertz (2006), and the possibility of dating after becoming a SMC is an issue covered in many of the support books

(Mattes, 1997; Sloan, 2007; Morrissette, 2008). Whether most SMCs do form a stable partnership and provide a social father for their children remains to be seen.

The children of single parents by choice

Despite research suggesting that SMCs endeavour to ensure their children have male role models and are open about the method of conception used, concern remains regarding the welfare of children conceived to single parents by choice. There has been a paucity of research regarding the development of children in SMC families and even fewer long-term follow-up studies following these children into adolescence and adulthood. Weissenberg *et al.* (2007) found that the socio-economic well-being of young children born to SMCs in Israel was within normal limits. Likewise, children conceived to single women via DI in the USA were found to be developing well at age 7 (Chan *et al.*, 1998). The cross-sectional study did not find any difference between DI-conceived children raised by single women, heterosexual or lesbian couples in terms of psychological adjustment, social competence or behavioural problems as reported by parents as well as teachers.

A long-term follow-up of a small sample of single-parent families in the UK (Golombok *et al.*, 1997; MacCallum and Golombok, 2004; Golombok and Badger, 2010) did not address SMCs per se, but single-parent families where the child had been raised since the first year of life without the presence of the father, or a father-figure, in a financially stable family home. The solo mother families were found to be similar to lesbian mother and traditional families in a range of measures assessing quality of parenting and child psychological adjustment at age 6 (Golombok *et al.*, 1997), 12 (MacCallum and Golombok, 2004) and 18 (Golombok and Badger, 2010). In early adulthood those from solo mother households showed lower levels of anxiety, depression, hostility and problematic alcohol use than their counterparts from traditional families and the same levels as those brought up in lesbian-couple families. Not all these women had actively chosen to parent alone, however, and nor had they all used ARTs. Therefore, although the results from this small sample may be applicable to children raised by SMCs, additional issues faced by being donor-conceived, that is the father being a sperm donor rather than a man the mother had a relationship with, may have an impact upon children, and subsequently adults, conceived to single women using donor sperm.

Longitudinal studies specifically exploring the parenting and psychological development of children born to single British women who have used DI (Murray and Golombok, 2005a, 2005b) have only followed children until 2 years of age. At this time the children were found to be functioning well, showing fewer emotional and behavioural problems than a matched comparison group of DI children with two heterosexual parents. The single mothers were also found to show greater joy and pleasure in their child and lower levels of anger than mothers who used DI while in a heterosexual relationship. How the children will fare as they grow up and understand the choice their mother made remains to be seen, however.

There is currently no research relating to SFCs and, consequently, there is only clinical anecdote at this time. Research is therefore needed to understand the motivations of, and issues faced by, SFCs. Moreover, long-term follow-up studies of both single father and mother by choice families are needed. Very little is known about the offspring raised in these family forms, their experiences, thoughts and feelings and how these might change over time. Although initial data from studies exploring adolescents' experiences of being donor-conceived (see Scheib et al., 2005; Jadva et al., 2009b) show that the majority of those with single mothers learnt about their origins early on and were comfortable with their donor-conceived status, it is important to bear in mind that others feel quite upset by the nature of their conception. As one donor-conceived young adult stated, 'The fact that my mother wanted a genetic connection with a child but didn't mind that she was denying me my connection to my father makes me very upset' (Jadva et al., 2009b: 1914). How do the offspring of SPCs feel about the decisions their parents made? What do they think about the sperm donor and how do they feel about not having a father in the traditional sense? How do they feel about the prospect of meeting this man at age 18, or in the case of truly anonymous donors never being able to meet him at all? How would a child feel knowing that their father had used an egg donor and a surrogate to conceive them and paid vast amounts of money for the process? These are all important questions to be taken into consideration when considering the welfare of offspring born to single parents by choice.

Issues for the future

Although studies concerning single parenthood by choice are small in number and limited in scope, there is currently no evidence to suggest that these single parents cause undue burden or harm to their children.

The Ethics Committee of the American Society for Reproductive Medicine's (2009) summary of their position is clear that single persons should not be discriminated against with regard to ARTs:

- 'Single individuals, unmarried heterosexual couples, and gay and lesbian couples have interests in having and rearing children.
- There is no persuasive evidence that children are harmed or disadvantaged solely by being raised by single parents, unmarried parents, or gay and lesbian parents.
- Data do not support restricting access to assisted reproductive technologies on the basis of a prospective parent's marital status or sexual orientation.'

It is therefore possible for single people to access ARTs in the USA. However, availability and legality varies tremendously across countries and can differ for single women and men. In the UK, for example, single women can access treatment with donor sperm. However, men in the UK would currently encounter problems becoming SFCs via surrogacy: a single person cannot apply for the parental order needed to grant parenthood to them and extinguish the legal mother status of the surrogate mother.

Even if ART availability becomes unproblematic for single people, arguments about the built-in bias of financial discrimination may well continue to exist. The high costs encountered in treatment, especially with regard to SFCs, mean that clinic-based ARTs are only available to well-off single men and women. Single parenthood by choice, therefore, becomes a stratified possibility. A single person may have adequate financial capacity to raise a child but not to pay the vast sums in order to conceive through clinic-based ARTs and the legal and safety benefits that the clinic provides. In the UK, single women may find themselves considering home insemination with a known donor, or sperm procured from internet matching sites in order to avoid the high costs involved in clinic-based ARTs, but then find themselves negotiating the donor's legal position and contact with the child. Public funding of ARTs, especially in the current economic climate, is likely to remain problematic. With scarce resources, monetary-wise as well as the shortage of donated gametes, issues of rationing come into play. Is becoming an SPC a lifestyle choice that should therefore only be available in the private market? Or do single people have as much right to be helped in their desire to have children as those individuals who are part of a heterosexual couple and have found that they have difficulty conceiving? These are issues that remain unresolved.

Regardless of access and affordability, as single parenthood by choice continues to grow as a family-building option, long-term follow-up of such children is greatly needed for a genuine discussion about the ethics of this choice, especially from the child's own perspective. As our ideas about motherhood, fatherhood and family formation evolve over time, with and without the aid of ARTs, so too are the issues we feel are at stake in these emerging family forms. In the interim, it is important to note that these parents by choice are bringing children into the world that are wanted and loved.

REFERENCES

Amato, P. (2005). 'The impact of family formation change on the cognitive, social, and emotional well-being of the next generation'. *Future of Children*, 15, 75–96.

Bhattacharya, S. (2006). 'Surrogacy and the single dad. The hunt for a family can take some unexpected turns'. *Boise Weekly*. Available at: www.boiseweekly.com/gyrobase/surrogacy-and-the-single-dad/Content?oid=930284 (accessed 15 June 2010).

Biblarz, T. and Stacey, J. (2010). 'How does the gender of parents matter?' *Journal of Marriage and Family*, 72, 3–22.

Blankenhorn, D. (1995). *Fatherless America: Confronting our Most Urgent Social Problem*. New York: Basic Books.

Bock, J. (2000). 'Doing the right thing? Single mothers by choice and the struggle for legitimacy'. *Gender and Society*, 14, 62–86.

Boivin, J. and Pennings, G. (2005). 'Parenthood should be regarded as a right'. *Archives of Disease in Childhood*, 90, 784–5.

Brewaeys, A. (2001). 'Review: parent-child relationships and child development in donor insemination families'. *Human Reproduction Update*, 7, 28–46.

Bridge (2011). *IVF, fertility and infertility treatment by the London Bridge fertility, gynaecology and genetic centre. Prices*. Available at: www.thebridgecentre. co.uk/06_prices/prices.htm#ivficsi (accessed 2 March 2011).

Buchanan, C., Maccoby, E. and Dornbusch, S. (1992). 'Adolescents and their families after divorce: three residential arrangements compared'. *Journal of Research on Adolescence*, 2, 261–91.

Chan, R. W., Raboy, B. and Patterson, C. J. (1998). 'Psychosocial adjustment among children conceived via donor insemination by lesbian and heterosexual mothers'. *Child Development*, 69, 443–57.

Coleman, L. and Glenn, F. (2009). *When Couples Part: Understanding the Consequences for Adults and Children*. London: One Plus One.

Correia, H. and Broderick, P. (2009). 'Access to reproductive technologies by single women and lesbians: social representations and public debate'. *Journal of Community and Applied Social Psychology*, 19, 241–56.

Davies, B. (2009). 'Daddies be Damned!' *The Daily Mail*, 31 October.

Dunn, J., Deater-Deckard, K., Pickering, K. and O'Connor, T. (1998). 'Children's adjustment and prosocial behaviour in step-, single-parent and non-stepfamily settings: findings from a community study'. *Journal of Child Psychology and Psychiatry*, 39, 1083–1095.

Ethics Committee of the American Society for Reproductive Medicine (2009). 'Access to fertility treatment by gays, lesbians and unmarried persons'. *Fertility and Sterility*, 92, 1190–3.

Ferri, E. (1976). *Growing Up in a One-Parent Family.* Windsor: NFER Publishing Company.

Gamble, N. (2009). 'Considering the need for a father: the role of clinicians in safeguarding family values in UK fertility treatment'. *Reproductive Biomedicine Online* 19, 15–18.

Golombok, S., Tasker, F. and Murray, C. (1997). 'Children raised in fatherless families from infancy: family relationships and the socioemotional development of children of lesbian single and heterosexual mothers'. *Journal of Child Psychology and Psychiatry*, 38, 783–91.

Golombok, S. and Badger, S. (2010). 'Children raised in mother-headed families from infancy: a follow-up of children of lesbian and single heterosexual mothers, at early adulthood'. *Human Reproduction*, 25, 150–7.

Grill, E. A. (2005). 'Treating Single Mothers by Choice', in A. Rosen and J. Rosen (eds.), *Frozen Dreams: Psychodynamic Dimensions of Infertility and Assisted Reproduction.* Hillsdale: The Analytic Press.

Haimes, E. and Weiner, K. (2000). 'Everybody's got a dad ...'. Issues for lesbian families in the management of donor insemination'. *Sociology of Health and Illness*, 22, 477–99.

Hall, L., Walker, A. and Acock, A. (1995). 'Gender and family work in one-parent households'. *Journal of Marriage and the Family*, 57, 685–92.

Hawkins, D., Amato, P. and King, V. (2006). 'Parent-adolescent involvement: The relative influence of parent gender and residence'. *Journal of Marriage and Family*, 68, 125– 36.

Hertz, R. (2002). 'The father as an idea: a challenge to kinship boundaries by single mothers'. *Symbolic Interaction*, 25, 1–31.
  (2006). *Single by Chance, Mothers by Choice. How Women Are Choosing Parenthood without Marriage and Creating the New American Family.* New York: Oxford University Press.

Hertz, R. and Ferguson, F. (1997). 'Kinship strategies and self-sufficiency among single mothers by choice: post modern family ties'. *Qualitative Sociology*, 20, 187–209.

Human Fertilisation and Embryology Authority (HFEA) (2010). *Human Fertilisation and Embryology Authority Statistics.* London: HFEA.

Jadva, V., Badger, S., Morrissette, M. and Golombok, S. (2009a). '"Mom by choice, single by life's circumstance..." Findings from a large-scale survey of the experiences of single mothers by choice'. *Human Fertility*, 12, 175–84.

Jadva, V., Freeman, T., Kramer, W. and Golombok, S. (2009b). 'The experiences of adolescents and adults conceived by sperm donation: comparisons by age of disclosure and family type'. *Human Reproduction*, 24, 1909–19.

Johnson, S. and O'Connor, E. (2002). *The Gay Baby-Boom: The Psychology of Gay Parenthood*. New York University Press.

Kirkman, M. (2004). 'Saviours and satyrs: ambivalence in narrative meanings of sperm provision'. *Culture, Health and Sexuality*, 6, 319–35.

Klock, S. C., Jacob, M. C. and Maier, D. (1996). 'A comparison of single and married recipients of donor insemination'. *Human Reproduction*, 11, 2554–7.

London Sperm Bank (2011). *Looking for Donated Sperm?* Available at: www. londonspermbankdonors.com (accessed 2 March 2011).

MacCallum, F. and Golombok, S. (2004). 'Children raised in fatherless families from infancy: a follow-up of children of lesbian and single heterosexual mothers at early adolescence'. *Journal of Child Psychology and Psychiatry*, 45, 1407–19.

Mallon, G. (2004). *Gay Men Choosing Parenthood*. New York: Columbia University Press.

Mannis, V. S. (1999). 'Single mothers by choice'. *Family Relations*, 48, 121–8.

Mattes, J. (1997). *Single Mothers by Choice. A Guidebook for Single Women Who Are Considering or Have Chosen Motherhood*. New York: Three Rivers Press.

Morrissette, M. (2008). *Choosing Single Motherhood. The Thinking Woman's Guide*. New York: Houghton Mifflin Company.

Murray, C. and Golombok, S. (2005a). 'Going it alone: solo mothers and their infants conceived by donor insemination'. *American Journal of Orthopsychiatry*, 2, 242–53.

Murray, C. and Golombok, S. (2005b). 'Solo mothers and their donor insemination infants: follow-up at age 2 years'. *Human Reproduction*, 20, 1655–60.

Popenoe, D. (1996). *Life Without Father: Compelling New Evidence that Fatherhood and Marriage Are Indispensible for the Good of Children and Society*. New York: Free Press.

Robinson, B. (1997). 'Birds do it. Bees do it. So why not single women and lesbians?' *Bioethics*, 11, 217–27.

Sacks, D. (2009). 'And now, single fatherhood by choice'. Available at: http://deanesmay.com/2009/01/05/and-now-single-fatherhood-by-choice/ (accessed 30 June 2010).

Scheib, J. E., Riordan, M. and Rubin, S. (2005). 'Adolescents with open-identity sperm donors: reports from 12–17 year olds'. *Human Reproduction*, 20, 239–52.

Sloan, L. (2007). *No Man? No Problem! Knock Yourself Up. A Tell-All Guide to Becoming a Single Mom*. New York: Penguin Group.

Soiseth, A. (2008). *Choosing You. Deciding to Have a Baby on my Own*. Berkley: Seal Press.

Velleman, J. D. (2005). 'Family history'. *Philosophical Papers*, 34, 357–78.

Weathers, H. (2007). 'Dads? Who needs them?' *The Daily Mail*, 29 November 2007.

Weissenberg, R., Landau, R. and Madgar, I. (2007). 'Older single mothers assisted by sperm donation and their children'. *Human Reproduction*, 22, 2784–91.

Whitney, A. (2001). 'Single father of triplets defends surrogacy deal'. *The Independent*, 18 September 2001.
Yeung, W. J., Sandberg, J. F., Davis-Kean, P. E. and Hofferth, S. L. (2001). 'Children's time with fathers in intact families'. *Journal of Marriage and Family*, 63, 136–54.

LEGISLATION

Human Fertilisation and Embryology Bill 1990
Human Fertilisation and Embrylogy Act, as amended 2008
Welfare Reform Act 2009

12 Reproductive donation and justice for gay and lesbian couples

John B. Appleby, Sarah Jennings and Helen Statham

Introduction

Lesbian women and gay men become parents via a number of routes depending on national regulatory legislation, access to health care and the implementation of social policies affecting parenting. Obtaining gametes or embryos from a third party is not always an issue. Both men and women can have conceived children within heterosexual relationships; can adopt where it is legal; and can become the same-sex partner of someone who has a child conceived within a heterosexual relationship, and are therefore considered a co-parent or step-parent. Reproductive donation is involved when lesbians become mothers using sperm, eggs or embryos (the latter two usually only if the woman is infertile) from a donor who is anonymous, known or open-identity. Recent legislative changes in the UK now allow both women of a couple to be named on their child's birth certificate. Lesbians and gay men can donate eggs and sperm, respectively, to lesbian or straight women and conceive a child with the intention of having or not having a parenting role. For a gay man to become a parent using reproductive donation he needs both a surrogate and a source of eggs (or possibly embryos), which may or may not be donated by the surrogate.

In this chapter we discuss some of the ethical debates surrounding same-sex parenting, which we define as gay or lesbian couples becoming joint parents using gametes or embryos from a third party. We are not considering issues for those of other sexual orientations. Our discussion is confined to the context of countries where same-sex relations are legal and where lesbian women and gay men have at least some access to parenthood through donation. The legal and social implications for same-sex parenting outside of this context, as well as lesbian and gay (L&G) rights more generally, are beyond the scope of this chapter.

In discussing issues arising for L&G couples who wish to become parents using assisted reproductive technologies (ARTs), it is important

to be aware that many dilemmas are similar to those faced by heterosexual couples and single women wishing to become parents. These
include legal constraints and the shortages of gametes, embryos and
surrogates. We argue that there may be additional constraints placed
on same-sex parents because of social stigma.

This chapter will argue that parenting is typically considered a virtuous life project for individuals in society, and that includes L&G couples. Where 'health needs' include reproductive health care services
(such as maternal care and donated gametes) that are provided to the
public, then equal access to such resources must be provided to same-
sex couples. In this case, distributive justice ensures equal opportunity
for same-sex couples to become parents. We will therefore argue that
same-sex couples have a positive claim right (a right that someone else
has an obligation to fulfil) to social goods meant to satisfy health needs,
as well as a negative liberty right (a right not to be interfered with by
others) to carry out plans to become parents. We will draw on three
different modes of ethical reasoning: consequentialism, deontology and
virtue ethics. Consequentialists are interested in the *outcomes* of parenting for same-sex couples and their children. Deontologists focus on
whether the *act* of parenting is good in and of itself. Virtue ethicists
argue that it is the *intent* to parent that displays moral character and
this exhibition of character is of primary value. Drawing on these three
theories can tell us something about why parenting is, more often than
not, considered normatively important for those who wish to do it.

Based on evidence and ethical analysis we will discuss three key questions: first, is the welfare of the child affected by same-sex parenting;
second, should society help prospective parents have an opportunity to
parent; and third, what is required to provide gay and lesbian couples
with the means to become parents.

Is the welfare of the child affected by same-sex parenting?

Prior debate about same-sex parenting has focused on the consequences
for children raised within these family forms. There is a large body of
empirical evidence about the well-being of children raised by same-sex
parents, which addresses a number of the concerns (outlined below) of
both those who object to same-sex parenting and those who support it.

Most research to date on outcomes for children in same-sex parent families has been with lesbian mother families, rather than gay
fathers. Research beginning in the 1970s focused on divorced women
who had 'come out' as lesbian after having conceived children within

heterosexual relationships. Studies have since focused on women in same-sex relationships who have conceived children by donor insemination. Limited empirical evidence exists about outcomes for children in gay father families, both for those conceived within heterosexual relationships and those who have been born or adopted into a same-sex parent family. Despite often playing a significant role in their children's lives, gay fathers are less likely than lesbian mothers to have legal custody of their children following the break-up of a heterosexual relationship. Furthermore, gay men need more biological resources than lesbian women for reproduction (i.e. eggs and surrogates) to create their own families within a same-sex relationship. However, there are increasing numbers of families being formed within male same-sex relationships. These families are being achieved via adoption, but also through gamete donation, embryo donation and surrogacy where it is legal and affordable.

There have recently been significant contributions to the body of evidence concerning the development of children adopted by gay fathers. Unfortunately, there are currently no published studies of children conceived into gay father families via assisted reproduction. However, we can still draw inferences about access to assisted reproduction techniques based upon currently available evidence and theories. Research with children who have same-sex parents has focused on three main areas: psychological well-being; gender development; and peer relationships.

Psychological well-being

Studies of lesbian mother families have assessed a wide variety of aspects pertaining to children's personal development, such as social competence and academic outcomes, behaviour and self-esteem (Patterson, 2006). Early studies of children born into heterosexual relationships, as well as more contemporary studies of children born into same-sex relationships, have illustrated that, as a group, children with same-sex parents do not differ significantly from their peers from opposite-sex parent families. This conclusion is drawn from looking across the range indices of personal development and well-being for children raised by both types of parents (Tasker, 2005; Patterson, 2006). These findings have been replicated internationally (e.g. Brewaeys and Van Hall, 1997) and by studying children, adolescents and young adults (Patterson, 2006). Most importantly, these findings have been replicated by studies using representative samples (Golombok et al., 2003; Wainright and Patterson, 2006) and multiple informants (Golombok et al., 2003). Some studies have reported negatively on the welfare of children in same-sex parent families, although these studies are broadly considered to be based on subjective bias and lacking in academic rigour (Stacey and Biblarz, 2001).

There are no studies at present of the psychological development of children born into male same-sex families. Early studies of children who live with their mothers but have contact with their gay fathers have not indicated that these children are at risk of emotional or behavioural problems (Golombok and Tasker, 2010). With regard to gay men as parents, early studies indicate that gay fathers gave similar reasons for wanting children (Bigner and Jacobson, 1989a) and had similar parenting practices (Bigner and Jacobson, 1989b) to heterosexual fathers. Studies of adoptive parenting have found the children of male and female same-sex couples to be equally as well adjusted as those with heterosexual parents (Erich *et al.*, 2005, 2009; Leung *et al.*, 2005). Although these first studies use less-rigorous methodologies, this finding has been replicated by a more robust US-based study of children adopted in early infancy by male same-sex parents. Farr *et al.* (2010) found that the children adopted by male couples showed no significant differences in their development compared to their peers adopted by female or heterosexual couples.

Psychosexual development

Our examination of psychosexual development focuses on three dimensions of sexual identity: core gender identity – whether one identifies as a male or female; gender role – whether one exhibits the behaviour 'typical' of the gender group; and finally sexual orientation – the gender(s) to which one is sexually attracted. Of the three, only having a gender identity opposite to one's biological sex is clinically defined as a psychological disorder. Variation in gender behaviour and sexual orientation are not clinically defined disorders, but these dimensions of psychosexual development are still explored in research.

Neither early nor more recent studies have found any evidence of gender identity confusion amongst children of same-sex parents (Golombok and Tasker, 2010). Although these studies were of lesbian mother families, the recent study by Farr *et al.* (2010) has found that children adopted by gay fathers also show typical gender development. Less stereotypical gender behaviour and attitudes have been reported by some authors; for example, children of lesbian mothers were less likely than their peers from heterosexual parent families to regard their own gender as superior (Bos and Sandfort, 2010) and were more tolerant of gender transgressions committed by boys – for example, wearing nail polish (Fulcher *et al.*, 2008). However, these modest differences have not been replicated across all studies. In this chapter we will not explore such differences as they have not been evidenced as being associated adversely with children's psychological well-being.

Less is known about sexual orientation given that most studies to date have focused on children. However, research suggests that children of lesbian mothers are no more likely than their peers to form a non-heterosexual identity in adulthood (Tasker and Golombok, 1997). Children are, however, less likely to be certain that their future romantic relationships will be heterosexual (Bos and Sandfort, 2010), and are more open to exploring non-heterosexual relationships as young adults (Tasker and Golombok, 1997).

Peers

Concerns for children's well-being often focus upon whether children will be stigmatized and victimized on account of their parents' sexual orientation and/or relationship (Patterson, 2009). Evidence regarding victimization has been mixed. While studies have found no difference in the extent of victimization between children parented by same-sex parents in contrast to their peers with heterosexual parents, many children do experience homophobia from their peers (Tasker and Golombok, 1997; Ray and Gregory, 2001; Wainright *et al.*, 2004; Gartrell *et al.*, 2005; Rivers *et al.*, 2008; Guasp, 2010). Therefore, while children with same-sex parents may experience homophobic victimization by peers, it is not the case that these children are systematically bullied or unable to form positive friendships.

Victimization of children is not a sufficient reason to deny same-sex couples the opportunity to be parents. First, victimization is moderated by the social context in which children live. For example, a cross-cultural study by Bos *et al.* (2008) found that children in the USA were twice as likely to experience homophobia from their peers than children in the Netherlands, despite being less open to their peers about their families than the Dutch children, perhaps reflecting more favourable legislation and social attitudes in the Netherlands for same-sex parents than in the USA. We suggest that instead of limiting the liberty of same-sex couples to be parents, society should instead emphasize the duty to treat children of same-sex parents with equal dignity and respect.

Assessing the research

Earlier criticisms levelled at research on same-sex parenthood, which cited weak methodology and liberal agendas, have largely been addressed by the more recent and robust research discussed above. Evidence and ethical reasoning demonstrates that L&G individuals should not be treated differently in their pursuit of parenthood, because of unfounded concerns for the well-being of their children. Furthermore, research evidence challenges the heteronormative assumptions that underlie theories about what children need from their families. The research community has moved towards the perspective that child well-being depends on family processes and parenting abilities that are not limited according to parent gender or sexual orientation (Stacey and Biblarz, 2001; Patterson, 2009; Golombok and Tasker, 2010). Thus, despite limited evidence of the outcomes for children in gay-father families, we argue that there is little reason to assume that gay fathers cannot provide what is important for their children's well-being.

Gay fathers may be subject to greater stigma and prejudice than lesbian mothers. It may be relevant to examine cultural assumptions and fears held about men being parents. These assumptions and the feelings of concern they inspire may lead to greater reluctance to provide gay men the opportunity to parent than lesbian women.

Popular portrayals of men include that of 'imposter' parents, such as the 'mother's helper' (Lamb and Oppenheim, 1989); or as bearers of a dangerous sexuality posing a threat to children (Freeman, 2003). If concerns about men as parents still penetrate popular opinion, as suggested by the media (Freeman, 2003), we must assess whether there is any evidence to substantiate these concerns.

With regard to men acting only as 'mother's helper', studies of heterosexual families indicate that, on average, men do parent differently from their female partners. However, on closer inspection it is married heterosexual fathers who show lowest parental involvement and skills. Fathers in other family arrangements, such as single-parent families, can and do take over the typical 'maternal' role (Stacey and Biblarz, 2001). Moreover, men are just as capable as women of being the primary carer (Parke, 1996; Lamb, 1997), and children can form attachments to their male parents just as well as to their female parents (van IJzendoorn and De Wolff, 1997). Given the findings of Farr *et al.* (2010) that male same-sex parents did not differ significantly in parenting practices compared to female parents, this suggests, as before, that parenting skills are not limited by gender, but may be moderated by social context.

Assumptions are often held that men pose a sexual danger to children, because there is more reported child abuse by men than by women. Despite the reality that abusive males make up a very small fraction of the population, awareness of it is inflamed by the media, creating suspicion of men who wish to be close and loving caregivers to their children (Freeman, 2003). Gay men may be under even more suspicion as it has also been argued by some critics of gay father families (e.g. Morgan, 2002; Cameron, 2009) that gay men are more likely than heterosexual men to abuse children. There is no evidence to substantiate this claim (American Psychological Association, 2005). Evidence provided by Cameron (2009) and Morgan (2002) is highly suspect (Hicks, 2005), for example in labelling men who abuse boys as gay, despite research evidence indicating that acts of child abuse do not reflect adult sexual orientation (Jenny et al., 1994). Second, this perspective is associated with the belief that homosexuality is a pathology that will lead to other deviant sexual practices. This has been condemned by the American Psychiatric Association and American Psychological Association since the mid 1970s (American Psychological Association, 2005).

Research evidence has nullified the heterosexist and homophobic assumptions of 'psychological theory, judicial opinion, and popular prejudice' (Patterson, 1992) with regard to female same-sex parents. Moreover, the evidence outlined above must lead to a reassessment of the cultural assumptions and fears that are held with regard to male same-sex parents. The burden of evidence is no longer on same-sex families to prove their abilities, but instead rests with critics to substantiate their claims.

To summarize, there is no evidence to support the claim that child well-being will be adversely affected by having a lesbian or gay parent. What does appear significant for the well-being of children is to be protected from bullying and homophobia, and this aversion of harm must be seen as part of our social duty to provide security to all persons. Children's security may also be left vulnerable when only their biological, rather than social parent, is recognized as a legal parent. For example, should a biological parent be taken ill, the social parent may have no legal rights to make decisions on behalf of their child, or to take custody of their child should a biological parent die (Elliot, 2010). Legal parenthood is of much greater concern when considering child well-being, in contrast to psychological harm for which there is no evidence.

While research evidence may alleviate concerns arising from heteronormative assumptions, there are of course objections to same-sex parenting on other grounds, such as religious beliefs. Such views cannot be addressed by psychological research (Herek, 2006). It is important to acknowledge the existence of such beliefs about the propriety of same-sex parenting, but they derive from a different ethical perspective to the one asserted here.

Should society help prospective parents have an opportunity to parent?

Asking whether or not society should provide people with an opportunity to parent presupposes that we know why being a parent matters. Does parenting matter? What is it about parenting that makes it good and something in which we would want everyone to be able to participate in if they so desired? Anja Karnein has discussed the universal right (entailing both a claim and liberty right to reproduce and raise children) to parenthood in Chapter 4. We will briefly summarize why parenting is an important activity for many individuals in society.

In liberal democratic societies we place a great deal of value on individuals being given the opportunity to carry out the life projects that they deem to be important in the narratives of their lives. Looking back on our lives to date we can review the projects in which we have been engaged so far. Similarly, we can look forward in time with projects in mind that we might like to initiate or continue because they may be of prudential value to us (Sumner, 1999). The ongoing and potential existence of these projects tells us something about how well our individual lives are going for us (Sumner, 1999). Parenting children may be one of the life projects a same-sex couple chooses to undertake because it is of value to them.

Parenting is a very popular life project and one often considered to be virtuous because of what it entails. Some argue that being a parent is good because it fosters maturity, responsibility, leadership and other qualities that society recognizes to be virtuous in character (Ruddick, 1979; Brighouse and Swift 2009). Parenting may therefore be considered good because it contributes to the human flourishing of the parents and their children (Velleman, 2008). If we agree that parenting is virtuous and that it is an activity society should support, then the next step would be to provide those who wish to become parents with the necessary means to have an opportunity to become a parent; however, individuals deemed to be a danger to children, e.g. paedophiles, could be excluded from this provision (Lafollette, 1980).

In order to have the opportunity to undertake (or at least reasonably aspire to undertake) projects in our lives, we recognize that individuals in society need to be assured of some basic goods. Such goods should provide individuals with the opportunity to form reasonable life prospects. What might constitute unreasonable life prospects that everyone could be expected to be able to enjoy might include becoming a professional athlete, a pop singer or a supermodel – all of which require innate talents or traits that are beyond the scope of what society can reasonably provide all people. In respect to parenting, the full extent of what such a list of basic goods might entail is difficult to ascertain. However, we will explain that the satisfaction of health needs (Daniels, 2008) and the provision of liberty to carry out life projects (in the UK a claim right to health needs is afforded to all members of society) are at least two of the most important kinds of goods. Basic goods like these serve to provide autonomous members of society with the necessary means to go about putting their plans for parenthood into action.

What is required to provide gay and lesbian couples with the means to become parents?

Assisting L&G couples to have the opportunity to become parents has implications for society at large, as well as for gamete donors and clinicians more specifically. As discussed, gay and lesbian couples cannot become parents without third-party assistance. For all couples who want children, the biological requirements are the same: sperm, an egg and someone to carry the child. A variety of arrangements to procure these biological goods and services exist depending on the wishes and desires of the potential parents and the availability of the resources.

The procurement and provision of reproductive tissue and labour can entail risks to those offering their services. For example, lesbians are also becoming egg donors in clinics that they may have initially approached with the sole intention of seeking donor insemination. However, in the absence of empirical evidence about their motivations and experiences, it is not clear that lesbians are a group at any more risk of coercion than heterosexual women. Ideally, society would provide an equal opportunity for same-sex couples to access donated reproductive tissues, such as gametes, with the requirement that the autonomy and liberty of the donors is not compromised (see Chapter 9, Pennings, Vayena and Ahuja). On the other hand, in the UK the law allows two men to be named as parents of a child, but surrogacy is not provided by the National Health Service (NHS) to anyone (see Chapter 16, Braverman, Casey and Jadva). Surrogates cannot be provided by the NHS for a number of reasons but especially because there is a need to protect surrogates from 'slavery of the talented' (Dworkin, 1981) whereby those with certain talents or capabilities are forced to share the fruits of their labour with others.

Health needs are central to this discussion and perhaps the most well-known account of health needs is the one given by Norman Daniels in *Just Health* (2008). He suggests that a broad notion of health needs must be taken into account in order to provide for our well-being (discussed in greater detail as 'Normal Species Functioning'; see Daniels, 2008). Daniels describes health needs using a six-point list, although we will focus on only two points. Point five suggests '[p]reventative, curative, rehabilitative, and compensatory personal medical services and devices' are 'healthcare needs' (Daniels, 2008: 42–3), and point six emphasizes the importance of the just distribution of 'other social determinants of health' (Daniels, 2008). For same-sex couples the fertility treatment needed to have the opportunity to parent would be associated with Daniels' fifth point and the fair delivery of those health care services is encompassed in his sixth point. Our account of health needs follows that of Daniels (leaving aside his use of 'Normal Species Functioning'), but we place increased emphasis on how health needs include fertility treatment and maternal care, which we argue must be equally provided to same-sex couples.

If society does provide the social infrastructure to address the health needs of its population, fertility treatment may be offered in that range of services. In the case of the NHS in the UK, the National Institute for Health and Clinical Excellence (NICE) recommends that NHS fertility clinics offer 3 cycles of IVF (although regions vary in what is offered, and could be anywhere between 0 and 3 cycles) to infertile patients who meet specified criteria, such as age requirements. If gametes from a third party are needed, patients can be put on a waiting list. In the NHS these are resources paid for by public funds and made available to the public on an as-needed basis. L&G couples will always need donated gametes in order to become parents. Ensuring that equal access to publicly funded gamete banks exists for both heterosexual couples and same-sex couples would be part of fulfilling society's mandate of fairly satisfying one aspect of an individual's health needs.

Infertility is one reason a couple might need ARTs in order to try and become parents, but not the only reason. Most L&G couples have no evidence of infertility, but as a couple they cannot physically conceive a child. Whether an infertile heterosexual couple or a fertile L&G couple, the end goal of becoming parents is the same and the same resources are needed. If either an L&G or heterosexual couple need access to reproductive resources to have an opportunity to become parents, their access to these resources should not be limited according to their fertility status. Where reproductive resources (e.g. donated gametes) are scarce, they should be distributed fairly amongst those individuals who share an equal claim to them.

Gay men also require a surrogate mother to carry their child. A claim against society to provide surrogates could only be made if society deemed it necessary to offer surrogacy services to all members of society who needed them. This would potentially imply that the state would have to provide women to fulfil the parenting dreams of individuals who cannot give birth to their own children. Given debates about payment and concerns about coercion of women into surrogacy, this is not an acceptable course of action and is why affording individuals a claim right to parenthood is not an acceptable option. It is difficult to satisfy claim rights to surrogates without also violating the liberty rights of women (see Braverman, Casey and Jadva, Chapter 16). Similarly, it is also difficult to satisfy the demand for gametes and embryos because individuals have a liberty right to abstain from donation.

While not fulfilling the desire of individuals to reproduce, adoption is also a means by which L&G couples can become parents, and is perhaps an option with greater success given the technical difficulties involved with IVF and surrogacy, which may not result in pregnancy. An argument can be made that there is a duty to parent existing children (i.e. children in need of adoption) before bringing additional children into the world. This argument would assume that the need for existing children to have parents morally outweighs the desire individuals have to create a child, genetically related or otherwise. In relation to providing same-sex couples with the opportunity to parent, this duty could only apply where these couples are considered acceptable parents and where children are available for adoption. Also, it could not be specific to same-sex couples and would have to apply to anyone considering parenthood, including those who can conceive without the use of ARTs.

We have so far only considered the welfare of children and the perspective of same-sex couples who wish to avail themselves of donated gametes. Now we turn to the perspective of other individuals involved, specifically donors and clinicians.

Pennings commented in 1995 that a strategy was needed to improve what was even then a 'meagre supply of gametes'. He suggested that the scarcity of available donors might be changed if the donation procedure were adapted to meet the wishes and desires of the donors. It was argued that giving donors the liberty right to direct their gametes to certain groups of recipients went against the general rule that donors relinquish all rights, duties and allocation of their gametes by donating. Alternatively, a donor's positive and negative right to be involved in the allocation is supported by the donor's autonomous interest in and contribution to the process. Pennings (1995) concluded that donors should have the negative (liberty) right to direct their gametes to categories accepted as relevant by the different moral communities in their society. They should not be given the positive right to add their own categories to the exclusion list (Pennings, 1995). If donors are not allowed to allocate their gift, they should at least be informed as to which categories of recipients are treated by the hospital to enable them to decide whether they want to donate gametes (Pennings, 1995).

At the time of Penning's writing (1995), attitudes to the use of gametes by single and lesbian women were less favourable than today and legislation largely prohibited medically assisting same-sex couples to become parents. However, we still know little from research about the views of donors themselves about choosing who will use their gametes or embryos. The SEED evaluation (HFEA, 2009) has reported that it is 'relatively common for donors to restrict the use of their donor gametes or embryos to specific family types or religions, for example, to married heterosexual couples'. Attitudes to this position of donors can be pragmatic, that is donation is a gift in the hands of the donor, and in an era of open-identity donation the donor may have a role in a future child's life and with his or her family. An alternative perspective is that the wish to control who receives the donation of gametes endorses unfair discrimination. Nevertheless, reproductive donation necessitates a different look at *how* we choose *who* has priority to receive scarce resources. The difference is that, in reproductive decision-making, life is being created, as opposed to other health care decisions where life is being maintained or improved, or suffering is being minimized. Without entering into a priority-setting discussion that extends beyond donation and same-sex parenthood, we will reiterate that while donors may wish to restrict the use of their gametes to certain kinds of prospective parents, the distribution of unrestricted donated gametes (i.e. where donors have no preference about the recipients) should not be subject to further restrictions that could be deemed unfair.

The final question focuses on the role of clinicians in helping same-sex couples become parents. To what extent should they act as gatekeepers to services and should they be able to choose what kind of family they will treat?

One argument is that physicians should only be able to deny fertility treatment if they have evidence to justify that the child's welfare would be at risk because of unfit parent(s) or for another reason. Physicians should not be able to discriminate against patients because of their sexual orientation. There is debate about whether fertility treatment should be provided to individuals from public health care schemes: a number of jurisdictions are restricting access, for example Denmark (Ziebe, 2010) and the Isle of Man (Zorlu, 2010). There is further debate about areas of medicine where individual clinicians may have particular views about providing particular services, including physician-assisted death (currently illegal in the UK) and abortion. It is interesting to consider the use of ARTs generally, and for L&G individuals specifically, within this framework.

The right of clinicians to act according to conscience is well established within reproductive medicine, specifically concerning abortion provision. In countries such as the UK where abortion is legal under certain criteria, doctors and other health professionals can assert a conscientious objection to participation in any aspect of abortion care (except in an emergency where the mother's life is at risk). Conscientious objection arises most commonly because of religious beliefs. Beyond unwavering conscientious objection, clinicians can also exercise professional discretion about specific abortions. For example, they may refuse to offer the operation at a particular gestation or for a particular reason or a combination of these (Statham *et al.*, 2006).

There is little empirical evidence about fertility doctors' attitudes towards providing treatment to same-sex couples, but it must be remembered that clinicians who choose to work in specialist fertility services are unlikely to adhere to a belief that assisted reproduction is fundamentally wrong. While little is known for lesbian couples, who mostly require only donated sperm, there is even less evidence about the provision of more complex surrogacy services to gay men. Lampic and colleagues (2009) surveyed 117 doctors at the 2005 Nordic IVF conference, and the majority of respondents supported lesbian couples' access to sperm donation, especially in Denmark and Finland where the treatment option was available at the time of the survey. Attitudes of IVF doctors in Sweden were similar to those found for the broader population of gynaecologists, with both younger and female gynaecologists being more supportive of treatment for lesbian women (Skoog Svanberg *et al.*, 2008). In a US study of the directors of the 369 Society for Assisted Reproductive Technology-associated ART programmes, representing 95% of all ART programmes in the USA, Gurmankin and colleagues (2005) found that 66% of clinics collected information about patients' sexual orientation, with 17% reporting that they were likely or very likely to turn away a lesbian couple who wanted donor insemination and 48% to turn away a gay couple who wanted to use surrogacy. A recent paper reporting on practising US obstetricians-gynecologists (Lawrence *et al.*, 2010) found 14% would discourage a woman with a female sexual partner from using ARTs and 13% would not help such a woman obtain the service. Doctors who were older, male and more deeply religious (especially Muslim and evangelical protestant) were more likely to be unsupportive of lesbian women.

The limited data available suggest that there are a small number of individual providers who do not support L&G access to ARTs. The impact on women appears small, with limited evidence that lesbians are failing to obtain treatment. Three cases have received significant publicity, two in the UK and one in the USA. One UK case centred on the issue of access to NHS-funded infertility services by women who were not necessarily biologically infertile (Roberts, 2009). The original decision by a Scottish Health Board 'to consider homosexual couples ineligible for fertility treatment because neither partner is medically infertile and they have not tried to conceive "in the normal way" for the requisite minimum of two years' was reversed after the couple claimed that exclusion of same-sex couples from necessary medical assistance to conceive constituted 'indirect discrimination' in breach of the Equality Act (Sexual Orientation) Regulations 2007 and violated their human rights. This couple had previously been told by a general practitioner that they had to access care privately and little is known about the extent to which other lesbian women are still advised that this is their only option.

The other UK case was more obviously discriminatory: the lesbian woman seeking treatment had become infertile (Blackburn-Starza, 2009). The NHS Trust involved reversed its decision not to provide treatment after arguments were made that discrimination on the grounds of sexual orientation was contrary to the Human Rights Act 1998 and the Equality Act 2010, and also because the discriminatory 'need for a father' originally specified in the Human Fertilisation and Embryology (HFE) Act 1990 was due to be replaced via the 2008 amendment. The amendment would specify a required assessment of the ability of the parent(s) to offer 'supportive parenting'.

The US case of Guadalupe Benitez and her spouse, Joanne Clark, against a clinic took eight years to resolve. Doctors had treated Ms Benitez with fertility drugs and provided guidance about self-insemination but had allegedly told her they would not inseminate her, due to their religious objections (Satkunarajah, 2009). Although the couple were referred to another clinic, where they were treated, their case for discrimination was upheld by the California Supreme Court, which barred Christian doctors denying treatment to patients on the grounds of sexual orientation. The ruling stated that laws preventing discrimination based on sexual orientation extended to the medical profession. In commentaries on the case, Appel (2006), while not in any way supporting discrimination, suggested that few prospective patients will suffer a great deal of embarrassment if a few physicians opt out. Furthermore, the overt expression of clinicians' 'strongly held biases' would 'do a service to prospective patients' by 'giving them a chance to avoid such providers' (Appel, 2006: 21) However, Appel's logic is based on the assumption that physicians only treat those of whom they approve. A non-sequitur such as this seems only to reinforce prejudicial cultures (whether intentional or not) rather than to encourage the fair treatment of L&G couples who would like to become parents.

Beyond the practice of individual doctors, it is important to bear in mind institutional constraints; for example, in countries where clinical services are controlled by religious institutions it may be more difficult for lesbians to obtain treatment. In such circumstances the opportunity for individuals to cross state or national borders can enable them to achieve a pregnancy (see Chapter 5 and Chapter 8). It may also be that even when a lesbian woman becomes pregnant in a relationship with another woman who intends to parent the child, legislation prevents both women from being recognized as mothers and only the biological mother has any rights to parenthood, as is the current situation in the Republic of Ireland (Elliott, 2010).

Where issued, professional guidance is clear. In the USA the Ethics Committee of the American Society for Reproductive Medicine finds 'no sound ethical basis' for a physician to deny reproductive services to unmarried, gay or lesbian patients (Ethics Committee of the American Society for Reproductive Medicine, 2009). Within the UK the British Medical Association (BMA) (Policy group: Annual Representative Meeting, 2008) reiterated support for the rights of doctors and other health care professionals to conscientiously object to carrying out certain non-emergency lawful procedures, where such conscientious objection is recognized in statute, as in abortion and IVF. If seeing patients seeking advice on such a procedure, the doctor should tell them immediately of his/her conscientious objection and of their right to see another doctor. It can be hoped that most health care providers would support the view of Greenfeld that the increasing number of gay male couples who are concluding that their sexuality need not prevent them becoming fathers, planning a family together, and turning to reproductive medical centres for help in becoming fathers. These couples deserve 'the same attention (and lack of discrimination) in their care that other couples, lesbian and heterosexual, receive in fertility centers around the country' (Greenfeld, 2007: 18).

Conclusion

In exploring same-sex parenthood we have discussed the welfare of children, whether we should provide same-sex couples with the means to become parents, and parenting as an important life project for those who aspire to take part in it. The nature of being a parent is often considered morally virtuous in society and this may be good reason for society to help individuals pursue their goals to become parents.

Our survey of empirical evidence concerning the well-being of children raised by same-sex couples confirms that there is nothing unusual about the development of these children or their welfare. The burden of proof is now on critics of same-sex marriage to provide evidence as to why the welfare of children would be at risk as a result of this family form.

An important point that we have argued is that if parenting requires certain health needs to be provided for (i.e. maternal care or fertility treatment), then there is an obligation to ensure that publicly funded health care resources are distributed fairly. Where same-sex couples are legally permitted to become parents, they must be able to exercise their liberty in order to realize those desires. Where same-sex couples are not legally permitted to become parents, we hope this injustice will be corrected.

We have also discussed cases where same-sex couples' liberty to become parents could be frustrated by physicians acting as gatekeepers to fertility treatment, and donors prejudiced against providing these couples with gametes. Educating the public about same-sex parenting may increase their acceptance of this increasingly prominent family form. Furthermore, stricter enforcement of anti-discrimination laws may improve L&G access to the goods required to satisfy their health needs, especially in relation to fertility treatment. Finally, we recognize that because same-sex couples require donated gametes and often a surrogate, it will commonly be difficult for them to get the necessary resources in place in order to become parents. Regardless of these inherent difficulties, society should endeavour to help same-sex couples in their pursuit of parenthood.

REFERENCES

American Psychological Association (2005). *Lesbian and Gay Parenting.* Washington: American Psychological Association.

Appel, J. M. (2006). 'May doctors refuse infertility treatments to gay patients?' *Hastings Center Report*, 36, 20–1.

Biblarz, T. J. and Stacey, J. (2001). '(How) does the sexual orientation of parents matter?' *American Sociological Review*, 66, 159–83.

Bigner, J. and Jacobsen, R. B. (1989a). 'The Value of Children to Gay and Heterosexual Fathers', in F. W. Bozett (ed.), *Homosexuality and the Family*. New York: Harrington Park.

Bigner, J. (1989b). 'Parenting Behaviors of Homosexual and Heterosexual Fathers', in F. W. Bozett (ed.), *Homosexuality and the Family*. New York: Harrington Park.

Blackburn-Starza, A. (2009). 'Lesbian couple fight NHS over fertility treatment'. *BioNews*, 518. Available at: www.bionews.org.uk/page_45634.asp.

Bos, H. and Sandfort, T. (2010). 'Children's gender identity in lesbian and heterosexual two-parent families'. *Sex Roles*, 62 (1–2), 114–26.

Bos, H. M. W., Gartrell, N. K., van Balen, F., Peyser, H., *et al.* (2008). 'Children in planned lesbian families: a cross-cultural comparison between the United States and the Netherlands'. *American Journal of Orthopsychiatry*, 78, 211–19.

Brewaeys, A. and Van Hall, E. V. (1997). 'Lesbian motherhood: the impact on child development and family functioning'. *Journal of Psychosomatic Obstetrics & Gynecology*, 18(1), 1–16.

Brighouse, H. and Swift, A. (2009). 'Legitimate parental partiality', *Philosophy & Public Affairs*, 37, 43–80.

British Social Attitudes (1993). Available at: www.britsocat.com/Body.aspx?control=BritsocatMarginals&AddSuperMap=LBFGAYADPT&JumpCrossMarginals=yes (accessed 25 August 2010).

Cameron, P. (2009). 'Gay fathers' effects on children: a review'. *Psychological Reports*, 104, 649–59.

Daniels, N. (2008). *Just Health: Meeting Health Needs Fairly*. Cambridge University Press.

Dworkin, R. (1981). 'What is equality? Part 2: equality of resources'. *Philosophy and Public Affairs*, 10, 283–345.

Elliott, I. (2010). *Voices of Children*. Dublin: Marriage Equality.

Erich, S., Leung, P. and Kindle, P. (2005). 'A comparative analysis of adoptive family functioning with gay, lesbian and heterosexual parents and their children'. *Journal of GLBT Family Studies*, 1, 43–60.

Ethics Committee of the American Society for Reproductive Medicine (2009). 'Access to fertility treatment by gays, lesbians, and unmarried persons'. *Fertility and Sterility*, 92, 1190–3.

Farr, R. H., Forssell, S. L. and Patterson, C. J. (2010). 'Parenting and child development in adoptive families: does parental sexual orientation matter?' *Applied Developmental Science*, 14, 164–78.

Freeman, T. (2003). 'Loving Fathers or Deadbeat Dads? The Crisis of Fatherhood in Popular Culture', in S. Earle. and G. Letherby (eds.). *Gender, Identity and Reproduction: Social Perspectives*. Basingstoke: Palgrave Macmillan.

Fulcher, M., Sutfin, E. L. and Patterson, C. J. (2008). 'Individual differences in gender development: associations with parental sexual orientation, attitudes and division of labor'. *Sex Roles*, 58, 330–41.

Gartrell, N., Deck, A., Rodas, C., Peyser, H., *et al.* (2005). 'The National Lesbian Family Study, 4. Interviews with the 10-year-old children'. *American Journal of Orthopsychiatry*, 75, 518–24.

Golombok, S. and Tasker, F. (2010). 'Gay Fathers', in M. Lamb (ed.), *The Role of the Father in Child Development*. Hoboken: John Wiley & Sons.

Golombok, S., Perry, B., Burston, A., Murray, C., *et al.* (2003). 'Children with lesbian parents: a community study'. *Developmental Psychology*, 39, 20–33.

Greenfeld, D. A. (2007). 'Gay male couples and assisted reproduction: should we assist?' *Fertility and Sterility*, 88, 18–20.

Guasp, A. (2010). *Different Families*. London: Stonewall.

Gurmankin, A. D., Caplan, A. L. and Braverman, A. M. (2005). 'Screening practices and beliefs of assisted reproductive technology programs'. *Fertility and Sterility*, 83, 61–7.

Herek, G. (2006). 'Legal recognition of same-sex relationships in the United States: a social science perspective'. *American Psychologist*, 61, 607–21.

Hicks, S. (2005). 'Is gay parenting bad for kids? Responding to the "very idea of difference" in research lesbian and gay parents'. *Sexualities*, 8, 153–68.

Human Fertilisation and Embryology Authority (HFEA) (2009). Paper re SEED, page 24. Release date: 12 December 2009. TRIM reference: 2009/09198 Version: 1 Doc name: Authority Paper – Sperm Egg and Embryo Donation.

Jenny, C., Roesler, T. A. and Poyer, K. L. (1994). 'Are children at risk for sexual abuse by homosexuals?' *Pediatrics*, 94, 41–4.

Lafollette, H. (1980). 'Licensing parents'. *Philosophy and Public Affairs*, 9, 182–97.

Lamb, M. (ed.) (1997). *The Role of the Father in Child Development*. New York: John Wiley & Sons.

Lamb, M. E. and Oppenheim, D. (1989). 'Fatherhood and Father–Child Relationships: Five Years of Research', in S. H. Cath *et al.* (eds.), *Fathers and their Families*. Hilldale: Analytic.

Lampic, C., Skoog Svanberg, A. and Sydsjö, G. (2009). 'Attitudes towards gamete donation among IVF doctors in the Nordic countries – are they in line with national legislation?' *Journal of Assisted Reproduction and Genetics*, 26, 231–8.

Lawrence, R. E., Rasinski, K. A., Yoon, J. D. and Curlin, F. A. (2010). 'Obstetrician-gynecologists' beliefs about assisted reproductive technologies'. *Obstetrics and Gynecology*, 116, 127–35.

Leung, P., Erich, S. and Kanenberg, H. (2005). 'A comparison of family functioning in gay and lesbian, heterosexual and special needs adoptions'. *Children and Youth Services Review*, 27, 1031–44.

Morgan, P. (2002). *Children as Trophies? Examining the Evidence on Same-Sex Parenting*. Newcastle-upon-Tyne: The Christian Institute.

Parke, R. D. (1996). *Fatherhood*. Cambridge, MA: Harvard University Press.

Patterson, C. J. (1992). 'Children of lesbian and gay parents'. *Child Development*, 63, 1025–42.

(2006). 'Children of lesbian and gay parents'. *Current Directions in Psychological Science*, 15, 241–4.

(2009). 'Children of lesbian and gay parents: psychology, law and policy'. *American Psychologist*, 64, 727–36.

Pennings, G. (1995). 'Should donors have the right to decide who receives their gametes?' *Human Reproduction*, 10, 2736–40.

Ray, V. and Gregory, R. (2001). 'School experiences of the children of LG parents'. *Family Matters*, 59, 28–34.

Rivers, I., Poteat, V. P. and Noret, N. (2008). 'Victimization, social support, and psychosocial functioning among children of same-sex and opposite-sex couples in the United Kingdom'. *Developmental Psychology*, 44, 127–34.

Roberts, M. (2009). 'Lesbian couple win battle to have Scottish NHS provide IVF'. *Bionews*, 497. Available at: www.bionews.org.uk/page_13703.asp.

Ruddick, W. (1979). 'Parents and Life Prospects', in O. O'Neill and R. Ruddick (eds.), *Having Children: Philosophical and Legal Reflections on Parenthood*. New York: Oxford University Press.

Satkunarajah, N. (2009). '8-year lawsuit settled over US lesbians denied IVF'. *BioNews*, 528. Available at: www.bionews.org.uk/page_49295.asp.

Skoog Svanberg, A., Sydsjö, G. K., Selling, E. and Lampic, C. (2008). 'Attitudes towards gamete donation among Swedish gynaecologists and obstetricians'. *Human Reproduction*, 23, 904–11.

Stacey, J. (2010). 'How does the gender of parents matter?' *Journal of Marriage and Family*, 72, 3–22.

Statham, H., Solomou, W. and Green, J. M. (2006). 'Late termination of pregnancy for fetal abnormality: law, policy and decision-making in four English fetal medicine units'. *British Journal of Obstetrics and Gynaecology*, 113, 1402–11.

Sumner, L. W. (1999). *Welfare, Happiness, and Ethics*. New York: Oxford University Press.

Tasker, F. (2005). 'Lesbian mothers, gay fathers, and their children: a review'. *Developmental & Behavioural Pediatrics*, 26, 224–40.

Tasker, F. and Golombok, S. (1997). *Growing Up in a Lesbian Family*. New York: Guildford Press.

van IJzendoorn, M. H. and De Wolff, M. S. (1997). 'In search of the absent father – meta-analyses of infant–father attachment: a rejoinder to our discussants'. *Child Development*, 68, 604–9.

Velleman, J. D. (2008). 'Persons in prospect'. *Philosophy and Public Affairs*, 36, 221–88.

Wainright, J. and Patterson, C. (2006). 'Delinquency, victimization, and substance use among adolescents with female same-sex parents'. *Journal of Family Psychology*, 20, 526–30.

Wainright, J., Russell, S. and Patterson, C. (2004). 'Psychosocial adjustment, school outcomes and romantic relationships of adolescents with same-sex parents'. *Child Development*, 75, 1886–98.

Ziebe, S. (2010). 'The death of Denmark's public ART funding'. *Bionews*, 564. Available at: www.bionews.org.uk/page_65111.asp.

Zorlu, G. (2010). 'Isle of Man "halves" fertility treatment funding'. *Bionews*, 570. Available at: www.bionews.org.uk/page_68004.asp.

LEGISLATION

Equality Act (Sexual Orientation) Regulations 2007
Equality Act 2010
Human Rights Act 1998
Human Fertilisation and Embryology Act 1990

13 Is disclosure in the best interests of children conceived by donation?

John B. Appleby, Lucy Blake and Tabitha Freeman

Introduction

In families in which parents conceived using donated sperm or donated eggs, only one parent will be the genetic parent of the child: the mother in the case of sperm donation and the father in the case of egg donation. Parents can choose to tell or not to tell their child about their donor conception. In families in which parents choose not to tell, children will grow up unaware that the person that they think of as their mother or father is not, in fact, their genetic parent. Furthermore, families in which children were conceived using an anonymous donor will likely never be able to know detailed or identifying information about their donor. In countries where donor anonymity has ended and donor-conceived adults are able to access information about their donor, it is still the case that if someone does not know they were donor conceived they will have no reason to access information about their donor. Therefore, is it in the child's best interests to be told about their donor conception?

This chapter outlines empirical research and ethical reasoning to discuss whether disclosure of donor origins is in a child's best interests. Our discussion considers deontological (duty-based) and consequentialist (outcome-based) ethics in relation to disclosure. We hold that the question of whether to disclose can best be answered by reviewing at least three types of considerations for each child: (1) medical welfare; (2) family welfare; and (3) rights. These considerations build on the established empirical evidence presented in the first half of this chapter. Our intention is to clarify reasons why telling or not telling may be the best decision.

This chapter has four sections. First, a historical introduction explains the changing culture of gamete donation in the UK. Next, topics of particular ethical importance to the child's best interests are discussed, such as security, autonomy, liberty, deception and well-being. The following section evaluates the outcomes of existing research that has explored the quality of parent–child relationships and the psychological well-being of parents and children in gamete donation families. Finally, the review of the empirical evidence will be developed with an ethical analysis of the kinds of considerations that should be made before deciding if disclosure is best for the child.

A brief history of the changing culture of gamete donation in the UK

One of the first medical papers about the process, success rates and secrecy of donor insemination (DI) of humans appeared in the British Medical Journal in 1945 (Barton *et al.*, 1945). Donor insemination (or artificial insemination by donor, AID, as it was referred to at this time) was an unregulated procedure that was practised by a handful of doctors and widely condemned. Donors were recruited through personal contacts and medical students were frequently used. For Dr Mary Barton and her colleagues the donor remained anonymous and they recommended that the parents told no one about the procedure and that they should register the birth as a child of their marriage (Barton *et al.*, 1945).

The legal context of donor insemination did not change until 1987 when the Family Law Reform Act made the (gamete) recipient mother and her partner the legal parents of a donor child, at which point all the rights and duties of parenthood were removed from the donor. Following the UK Human Fertilisation and Embryology Act in 1990, donor insemination became a legally regulated procedure, as opposed to being professionally regulated. However, it also remained the subject of private arrangements between two partners. In clinics some non-identifying information about the donor was recorded and made available to donor offspring at age 18 upon request (HFE Act, 1990). Studies conducted in the 1980s and 1990s found that the majority of gamete donation parents did not tell their child about their donor conception and did not intend to tell them in the future (Klock and Maier, 1991; Nachtigall *et al.*, 1997; Golombok *et al.*, 1999).

In April 2005 donor anonymity was removed in the UK. Children born through assisted reproduction involving donated gametes (sperm, egg or embryos) were given the right to access *identifying* information about their donor(s) upon reaching age 18 (HFEA, 2004). The identifying information about the donor includes name and last known address (HFEA, 2004). At the age of 16, children can access some non-identifying information about their donor, including: physical description; year and country of birth; ethnicity;

number and gender of their children; marital status; and medical history (HFEA, 2004).

More gamete donation parents than ever before are choosing to disclose. The following studies have found rates of disclosure or intentions to disclose as being 50 per cent or above in Sweden (Lalos *et al.*, 2007), New Zealand (Hargreaves and Daniels, 2007), America (MacDougall *et al.*, 2007) and Australia (Godman *et al.*, 2006; Hargreaves and Daniels, 2007; MacDougall *et al.*, 2007). A recent study in Belgium by Laruelle *et al.* (2011) found that parents using egg donors were no more or less likely to tell their children of their donor origin whether using an anonymous or known donor. While disclosure may be increasing in some countries, there is still no conclusive evidence linking parents' decisions to disclose and their use of a known donor.

In the UK the rate of disclosure is still relatively low, but seems to be rising. In the most recent study of gamete donation children in the UK, families were visited when children were seven years old. Parents had begun the process of telling their children that they were conceived using donor gametes in 28 per cent of cases using donor insemination and 41 per cent of cases using egg donation (Golombok *et al.*, 2011). It seems that the culture of gamete donation is in transition, changing from one of secrecy in which the anonymity of the donor was guaranteed, to one in which disclosure is encouraged and offspring are entitled to identifying information about the donor. Egg donation only became available in 1984 (Lutjen *et al.*, 1984) and so has a much shorter history than sperm donation. But like sperm donation, egg donation has also changed from a procedure that was characterized by secrecy to one about which there is now greater openness.

The practicalities of disclosure: how do parents disclose, and why?

What exactly is meant by disclosure? In most cases the term is used to refer to the process by which parents tell their offspring that they were conceived using donated sperm or eggs. Of course, it is always up to parents to decide how much or how little information is disclosed and an offspring's understanding of this information may vary according to their age. While not all parents inform children of their donor origins in the same way (or using the same amounts of information), the assumption is usually made that disclosure will lead to offspring becoming aware that (at least) one of their parents is not their biological progenitor. Why is this information considered important? Over recent decades there has been a growing emphasis on the importance of inheritance and an individual's right to know their genetic heritage. There is also the notion that secrecy in families is inherently bad when the truth about an individual's biological parentage is concealed (Smart, 2009). Research on adoption has found that being open about the adoption is beneficial for children (Palacios and Brodzinsky, 2010). This body of research has contributed to the notion that disclosure of donor origins within gamete donation families would also be in the best interests of the child.

The question of whether to disclose primarily affects heterosexual couples. High rates of disclosure have been found in lesbian mother families and single mother families, where some explanation has to be offered to explain the arrival of the child in the absence of a father. In heterosexual families this is not the case, and friends and family of the couple, and the child themselves, are likely to assume natural conception unless told otherwise.

Few studies have examined disclosure rates in both sperm and egg donation families. Some have found that a slightly higher proportion of egg donation parents disclose when compared to donor insemination families, yet differences between family types have not reached statistical significance (Lycett, *et al.*, 2004; Golombok *et al.*, 2005; Murray *et al.*, 2006; MacDougall *et al.*, 2007). It has been suggested that egg donation mothers may be more likely to disclose because they experience pregnancy and early mother–infant bonding, which may make them feel that this biological link overrides genetics and that the child is truly their own (Raoul-Duval *et al.*, 1992). Donor insemination fathers do not have a genetic or biological link with their child, and therefore may be more likely to keep their use of donated sperm secret. Yet contrary to this suggestion, studies have found that the biological link between egg donation mothers and their children is often given as a reason as to why mothers do not feel the need to disclose (Rumball and Adair, 1999; Hunter *et al.*, 2000; Golombok *et al.*, 2004; Shehab *et al.*, 2008).

One of the main reasons parents give when explaining why they chose to disclose is that they want to be honest with their children and that they feel that the child has the right to know about his or her origins. Other reasons include wanting to avoid their child finding out about the nature of their conception from a third party, and wanting to avoid the potentially damaging impact of secrecy within families (Rumball and Adair, 1999; Golombok *et al.*, 2004; Hargreaves and Daniels, 2007; Shehab *et al.*, 2008; Laruelle *et al.*, 2011).

How do parents tell their young children that they were donor-conceived? Disclosing parents have been found to take a 'seed-planting' approach, gradually giving their children information, typically starting when children are four or five years old (MacDougall *et al.*, 2007). Some parents begin disclosure using brief, story-like descriptions, such as 'we needed help to have a family'. Other parents give their young children a more detailed and scientific explanation of the basics of reproduction, and how they had needed either sperm or an egg from another person in order to have a child (Blake *et al.*, 2010). Children's reactions have been found to be that of curiosity, a neutral response or no response at all. Some parents report that their children expressed sadness, or asked: 'Does this mean you are not my real mother/ father?' However, parents found that the impact of such statements was not as painful as they had feared (Rumball and Adair, 1999; Scheib, 2003).

Although disclosure has become more common, it is still the case that many parents choose not to disclose. In the case of anonymous donation, parents may not want their children to feel frustrated or upset by the lack of information that is available about their donor. Alternatively, Laruelle *et al.* (2011) found that half of the parents in their study using anonymously donated eggs had chosen anonymous donors for the purpose of maintaining secrecy. Others fear that the child may have less love for a parent to whom they are not genetically related. Parents may also fear being subjected to public scrutiny and judgement if their use of donated gametes were to become widely known. Parents may also not know how and when to tell. Some parents believe that social parenting is more important than biology, and therefore feel that there simply is no need to tell.

Ethical overview

Consequentialist and deontological theories present two distinct ways of thinking about the interests of the child. If an action affecting a child's interests is in itself morally bad, regardless of the consequences, deontologists suggest that this action should not be taken. In cases where conflicting moral duties arise, the moral dilemma may not have a clear resolution and a compromise must be made. In this chapter, deontological reasoning is used at times to discuss the course of action that is most likely to fulfil the child's best interests. The child's interests do not only include current interests, but also future interests (life plans, priorities and desires). In contrast, consequentialism will also be discussed, as it equates the greatest good for the child with the best outcomes for the child's welfare. The greatest good is determined by identifying which potential course of action provides the most benefits.

In accordance with utilitarian theory, this would mean taking into account the benefits (and harms) to all individuals involved (e.g. parents and siblings).

Autonomy and liberty are important determinants of an individual's well-being. First, autonomy, the ability to make decisions about one's own life, is good for a person's well-being. Although children lack the same degree of autonomy as adults, providing a child with the means to maintain and develop the autonomy they have is necessary for them to be able to make increasingly sovereign decisions about their life projects and aspirations. Second, individuals require liberty in order to be able to carry out their intended plans and life projects, without the undue interference of others (Dworkin, 1997; Sumner, 1999). What a person knows about themselves and the world they live in allows them to make informed decisions about the way they live their lives. If donor-conceived individuals are deprived of information that could potentially hinder their perceived life projects, this would affect their well-being (Sumner, 1999).

In life, the basic good of security provides us with the means to rely upon and form reasonable expectations about the character of individuals and entities in the world around us. Once an individual has some form of security, trust can then be cultivated in relationships with others (Jones, 1996). Children usually trust their parents (except in cases where they believe it is prudent not to), because without parents children would not have the means to satisfy their own needs to survive, nor be adequately equipped to fulfil prospective goals. Children's trust in parents is important, because without it they might not have the same prospect of living a morally good life.

Parents' deception of their children can satisfy as well as frustrate a child's best interests (Bok, 1999). When considering whether or not children should be told about their donor conception, two main questions arise: (1) when children are not told, are they morally wronged; and (2) if children do find out later in life or by accident, do they then consider their earlier deception morally wrong. Deception can be understood in this chapter to imply the withholding of information in a manner that affects a person's capacity for self-determination. This is not to say the individuals are not still self-determining, but instead it means that they are without some information that would affect or improve their autonomy. Upon becoming adults, individuals may have a reasonable expectation not to have been deceived by parents whom they trust (Baier, 1986; Hardin, 1992) to tell them about information that is of practical value to their lives. Trust and deception are therefore important when deciding whether disclosure is in a child's best interests.

Families in which parents have
not disclosed donor origins

So what do we know of the psychological well-being of parents and children in families in which parents do not disclose, and children are unaware that their mother or father is not, in fact, their genetic parent? Findings from studies conducted in the 1980s and 1990s, in which the vast majority of parents had *not* disclosed, are described below in terms of parent psychological well-being, the quality of the parent–child relationship, and child psychological well-being.

Parents who conceive via gamete donation have been found to be psychologically well adjusted and no different to their naturally conceiving counterparts (Golombok *et al.*, 1996, 2002, 2004, 2005, 2006). In terms of levels of marital satisfaction, no significant differences have emerged in comparisons of gamete donation families and control groups of IVF, adoptive and natural conception families (Golombok *et al.*, 1996, 2002; 2004, 2005, 2006; Murray *et al.*, 2006). Low levels of parental psychological disorder and a secure relationship between the mother and father have been found to be beneficial to children's psychological development: therefore, it can be concluded that non-disclosing gamete donation families provide children with a positive family environment in which to grow.

Some studies have found evidence of superior parent–child relationships in gamete donation families when compared to natural conception families. For example, in the first phase of the European Study of Assisted Reproduction Families, families were recruited from Italy, the Netherlands, Spain and the UK when children were aged between 4 and 8 years old (Golombok *et al.*, 1996). Donor insemination and IVF mothers were found to express greater warmth to their child, to be more emotionally involved with their child, to interact more with their child, and to report less stress associated with parenting than natural conception mothers. Similarly, fathers in the assisted reproduction families were found to interact more frequently with their child, and to make a greater contribution to parenting. In the second phase of the study, mothers in assisted reproduction families showed greater enjoyment in parenting, and fathers showed greater warmth to their child and greater enjoyment in parenting (Golombok *et al.*, 2002). Assisted reproduction parents have made an enormous commitment and effort to have a family of their own; therefore, it is unsurprising that these families are characterized by positive relationships.

Yet not all research has found evidence of superior parenting in gamete donation families. An American study found that fathers who perceived higher levels of stigma surrounding male infertility and donor insemination reported less warmth and fostering of independence in their children (Nachtigall *et al.*, 1997). Differences in the quality of the father–child relationship between family types also emerged in the second phase of the European Study of Assisted Reproduction Families, conducted when children were 12 years old (Golombok *et al.*, 2002). Donor insemination fathers were found to be less involved in the disciplining of their children than natural conception fathers.

There is some evidence of assisted reproduction parents being emotionally over-involved and over-protective in their children's lives. A number of studies have found that gamete donation mothers, and in some cases fathers, are more over-involved and over-protective than parents in control groups of natural conception and/or adoptive families (Golombok *et al.*, 1996, 2002, 2004, 2005).

Perhaps the most important question to ask is: how do children fare in non-disclosing families? The majority of studies investigating family functioning in gamete donation families have found children to be functioning well (Kovacs *et al.*, 1993; Golombok *et al.*, 1996, 2002, 2004, 2005, 2006; Murray *et al.*, 2006). These findings are supported by a review of empirical research published between 1980 and 2000, which concluded that there are no significant differences in child functioning between assisted reproduction families and natural conception families in terms of emotions, behaviour, self-esteem or perceptions of the family relationship (Hahn, 2001). Similarly, a study of 769 children conceived via ARTs who were between 5 and 9 years old, found that regardless of whether they were donor-conceived, children did not differ in their levels of psychological adjustment (Shelton *et al.*, 2009).

In studies of non-disclosing families, one must bear in mind that the secrecy surrounding the child's donor conception in these families has been successfully maintained. We do not know how these families would fare if the child were to find out about their donor conception. Although non-disclosing families have been found to be functioning well, there is inevitably a risk of accidental disclosure, especially if parents have told family members and friends about their use of donated gametes. We do not have systematic research on the risks of accidental disclosure; however, there are some accounts of adults who inadvertently discover their donor origins and subsequently report feeling anger or distrust towards parents (Turner and Coyle, 2000).

Families in which parents have disclosed donor origins

What do we know about anonymous gamete donation families in which parents have disclosed and offspring are aware that they were conceived with donor gametes?

Some donor offspring find the experience of learning that they are conceived using an anonymous donor to be frustrating and upsetting. In a study of adult donor offspring recruited from donor conception support networks in the UK, USA, Canada and Australia, offspring described feeling shocked to learn of their donor conception, and felt that they could no longer trust their family (Turner and Coyle, 2000). They felt that they had a right to know their genetic origins, and wanted to search for their donor. Unfortunately there was little consistency as to how and when they were told about the nature of their conception, so it is difficult to draw conclusions about which aspects of disclosure were particularly upsetting. The recruitment of donor offspring via support networks may have lead to a biased sample of participants who had experienced difficulties and wanted to discuss them. Yet this study is valuable in revealing that some donor offspring struggle to accept their donor origins.

What factors affect how offspring feel about their donor conception? Offspring who had a good relationship with their mother, and who perceived their mother's overall mental health as good, have been found to have more positive attitudes towards their means of conception (Mahlstedt et al., 2009). Another factor which may affect how offspring feel about being donor-conceived is how old they were when they first learnt of their origins. Jadva et al. (2009) compared the views of donor offspring who were told about the nature of their conception in childhood to those who were told during adulthood. Those who had learnt of their donor conception in adolescence or adulthood were significantly more likely to have more negative attitudes towards their donor conception. Yet other studies have found that the age at which disclosure occurs does not affect how offspring will feel about their donor conception (Paul and Berger, 2007; Mahlstedt et al., 2009).

Some donor offspring struggle to come to terms with learning that they were donor-conceived and experience feelings of anger and betrayal. Future research needs to explore how offspring conceived via anonymous donor, in which disclosure occurred in early childhood, feel about their donor conception as adults. Research that assesses families when offspring enter adolescence and adulthood is required, as this will likely be a time when questions of identity and independence become particularly salient.

Comparative studies of disclosing vs. non-disclosing families

Who is faring better: families in which parents tell their child that they are donor-conceived, or those who do not? Comparisons of disclosing and non-disclosing families are only now becoming possible as more parents choose to tell their child about their donor conception.

Early attempts at comparative studies defined disclosing families as those who had disclosed and those who intended to, and non-disclosing families as those in which parents had decided never to tell, or were uncertain. Findings from these studies should be interpreted with caution, as those parents who intend to disclose may not actually do so. Some studies found no differences between disclosing and non-disclosing families (Brewaeys *et al.*, 1997, Golombok *et al.*, 2005). Yet Lycett *et al.* (2004) found a difference between family types in maternal discipline: mothers in disclosing families reported less frequent and less severe arguments with their children. Disclosing mothers also reported their children to be less of a strain and exhibit fewer conduct problems, and perceived themselves as more competent parents. The authors suggested that disclosure itself may not necessarily produce positive parent–child relationships, but rather that those mothers who are inclined to openness may adopt a more relaxed approach to parenting in general, and may be less likely to see their child's behaviour as troublesome.

Other studies have defined disclosing families as those who had actually done so, and non-disclosing families as those who had not done so. One study of this nature found no difference between family types (Nachtigall *et al.*, 1997), yet others have found differences between groups, which once again emerged in the domain of parental discipline. In the second phase of the European Study of Assisted Reproduction Families, mothers and children in disclosing families were found to have less frequent and less severe disputes, and mothers were found to be less strict, as rated by mothers and children independently (Golombok *et al.*, 2002). In a Lycett *et al.* (2004) study, a comparison of the six families who had disclosed and the twenty families who had definitely decided against disclosure found differences between groups only in the father's role in supervision, with non-disclosing fathers tending to be stricter.

The most recent comparative study of gamete donation families in the UK found slight differences between those families who had disclosed donor origins, those who had not done so and natural conception families (Golombok *et al.*, 2011). Families were assessed when children were 7 years old. Of these families 23 (34 per cent) had begun the process of disclosure. Differences between groups were found in observational ratings of mother–child interaction (interaction characterized by warmth, mutual responsiveness and cooperation) and interview ratings of maternal positivity (the level of warmth and sensitivity and the quality of interaction between parent and child). In this analysis, natural conception families fared the best and the non-disclosing families the worst. Yet when disclosing and non-disclosing groups were compared directly, no differences emerged. The study also found no differences in ratings of maternal negativity, suggesting that levels of conflict and hostility are no higher in non-disclosing than disclosing families. Most importantly, there were also no differences in children's psychological well-being: children in both disclosing and non-disclosing families were found to be functioning well.

What can we conclude from the comparative studies that have been conducted thus far? Some studies have found slightly better outcomes for those families who disclose donor origins, in terms of conflict, and others have no differences between groups. No studies have found differences in children's psychological well-being, suggesting that children in both disclosing and non-disclosing families are functioning well.

One should bear in mind the limitations of the studies outlined above. Sample sizes have typically been small and therefore analyses have had limited statistical power. Also of note is that most studies mentioned have explored family relationships in which offspring were under the age of 12. Studies of families in which offspring are entering adolescence and adulthood, and particularly longitudinal designs, are required in order to understand how non-disclosing and disclosing families function as children grow older and develop a more sophisticated understanding of their donor conception.

Ethical decision-making

The empirical evidence presented so far describes what is known about families who have and have not told their children that they were donor-conceived. In cases where children are told at a young age and in cases where children are not told and have not yet found out about their donor conception, children have been found to be functioning well. Although extremely valuable, this research is not sufficient grounds, in and of itself, to decide whether or not disclosure of donor origins is in the child's best interests.

In developing a bioethical perspective, we argue that it is necessary to evaluate the following types of considerations before drawing any conclusions about whether disclosure is in the child's best interests: (1) medical welfare; (2) family welfare; and (3) rights. This set of considerations is not exhaustive but rather exemplifies some of the most prominent and pressing concerns for which parents are accountable.

Medical welfare

When evaluating the medical welfare of donor-conceived individuals it is important to consider the social and psychological effects of any decision to disclose or not. For a donor-conceived person, knowing about the nature of their conception allows them to take the necessary steps (perhaps more commonly as adults) to understand the medical risks that they may be susceptible to because of their genetic backgrounds. If a person is conceived with donated gametes from an anonymous donor, it may be important for them to at least know who is *not* their genetic parent, since knowing about our genetic relationships with others can imply the presence or absence of certain health risks. For example, if you discovered that your family had a reliable history of cancer occurrence, it would be helpful if you knew whether you were genetically related or not to that high-risk group of people.

If a person knows whether they are the potential carrier of a genetic disease they may be better off than a person who does not know. Typically people do not need to take a genetic test to determine if they are at risk of being carriers, because they simply look at their genetic lineage and determine if anyone has had the disease before. When an individual who has not been told about their donor conception reflects on their social family histories and does not recognize a risk of inheritable diseases, they may obtain an incomplete assessment of the risks to their welfare. In cases of anonymous donation, donor-conceived individuals do not necessarily have access to a donor's genetic and medical information, but at the very least the individual would have the requisite information needed to make a decision to get screened for genetic health risks (regardless of their probabilities) if they wanted to. However, in the UK and USA clinics provide some screening of donors for genetically inheritable diseases and check their family histories. As a result more than half of would-be donors are rejected. This may, in turn, put donor-conceived children at less risk of inheritable genetic diseases than 'naturally' conceived children whose parents are not usually screened before conceiving. Regardless, ensuring that a donor-conceived person has the knowledge to make informed decisions about the management of their health, and then ensuring they are at liberty to follow through with their decisions, is a consideration that should weigh heavily when deliberating the best interests of that person.

Individuals are not always good candidates for learning about the nature of their conception. For example, if a person was depressed or mentally ill, their medical welfare may be put at further risk by disclosing a potentially traumatic fact about their lives. Individuals who are at risk of suffering grievous harm as a result of disclosure may be temporarily, or even permanently, considered inappropriate candidates to be informed. In cases where an individual has grown up with the knowledge that they are donor-conceived, and that their donor was anonymous, it is not yet known how the inability to find out more information about the donor will affect psychological well-being over the course of their lives. Potentially this could be frustrating and distressing. It is always necessary to weigh the proportion of risks when considering the consequences of disclosure. Consequentialists may argue that although it is important to give individuals information that is medically relevant to them, in cases where this information could cause disproportionate harm it may be necessary to conceal this information, at least temporarily.

Family welfare

When considering the best interests of the child, it is also necessary to take into account the welfare of the family. Disclosure of information to the child about the nature of their conception may affect the welfare of the social and genetic parents, as well as the welfare of siblings. A child's best interests are potentially co-dependent on the welfare of others in their family.

If telling a child about their donor conception would jeopardize the stability of the family, this could greatly affect the welfare of individuals in the family. Furthermore, if disclosure caused distress for the parents, then this could potentially affect the child. Potential harm could also be passed on to other siblings in the family. If disclosure presented the risk of serious harm as a result of disrupting family dynamics and relationships, then this could potentially outweigh any deontological principle that claims disclosure is always in a child's best interest. Consequentialists might argue that the greatest benefit to the child at this time, taking into consideration family welfare, would be derived from non-disclosure.

Rights

When considering whether it is in a child's best interests to be told about their donor conception, it is not uncommon to refer to the rights of the individuals involved in disclosure. Parents may argue for a negative liberty right to privacy (i.e. a right not to have their privacy interfered with). In contrast, critics might argue that the child has a positive claim right not to be deceived (and therefore to be told the truth) about issues that may impact on their welfare (i.e. physical, mental and moral). Indeed, there may be a number of both positive claim rights and negative liberty rights that are brought into the argument about disclosure and the child's best interests, but they can end up conflicting with one another. Determining the best interests of the child may involve reconciling conflicting claim and liberty rights belonging to the parents and to the child.

When parents choose to withhold information from their child about the genetic relationships they share (or do not share), the parents are not impeding the child from leading an autonomous or self-determining life (Dworkin, 1997). Instead, information that could improve a child's autonomy or self-determination is being withheld by the parents. The child likely trusts that what they are being told (or have been left to infer) is correct about the genetic relationships they have with their parents. Offspring are able to make self-determined choices with the information that they have. What has been infringed upon is their liberty to carry out any meaningful activities that are based on their genetic relationships as they understand them. If a child were informed that they had been deceived, then they would have the necessary information to revise their autonomous choices in light of this. They would then be at liberty to carry out their genetically relevant desires (e.g. creating a factually correct genetic family tree – although this may be to some degree impossible with anonymous donors). It could be argued that it is in the interests of children to be told of their donor origins, because doing so honours a right for persons to be at liberty to carry out their self-determined life projects. However, parents may want to keep their child's donor conception a secret in order to keep the truth about their biological ties or the reasons why they used a donor private. How does the child's claim right weigh against parents' liberty right to privacy?

We must first acknowledge that the basic act of reproduction involves the sharing of genetic substance to create another person; thus, creating a genetic relationship. Genetic exceptionalism refers to the belief that genetic information (e.g. knowledge that I carry a gene – perhaps one that has been linked to a particular inheritable disease) is different than other kinds of medical information (e.g. that I have a broken leg), and therefore warrants unique treatment (O'Neill, 2007). For example, if I know that one of my genetic parents carries a gene for an inheritable disease, this is sufficient information for me to assume that I *might* also carry the gene for the same disease. On the other hand, having know-ledge that one of my parents once had a broken leg does not give me sufficient information to assume that I might have a broken leg at some point as well. There is no clear causal relationship between the broken leg my parent had and my likelihood of breaking a leg. However, the knowledge of my parent having an inheritable disease tells me that, because I carry some of the same genes as they do, in this exceptional circumstance I can reasonably assume that I might also carry the same inheritable disease that they carry. The exceptional nature of genetic information may exclude it from the realm of what parents have the lib-erty right to consider private to begin with – after all, a child could take a genetic test to determine his own genetic make-up and this would not likely be considered a breach of the parents' privacy, but rather an exercise in the child's self-determination. Pennings (2001) suggests that while parents might claim that they have a right to keep facts about their genetic relationships private, this act of concealment may infringe on the privacy right of donor-conceived children not to be misinformed about their own genetic ties to their parents. However, parents could claim that using a sample of their tissue for a genetic test to identify genetic relatedness, without their permission, is a violation of their priv-acy. Furthermore, performing DNA tests on the tissue of another per-son without their consent is illegal in some countries, such as the UK (Human Tissue Act 2004). If we consider reproduction to be an act of exposure, which carries with it a truth about relatedness (because the genetic material we share carries biological information), then it is unclear whether parents have an inherent liberty right to privately conceal the truth about the genetic link that they do not have with their donor-conceived children. What can be said with certainty is that discussing the competing rights of parents and children is important in any deliberation about whether disclosure of donor origins is in the child's best interests.

Conclusion

This chapter has investigated the question of whether disclosure is in the best interests of children conceived using donated gametes. We have gone about this by first considering the historical context up until

Brewaeys, A., Golombok, S., Naaktgeboren, N., de Bruyn, J. K., et al. (1997). 'Donor insemination: Dutch parents' opinions about confidentiality and donor anonymity and the emotional adjustment of their children'. *Human Reproduction*, 12, 1591–7.

Dworkin, G. (1997). *The Theory and Practice of Autonomy*. Cambridge University Press.

Godman, K. M., Sanders, K., Rosenberg, M. and Burton, P. (2006). 'Potential sperm donors', recipients' and their partners' opinions towards the release of identifying information in Western Australia'. *Human Reproduction*, 21(11), 3022–6.

Golombok, S., Brewaeys, A., Cook, R., Giavazzi, M. T., et al. (1996). 'The European study of assisted reproduction families: family functioning and child development'. *Human Reproduction*, 11, 2324–31.

Golombok, S., Murray, C., Brinsden, P. and Abdalla, H. (1999). 'Social versus biological parenting: family functioning and the socioemotional development of children conceived by egg or sperm donation'. *Journal of Child Psychology and Psychiatry*, 40(4), 519–27.

Golombok, S., Brewaeys, A., Giavazzi, M. T., Guerra, D., et al. (2002). 'The European study of assisted reproduction families: the transition to adolescence'. *Human Reproduction*, 17, 830–40.

Golombok, S., Lycett, E., MacCallum, F., Jadva, V., et al. (2004). 'Parenting infants conceived by gamete donation'. *Journal of Family Psychology*, 18, 443–52.

Golombok, S., Jadva, V., Lycett, E., Murray, C., et al. (2005). 'Families created by gamete donation: follow-up at age 2'. *Human Reproduction*, 20, 286–93.

Golombok, S., Murray, C., Jadva, V., Lycett, E., et al. (2006). 'Non-genetic and non-gestational parenthood: consequences for parent-child relationships and the psychological well-being of mothers, fathers and children at age 3'. *Human Reproduction*, 21, 1918–24.

Golombok, S., Readings, J., Blake, L., Casey, P., Mellish, L., Marks, A., et al. (2011). 'Children conceived by gamete donation: psychological adjustment and mother–child relationships at age 7'. *Journal of Family Psychology*, 25(2), 230–9.

Hahn, C. S. (2001). 'Review: Psychosocial well-being of parents and their children born after assisted reproduction'. *Journal of Pediatric Psychology*, 26(8), 525–38.

Hardin, R. (1992). 'The street-level epistemology of trust'. *Analyse Kritik*, 14, 152–76.

Hargreaves, K. and Daniels, K. R. (2007). 'Parents' dilemmas in sharing donor insemination conception stories with their children'. *Children and Society*, 21, 420–31.

Human Fertilisation and Embryology Authority (HFEA) (2004). *Human Fertilisation and Embryology Authority (Disclosure of Donor Insemination Regulations)*. Available at: www.opsi.gov.uk/SI/si2004/20041511.htm.

Hunter, M., Salter-Ling, N. and Glover, L. (2000). 'Donor insemination: telling children about their origins'. *Child Psychology and Psychiatry*, 5, 157–63.

Jadva, V., Freeman, T., Kramer, W. and Golombok, S. (2009). 'The experiences of adolescents and adults conceived by sperm donation: comparisons by age of disclosure and family type'. *Human Reproduction*, 24, 1909–19.

Jones, K. (1996). 'Trust as an Affective Attitude'. *Ethics*, 107(1) October, 4–25.

Klock, S. C. and Maier, D. (1991). 'Psychological factors related to donor insemination'. *Fertility and Sterility*, 56, 489–95.

Kovacs, G. T., Mushin, D., Kane, H. and Baker, H. W. G. (1993). 'A controlled study of the psycho-social development of children conceived following insemination with donor semen'. *Human Reproduction*, 8(5), 788–90.

Lalos, A., Gottlieb, C. and Lalos, O. (2007). 'Legislated right for donor-insemination children to know their genetic origin: a study of parental thinking'. *Human Reproduction*, 22, 1759–68.

Laruelle, C., Place, I., Demeestere, I., Englert, Y., *et al.* (2011). 'Anonymity and secrecy options of recipient couples and donors, and ethnic origin influence in three types of oocyte donation'. *Human Reproduction*, 26, 382–90.

Lutjen, P., Trounson, A., Leeton, J., Findlay, J., *et al.* (1984). 'The establishment and maintenance of pregnancy using in vitro fertilisation and embryo donation in a patient with primary ovarian failure'. *Nature*, 307, 174–5.

Lycett, E., Daniels, K. R., Curson, R., Chir, B., *et al.* (2004). 'Offspring created as a result of donor insemination: a study of family relationships, child adjustment, and disclosure'. *Fertility and Sterility*, 82, 172–9.

MacDougall, K., Becker, G., Scheib, J. E. and Nachtigall, R. D. (2007). 'Strategies for disclosure: how parents approach telling their children that they were conceived with donor gametes'. *Fertility and Sterility*, 87, 524–33.

Mahlstedt, P. P., LaBounty, K. and Kennedy, W. T. (2009). 'The views of adult offspring of sperm donation: essential feedback for the development of ethical guidelines within the practice of assisted reproductive technology in the United States'. *Fertility and Sterility*, 93, 2236–46.

Murray, C., MacCallum, F. and Golombok, S. (2006). 'Egg donation parents and their children: follow-up at age 12 years'. *Fertility and Sterility*, 85, 610–18.

Nachtigall, R. D., Tschann, J. M., Szkupinski Quiroga, S., Pitcher, L., *et al.* (1997). 'Stigma, disclosure, and family functioning among parents of children conceived through donor insemination'. *Fertility and Sterility*, 68, 83–9.

O'Neill, O. (2007). *Autonomy and Trust in Bioethics*. Cambridge University Press.

Palacios, J. and Brodzinsky, D. M. (2010). 'Review: Adoption research. Trends, topics, outcomes'. *International Journal of Behavioral Development*, 34(3), 270–84.

Paul, M. S. and Berger, R. (2007). 'Topic avoidance and family functioning in families conceived with donor insemination'. *Human Reproduction*, 22, 2566–71.

Pennings, G. (2001). 'The right to privacy and access to information about one's genetic origins'. *Medicine and Law*, 20, 1–15.

Raoul-Duval, A., Letur-Konrisch, H. and Frydman, R. (1992). 'Anonymous oocyte donation: a psychological study of recipients, donors and children'. *Human Reproduction*, 7(1), 51–4.

Rumball, A. and Adair, V. (1999). 'Telling the story: parents' scripts for donor offspring'. *Human Reproduction*, 14, 1392–9.

Scheib, J. E. (2003). 'Choosing identity-release sperm donors: the parents' perspective 13–18 years later'. *Human Reproduction*, 18, 1115–27.

Shehab, D., Duff, J., Pasch, L. A., MacDougall, K., *et al.* (2008). 'How parents whose children have been conceived with donor gametes make their disclosure decision: contexts, influences, and couple dynamics'. *Fertility and Sterility*, 89, 179–87.

Shelton, K. H., Boivin, J., Hay, D., Den Bree, M. B. M. van, Rice, F. J., Harold, G. T. (2009). 'Examining differences in psychological adjustment problems among children conceived by assisted reproductive technologies'. *International Journal of Behavioral Development*, 33, 385–92.

Smart, C. (2009). 'Family secrets: law and understandings of openness in everyday relationships'. *Journal of Social Policy*, 38, 551–67.

Sumner, L. W. (1999). *Welfare, Happiness, and Ethics*. New York: Oxford University Press.

Turner, A. J. and Coyle, A. (2000). 'What does it mean to be a donor offspring? The identity experiences of adults conceived by donor insemination and the implications for counselling and therapy'. *Human Reproduction*, 15, 2041–51.

LEGISLATION

Family Law Reform Act 1987
Human Fertilisation and Embryology Act 1990
Human Tissue Act 2004

Tabitha Freeman, John B. Appleby and Vasanti Jadva

Introduction

The long-standing ethical and policy debate about whether gamete donors should remain anonymous or be identifiable has been conducted with very limited empirical evidence about the implications of open-identity donation for those involved. While there is a growing consensus that the use of identifiable donors is preferable to the secrecy that has traditionally surrounded gamete donation, there is uncertainty around the consequences of policy decisions to remove donor anonymity, particularly regarding potential outcomes should donor offspring wish to meet their donor or other families created using their donor's gametes. Open-identity donation is now available and is sometimes mandatory in several countries around the world, although it will be some years before the social effects of this regulatory change are realized. In the UK, for example, the entitlement of individuals conceived using donated gametes from 1 April 2005 onwards to receive identifying information about their donor at age 18 will not come into effect until 2023.

There are various types of identifiable donors. Clinics may use 'identity-release' donors whose identifying information is accessible once the child conceived with their gametes reaches a specified age; information may or may not be available to parents before this time. Alternatively, in instances where children have been conceived using anonymously donated gametes, the donor may choose to revoke their anonymity and make their identity known at a later stage. Lastly, the donor's identity may be known from the time of the child's conception, as is the case when prospective parents ask friends or relatives to donate their gametes, a practice that appears to be on the increase since the removal of donor anonymity. This chapter is primarily concerned with the first two types of open-identity donation, that is identity-release donation and formerly anonymous donation, and will focus on donations that occur within the context of the clinic (for a discussion of intra-familial donation, see Vayena and Golombok, Chapter 10).

Open-identity donation impacts upon every stage of reproductive donation and upon all the actors involved, from the early decisions of potential donors and recipients before giving or receiving gametes to the choices offspring may later make regarding contact with the donor. This chapter examines the consequences of open-identity donation for parents, offspring and donors after the birth of the resulting child; discussions of its impact 'pre-birth' can be found elsewhere in this book (see Pennings, Vayena and Ahuja, Chapter 9). The discussion predominantly refers to offspring conceived by sperm donation, although information about egg donation is included where possible (for a discussion of embryo donation, see MacCallum and Widdows, Chapter 15).

The main objective of the chapter is to address some of the 'unknown' implications of open-identity donation by drawing upon empirical research describing contact experiences between donor relations and developing a bioethical analysis of the issues raised by this phenomenon. As donor offspring can only seek information about their donor relations if they are aware of the nature of their conception, the impact of open-identity donation on parents' disclosure decisions and, conversely, on offspring's responses to disclosure are also considered. In looking at the consequences of open-identity donation for parents, offspring and donors separately, the ethical approach developed in this chapter acknowledges that the specific needs and desires of these groups may differ and indeed conflict, while remaining faithful to the prioritization of the best interests of the child. The analysis is also sensitive to potential differences within these groups, for example in terms of offspring's age and parent's sexual orientation and marital status, which may affect individuals' attitudes towards, and experiences of, open-identity donation.

Open-identity donation: social, policy and ethical context

The introduction of open-identity donation as a common practice in fertility clinics around the world has significantly changed the wider social, policy and ethical landscape in which gamete donation occurs. While not universal, various systems of open-identity donation have been established over the past few decades in several jurisdictions, including Sweden, the Netherlands, Norway, Austria, Switzerland, the UK, the USA, the Australian States of Victoria and Western Australia and New Zealand. These range from the mandatory use of identifiable donors in all registered clinics, as in the UK and the Netherlands, to 'double-track' systems of anonymous and non-anonymous donation, as in the USA. In situations where recipients have a choice about the type of donor they seek, it has been found that the use of open-identity donation is increasing (Brewaeys *et al.*, 2005; Scheib and Cushing, 2007). In some jurisdictions, such as the UK, New Zealand and the Australian State of Victoria, voluntary registers have been set up to facilitate contact between donor offspring and their formerly 'anonymous' donors for those conceived before the removal of donor anonymity.

Part of the explanation for the rise in open-identity donation is the increased availability of assisted conception for individuals and couples who were previously denied access due to their sexual orientation, marital status or age. Lesbian couples and solo mothers now constitute a significant proportion of the donor insemination (DI) parent population. Unlike infertile heterosexual couples, these 'non-traditional' parents are generally open with their children about their method of conception, in part due to the absence of a social father, and tend to be more favourably inclined towards having an identifiable donor (Brewaeys *et al.*, 2005). As an alternative to using identifiable donors recruited via a clinic, friends or relatives may be asked to donate gametes (Adair and Purdie, 1996; Baetens *et al.*, 2000), and recipients sometimes choose to form various types of co-parenting arrangements with these 'known donors'.

As these examples illustrate, there are multiple routes to parenthood in contemporary societies, with discourses around assisted conception both untying the bonds of genetic relatedness that were traditionally perceived to hold 'the family' together while contributing to the increased importance placed on genetic identity (Gollancz, 2001; Freeman and Richards, 2006). In particular, the 'medicalization' of genetic identity and family history has foregrounded the importance of knowing one's genetic origins (Finkler, 2001). As such, families created by assisted conception feed into wider demographic and cultural transitions in the nature of family life, with the diversification of family forms both challenging and reinforcing the ideology of the traditional nuclear family. This is evidenced by the proliferation of non-married and/or non-genetic parental relationships arising from changing patterns of childbearing, cohabitation, (re)marriage and divorce.

The policy debate around donor identification has also opened up the related issue of donor offspring's rights to knowledge of their 'donor siblings' (i.e. children conceived using the same donor growing up in different families). For example, in the UK the Human Fertilisation and

Embryology Act 2008 makes provision for donor-conceived individuals at age 18 to seek identifying information about any donor siblings they may have, provided all siblings consent to the disclosure. In the meantime, contact between donor siblings may be facilitated on a consensual basis through voluntary registers, such as the Donor Sibling Link in the UK. In the USA the Donor Sibling Registry (DSR), established in 2000 by a donor-conceived child and his mother, has put thousands of donor offspring and their parents in contact with other families who share the same donor and, in rarer instances, their donors. This privately run website bypasses donor anonymity by using the unique identification number ascribed to donors to connect donor relations.

Policy debates around the identification of donor siblings have primarily been limited to concerns about unwitting incest between genetic relations (Barton *et al.*, 1945; Department of Health and Social Security, 1984; Human Fertilisation and Embryology Act 1990). Similarly, policy for donor identification is based on pre-existing international law and UK adoption law that suggests individuals have a claim right (i.e. a right that someone else is obligated to satisfy for the claimant) to access information about their genetic origins. However, it is clear that the implementation of donor and donor sibling identification raises a host of new ethical questions concerning the rights and responsibilities of donor offspring, parents and donors as new paths of communication between them, and their families, are opened up.

From an ethical perspective, meetings between donor relations and their families occur when individuals decide to explore the possibility of social interaction with each other because it might be important. The previous chapter (Appleby, Blake and Freeman, Chapter 13) discussed reasons why knowing about one's donor might be important and what the consequences of donor anonymity are. Since knowing your genetic inheritance could in some cases benefit your well-being, it might be possible to extend this argument to include the claim that knowing your genetic family history is also important in this regard. At the very least, knowing could be important because you could find out about health or behavioural risks that run in your family that are heritable but may not be identifiable with genetic tests. In this case, does knowing an individual who is a part of your genetic history, by meeting them personally, make a difference ethically?

What are the ethical consequences of meetings that do take place? According to consequentialists, if a meeting is the best choice, then on balance the outcome (quantifiable or non-quantifiable) should leave the group as a whole better off. However, it is difficult to say whether meetings are always good or always bad because the interests of different groups of individuals, and the individuals themselves, are not always the same. For offspring, it may be argued that knowing and meeting one's genetic relations in person is morally important. For parents, enacting this benefit for their children may need to be countered by weighing the potential risks of harm involved. Likewise, for donors these meetings may raise ethical dilemmas concerning feelings of moral responsibility for their donor offspring. These ethical issues, alongside empirical evidence of potential outcomes, will be explored further below.

Implications of open-identity donation for parents

How does open-identity donation affect parents' disclosure decisions?

The introduction of identifiable donors will have little impact in practice if parents do not tell their children about the nature of their conception (Frith, 2001). As discussed in the previous chapter, there is strong and consistent evidence that, at least until relatively recently, the large majority of heterosexual parents have chosen not to tell their children about their donor origins (Golombok *et al.*, 1996, 2002; Brewaeys *et al.*, 1997; Nachtigall *et al.*, 1998; Gottleib *et al.*, 2000). While some studies report that a growing number of parents intend to disclose (Adair and Purdie, 1996; Rumball and Adair, 1999; Hunter *et al.*, 2000; Lycett *at al.*, 2004), intentions are not necessarily born out in practice and it has been found that the disclosure process can become increasingly difficult the older children become (Golombok *et al.*, 2002). Furthermore, these studies have by and large been conducted with parents who conceived using anonymously donated sperm, and disclosure patterns amongst those who use identifiable donors may not be directly comparable. Indeed, lack of knowledge about the donor has been identified as a key reason for parents deciding against disclosure in cases of anonymous donation, due to concerns about the potential frustration children may suffer from not knowing who their donor is (Cook *et al.*, 1995; Nachtigall *et al.*, 1998; Lindblad *et al.*, 2000; Lycett *et al.*, 2005).

There is some evidence that the use of identifiable donors and cultural attitudes favouring openness have increased disclosure rates among parents (Daniels and Lewis, 1996; Scheib *et al.*, 2003; Golombok *et al.*, 2004). While some research does not support this link (Baetens *et al.*, 2000; Greenfeld and Klock, 2004; Laruelle *et al.*, 2011), other studies have found an association between the use of identifiable donors and high rates of disclosure or intention to disclose (Greenfeld *et al.*, 1998; Godman *et al.*, 2006). For example, in a study of Dutch recipients' choices regarding the use of anonymous or identifiable sperm donors, those who opted for identifiable donors did not consider secrecy about the donor conception an option (Brewaeys *et al.*, 2005). High rates of intended and actual disclosure amongst parents who use identifiable donors can in part be explained by the high proportion of lesbian and solo mothers who choose this type of donor; in the Brewaeys *et al.* (2005) study, 98 per cent of lesbian parents interviewed used an identifiable donor compared to 63 per cent of heterosexual couples. More generally, it is perhaps reasonable to assume that parents who are open about DI will be more likely to choose identity-release donors; indeed, recent research has found parents who have had children in this way to be open and positive about their method of conception and the accessibility of the donor's identity (Scheib *et al.*, 2003; Leeb-Lundberg *et al.*, 2006). However, it must also be recognized that the availability of identifying information about the donor may equally act as a disincentive to disclose for some parents; for example, parents may perceive their child's possible knowledge of, and contact with, the donor as a threat to family relationships and the welfare of the child. Indeed, in cases of oocyte donation where recipients had a choice between known and anonymous donation, no link was found between parents' choice of donor and their disclosure intentions, with approximately half choosing to opt for secrecy overall (Baetens *et al.*, 2000; Laruelle *et al.*, 2011).

The impact of open-identity donation on parental disclosure decisions remains an open question, and perhaps at this stage it is only possible to conclude that having identifiable donors may influence parents' inclinations towards both secrecy and openness in different ways. It appears that a range of factors may impact on the decision-making process, including the type of donation (i.e. sperm, oocyte or embryo) and the type of 'identifiable' donor (e.g. identity-release donor selected at a clinic or known donor chosen from amongst family and friends) involved. Variation in the parents' personal background may also play a role in their disclosure decisions, including their sexual orientation and marital status, age and ethnic origin. Despite the policy and cultural embrace of openness around gamete donation, it seems that there is no guarantee that using identifiable donors will lead to parents informing their child about their conception. Indeed, while there are signs that disclosure rates may be on the increase overall, non-disclosure and donor anonymity may remain preferable to many parents, particularly those in heterosexual partnerships.

Why might parents wish to find out about their child's donor relations?

Through their disclosure decisions, parents implicitly act as gatekeepers concerning whether a child gains knowledge of their donor relations. It is therefore of interest to consider why parents might wish to find out about their child's donor relations, and the value they place on sharing this information with their child. Parents' motivations for seeking their child's donor relations were explored in a study of 791 parents (39% lone mothers, 35% lesbian couples, 21% heterosexual couples) recruited via the Donor Sibling Registry (DSR) who had conceived using anonymously donated gametes, of whom just under half were now seeking contact with the donor and the majority with their child's donor siblings (Freeman *et al.*, 2009). Parents' most common reasons for searching for donor relations were curiosity about their appearance and personalities, and wishing to give their child a better understanding of themselves. For those searching for donor siblings, wanting their child to have a sibling was also significant, particularly in cases where the child was a singleton. Parents in households without fathers were more curious about their child's donor origins than those in families headed by heterosexual couples. Lone mothers in particular highlighted that giving their child a secure sense of identity was a key motivation underpinning their search.

While parents were generally open to the idea of their child developing some kind of relationship with their donor siblings, many expressed reticence about their child being in contact with their donor, particularly those within heterosexual partnerships; knowing about the donor was generally considered more important than forming a relationship with him. This observation is in line with Scheib *et al.*'s (2003, 2005) study of families created with open-identity sperm donors, where parents emphasized their curiosity about the donor in relation to the impact on their child's identity rather than perceiving this man as a potential father figure.

What are parents' experiences of making contact with their child's donor relations?

If parents obtain identifying information about their child's donor or donor siblings, this opens up further decisions around whether to pursue contact with them. In the DSR study, a clear distinction was found between parents' motivations, expectations and experiences of searching for, finding and contacting their child's donor relations (Freeman *et al.*, 2009). Overall, parents' experiences of meeting donor relations far exceeded their expectations, with mutual feelings of warmth and affection overcoming their initial reservations. More than half of the families who had contacted donor siblings remained in regular contact and the large majority reported this to be a positive experience. Most notably, unanticipated feelings of relatedness developed between family members that were described in terms of close and lasting bonds of family and friendship. Of particular interest was the emotional closeness that arose between parents and their child's donor siblings, with mothers reporting strong 'maternal' feelings towards these children despite the lack of a direct genetic connection. Parents' sexual orientation and marital status did not appear to have a significant impact on the contact outcomes. Positive experiences were also reported in Scheib and Ruby's (2008) study of contact between families created by identity-release donation which included 14 families (50% lone mothers, 43% lesbian couples, 7% heterosexual couples).

Parents in the DSR study likewise reported unexpectedly positive experiences of contacting their child's donor (Freeman *et al.*, 2009). In particular, knowing, rather than simply knowing about, the donor was described as having a beneficial impact on the child's sense of self and family, with an enhanced knowledge of one's origins being directly linked to psychological well-being. As one mother described, my daughter 'has become a calm confident person, who relishes knowing who she is and why. Knowing her dad has completed her in some way and has allowed her to grow.' However, while the DSR study provides some insight, very little is known about the nature of the bonds that may develop between an offspring and their donor, and it is likely that contact outcomes will be highly variable according to the individual circumstances of both the child and the donor and their respective families.

The new forms of relatedness that may be created by reproductive donation are a significant consequence of open-identity donation about which very little is known. As yet, we do not have an adequate language to describe the connections between donor relations and their families, which defy conventional notions of familial bonds based on factors such as shared upbringing, family history or legal obligation. While the findings of the DSR study suggest that contact between donor relations may have a positive impact on those involved, significant caveats apply. Most pertinently, the sample in this study cannot be claimed to be representative of the population of donor conception families as a whole. In particular, by virtue of their membership of the DSR, the participants in this study were likely to be favourably disposed towards finding their donor relations. It is also important to note that not all parents' experiences of contacting their child's donor relations were positive. Problems may arise due to differences in families' expectations regarding establishing and maintaining contact, and negotiating the host of new disclosure issues this raises. For example, some young children had met and formed friendships with their donor siblings without being aware of their genetic connection, and in these instances parents could differ as to if, when and how they wished their child to be informed about their genetic relatedness.

Implications of open-identity donation for offspring

How does open-identity donation impact on donor offspring's responses to disclosure?

If told in an age-appropriate manner at a young age, children's responses to learning about their donor origins tend to be positive or neutral. In the case of anonymous donation, young children have been found to react to the discovery that an unknown donor exists with curiosity and a desire to know more about the donor, although some express little interest (Snowden, 1990; Rumball and Adair, 1999; Lindblad *et al.*, 2000; Vanfraussen *et al.*, 2001, 2003; Lycett *et al.*, 2004; Lycett, 2005; Scheib and Ruby, 2008). If the discovery that one was conceived by an anonymous donor occurs in late adolescence or adulthood, responses may be less positive, particularly if this revelation takes place under adverse circumstances such as parental divorce (Jadva *et al.*, 2009). In such cases, lack of information about one's genetic origins may become a source of deep frustration and upset (Turner and Coyle, 2000; Kirkman, 2004).

It is helpful to think of individuals' responses to disclosure as a process rather than a singular event, with feelings about one's donor origins potentially changing over the life course. Most pertinently, the majority of studies assessing the impact of disclosure have focused on young children who, by virtue of their age, are unlikely to comprehend the full implications of gamete donation regarding their lack of genetic relationship with one of their parents. Such an understanding will probably not occur until they achieve the abstract thinking associated with adolescence (Steinberg and Silk, 2002). Adolescence is also a time when issues of identity become salient (Erikson, 1968), which is likely to lead to an increased interest in one's donor conception. Similarly, events in adulthood, such as the death of one's parents, may trigger an interest in one's genetic origins, as is evident in studies of adopted people (Crawshaw, 2002).

So, how might offspring's responses to being told about their donor conception be affected by the knowledge that their donor is identifiable? Will knowing that they can find out about their donor make learning about their donor conception easier to integrate into their self-narrative? Will discovering that they were conceived using an identifiable donor intensify their interest in their genetic origins? How will offspring conceived with identity-release donors respond to discovering they will have to wait until a specified age to find out about their donor? Very little is known about these issues. However, Scheib's (2005) study of 29 adolescents conceived using open-identity sperm donors who learned of their origins at an early age found that most were comfortable with knowing about the nature of their conception. A further important question to ask is whether offspring conceived using open-identity donation will ultimately respond to disclosure by seeking identifying information about their donor relations. It is not possible to predict the proportion of offspring who will decide to access identifying information about their donor and donor siblings when presented with this choice. There is some indication that the majority will want to obtain their donor's identity; for example, over 80 per cent of the adolescents in Scheib's (2005) study felt that it was at least moderately likely that they would opt to contact their donor on reaching adulthood. However, other studies suggest greater variability. For example, offspring may decide against finding out about their donor in order to protect the feelings of their birth parents, and some may want non-identifying rather than identifying information (Vanfraussen et al., 2001, 2003; Lycett 2005).

Why might offspring wish to find out about their donor relations?

There are many reasons why offspring may wish to find out about their donor relations. The DSR study included 165 adolescent and adult sperm donor offspring (58% with heterosexual couple parents, 23% with single mother parents and 15% with lesbian couple parents), of whom the majority were searching for both their donor and donor siblings (Jadva et al., 2010b). Most offspring were searching for their donor and donor siblings out of curiosity, with a greater proportion of those from father-absent families wishing to meet their donor. Gaining a better understanding of oneself was also perceived as important, as were medical issues related to knowledge of the donor. The child's age when they were told about their donor conception was significant in this regard, with those who found out in adulthood being more likely to search for medical reasons and those who found out in childhood being more likely to search out of curiosity. These findings are in line with Scheib *et al.*'s (2005) study, with the main reasons given by adolescents conceived by identity-release donation for wishing to contact their donor relating to feelings of curiosity, with many believing this would help them learn more about themselves. Adult offspring in the DSR study also reported that their interest in their genetic background was triggered by having children themselves, illustrating that the importance of genetic identity goes beyond the donor–offspring relationship to include their wider family networks and future generations.

Over 90 per cent of the offspring in the DSR study who had found their donor siblings or donor went on to make contact with them. However, this was a sample of offspring with an active interest in their donor relations, and it is difficult to predict more generally whether offspring will pursue contact with their donor relations once identifying information has been accessed. Other similar voluntary registers that are state-run, for example in the Australian state of Victoria and the UK, have had far lower levels of take-up to date, with small numbers of donor relations having made contact in this way.

What are offspring's experiences of making contact with their donor relations?

The large majority of offspring in the DSR study who had been in contact with their donor siblings and donor reported this to be a positive experience. Many described their ensuing relationships with donor siblings in terms of the development of close family bonds. For those who had met their donor, this was likewise described as having a positive impact on their lives; as one adolescent boy describes: 'I am so glad I met [my donor], and would not trade the world for the experience I had … he is one of the most important people in my life to this day.' Indeed, as with the parents, a snowball effect was observed as offspring went from seeking, to finding, to contacting, to meeting and forming relationships with their donor relations, with their positive experiences heightening as their initial curiosity evolved into an emotional sense of family bonding.

Not all offspring's experiences are positive, however, and the risks involved in facilitating contact between donor relations were also highlighted in the DSR study. Contact experiences may lead to disappointment, bitterness and distress, particularly if the expectations of those involved are incompatible. As one donor conceived adult described, 'although [my donor] is glad that I was born, he is not proud to have participated in donor conception … It is a pretty bad feeling that my life has been such a source of shame and embarrassment, through no fault of my own, by the people who brought me into this world.'

What is the value of family history and ancestry for offspring?

J. David Velleman (2008) argues spending time with those with whom we share consanguine (genetic) relations is morally important because it gives us a window into understanding where we came from and what we came from. In other words, getting to know our *genetic* family history not only tells us something about our physical appearance, but also why we are who we are. For example, it is not just important to know who you got your blonde hair and blue eyes from; it is also important to know if a character trait you have runs in your genetic family history. He argues that there is also value in understanding how our lives fit into the narratives of our family histories (Velleman, 2005). Furthermore, this information is good, according to Velleman, because it gives us a foothold in the world from which to make sense of our lives, which consequently helps us lead a flourishing life (Velleman, 2008). Velleman's account places value on knowing our genetic family history first, and then places additional emphasis on knowing the way our genetic family history has played out socially to date. For Velleman, contact between parents, children and donors is of high moral priority.

Are the moral goods that can be obtained through new relationships with an unfamiliar genetic parent (and other members of a 'donor family') any more valuable, or additionally valuable, than the social relationships that are obtained between the donor-conceived child and a familiar non-genetic parent (and other members of their 'social family')? Contrary to Velleman's argument in favour of knowing family history (Velleman, 2005), Anja Karnein (see Chapter 4) argues that children would not be worse off without genetically related parents. Being born into a family with a non-genetic relation to one or both parents would still offer children a lineage of social relationships that have certainly played a unique causal role in their coming into existence; any other parental arrangement would have likely meant that *they* would never have been brought into existence. If knowing the narrative of events that played a role in your genesis is important, it appears that this good could be *almost* completely obtained (short of obtaining both a genetic and social narrative) without needing to meet a genetic relative. In other words, this argument claims that the family history of social parents is just as – if not more – important to the existence of a donor-conceived child as is the family history of the genetic donor (see also Wilson, 1997; Smart, 2010).

Implications of open-identity donation for donors

*How do donors feel about the children conceived using their
gametes? What impact does meeting these children have?*

Most research on donors has focused on their motivations for, and
attitudes towards, donating. Indeed, until the introduction of open-
identity donation, a donor's role was effectively perceived to end at the
point of their donation. While some studies have assessed donors' feelings towards any children conceived with their donated gametes (e.g.
Thorn *et al.*, 2008; Purewal and van den Akker, 2009), this was within
the context of anonymous donation where contact with any offspring
was extremely unlikely. Open-identity donation has opened up potentially greater involvement for donors beyond their genetic contribution,
meaning that donors' views about, and eventual experiences of, contact
with offspring have become of critical importance.

Due to the recent introduction of open-identity donation, the experiences of identifiable donors remain largely unknown. Nonetheless,
the DSR study of anonymous sperm donors who subsequently choose
to make their identity known to any offspring conceived with their
gametes may provide some insight (Jadva *et al.*, 2010a). This study of
63 sperm donors and 11 egg donors found that although most were
content about having donated, many were concerned about the well-
being of children created with their gametes and being unable to
contact them. Most wished to know how many offspring had been
conceived with their gametes, with half wishing to have identifying
information.

The donors' concerns had a clear moral component, with some
reporting a burden of responsibility towards any child their donation
helped to create. Indeed, although people who donate through clinics
are generally protected from any legal or financial duties to children
conceived as a result of their donation, the DSR study suggests that
donors may feel a sense of obligation to support their donor offspring
should they be in financial or emotional need; for example, if the child's
birth parent(s) should die. While it has yet to be tested whether donors
would act upon this sense of moral responsibility in practice, the possibility of this predicament arising can present an uncomfortable uncertainty in their lives. In the DSR study, donors generally presented a
positive sense of moral commitment towards their offspring and felt
that they were ethically justified in making themselves available for contact because they believed this to be in line with the rights of the child.
All of the donors who had met the families their gametes had helped

to create reported positive experiences, with the majority intending to maintain contact over time.

It has been suggested that open-identity donation will impact on the type of people who donate, both in terms of their demographic profile and motivations for donating. For example, identifiable sperm donors are described as being older and more likely to have had children themselves than anonymous ones. Several studies have reported anonymous egg and sperm donors' principal motivations for donation as being financial payment and altruism (Sauer *et al.*, 1989; Schover *et al.*, 1992; Cook and Golombok, 1995; Fielding *et al.*, 1998; Jadva *et al.*, 2010a; Kenney and McGowan, 2010). While altruism and payment remain important motives, it has been suggested that the introduction of open-identity donation may lead to the wish to procreate becoming more prominent, particularly among sperm donors (Janssens *et al.*, 2006). Although it is still early days, it is possible that identifiable donors' attitudes towards their offspring may reflect such a shift, in that they may be amenable to meeting and establishing relationships with their offspring. However, in many jurisdictions, such as the UK, offspring will not be able to contact their donor until reaching adulthood and it is likely that this could have a significant impact on the nature of any relationships that may be formed.

How does open-identity donation impact on the responsibilities and rights of donors?

If a donor agrees to meet with parents and their donor offspring, it is difficult to infer what the outcome will be. The donor likely recognizes that there is something good about meeting the parent(s) and child(ren). There is always the risk that this exposure will be traumatic for the donor, parents or child, and it is difficult to ascertain what degree of responsibility (if any) the donor may feel toward the child. Donors may have no legal obligation to associate with the parents or children yet, as the DSR study suggests, donors might feel morally bound to fulfil some newly perceived responsibility for those individuals (particularly the child). If the parent eliminates contact between the child and the donor, does the donor's newly inferred moral responsibility then become frustrated (perhaps indefinitely)? Such harms may be difficult to avert in all cases.

What are the consequences of donors meeting parents and their donor-conceived children if the donors themselves have children and family who are unaware of their existence? Do donors have a right to protect their families from the potential shock of learning that they have donor relations? Conversely, does a donor-conceived child have a right to knowledge of the donors' own children, to whom they are genetically related as half-siblings? Eighteen may be the age at which a person is legally an adult in the UK, but aside from adulthood, why is this necessarily the best time to inform the child about the identity of their donor? Over the course of eighteen years, a donor's life will change, and some changes might be significant in terms of the consequences of meeting a genetically related child. In could be in the interests of both donor and child to have the opportunity to make contact at an earlier stage.

Conclusions: ethical and policy considerations in open-identity donation

While some have argued that, at least in principle, open-identity donation is likely to be in the best interests of a child because it upholds an individual's right to knowledge of their 'genetic origins', the practical and ethical consequences of putting such a system into practice are only now unfolding. This chapter has drawn upon empirical evidence and moral reasoning to examine some of the complexities of open-identity donation for all those involved, particularly concerning the implications should donor-conceived offspring and their families seek contact with their donors and with other families created using their donor's gametes. In particular, the discussion has highlighted potential conflicts between the interests, rights and responsibilities of parents, offspring and donors, as well as between individual perspectives and wider cultural, ethical and policy norms. For example, parents may maintain a preference for non-disclosure despite the mandatory use of open-identity donation in clinical practice, thus effectively 'anonymising' the donor by not informing the child about their donor origins.

The discussion has also explored how open-identity donation may lead to new forms of kinship and relatedness in situations where donor offspring and their families make contact with their donor relations. The new concepts of family relatedness that are emerging are being created through an ongoing process of negotiating and defining experiences of 'sharing' gametes with relative strangers. As one mother describes, her child and his donor sibling 'call each other "brother" and "sister" – not half-brother or half-sister. There is an indescribable relationship there. Much more than distant relatives but different than if they had grown up together as full siblings. The kids will be better defining this relationship as they move forward.' Furthermore, while the focus has been on genetic relationships between a donor-conceived individual and their donor and donor siblings, it is clear that their wider families are involved. If concerns about genetic identity and relationships underpin ethical and policy arguments for open-identity donation, it is thus necessary to re-evaluate where and how the lines of relatedness are drawn.

The policy focus on the relationship between the donor-conceived individual and their donor and donor siblings has also created inconsistencies in current policy on donor identification. For example, a donor-conceived individual's claim right to identifying information about the donor's own offspring has not been addressed and yet these are also their genetic half-siblings. Identity-release donation, where donor offspring must reach a specified age before gaining access to identifying information about their donor, gives rise to further complications. For example, if a donor-conceived individual has younger birth siblings created with the same donor, their siblings could potentially find out their donor's identity before reaching the specified age. More significantly, the identity-release principle may lead to disappointment and frustration if the donor is unable or unwilling to be traced when access is sought; for example, if the donor's feelings about making contact change as their own personal and family circumstances change or if indeed, they die before this time. A further policy concern raised by open-identity donation is how to maintain an adequate supply of donors in light of fears that open-identity donation will significantly lower recruitment levels. One proposal has been to raise the number of children who can be created from the gametes of any one donor. As yet, little is known about the psychological impact of finding a large number of donor siblings or donor offspring for donor offspring and donors respectively, as well as for members of their families. However, at the very least it would be judicious to acknowledge that this carries risks of potentially negative outcomes (Janssens et al., 2006; Sawyer, 2010).

As with any system, open-identity donation may raise as many problems as it solves, while still remaining preferable to the alternatives. The introduction of open-identity donation has developed alongside, and indeed may have partially contributed to, increasing numbers of individuals and couples seeking alternative forms of reproductive donation. These alternative forms include using gametes donated by known donors which may or may not take place in a clinic, or by donors advertising their services on dedicated websites. Donated gametes may also be purchased from clinics in other countries operating under different systems. While ethicists and policy makers grapple with refining the moral and regulatory frameworks in which reproductive donation takes place and empirical researchers attempt to gain evidence about the psychological outcomes for those involved, one thing remains certain: those who wish to have children using reproductive donation will endeavour to find the means to do so on their terms and within the emotional, ethical and practical constraints of their everyday lives, which may or may not be amenable to open-identity donation.

REFERENCES

Adair, V. and Purdie, A. (1996). 'Donor insemination programmes with personal donors: issues of secrecy'. *Human Reproduction*, 11, 2558–63.

Baetens, P., Devroey, P., Camus, M., Van Steirteghem, A. C., *et al.* (2000). 'Counselling couples and donors for oocyte donation: the decision to use either known or anonymous oocytes'. *Human Reproduction*, 15, 476–84.

Barton, M., Walker, K. and Weisner, B. P. (1945). 'Artificial insemination'. *British Medical Journal*, 1, 40–2.

Brewaeys, A., Golombok, S., Naaktgeboren, N., de Bruyn, J. K., *et al.* (1997). 'Donor insemination: Dutch parents' opinions about confidentiality and donor anonymity and the emotional adjustment of their children'. *Human Reproduction*, 12, 1591–7.

Brewaeys, A., de Bruyn, J. K., Louwe, L. A. and Helmerhorst, F. M. (2005). 'Anonymous or identity-registered sperm donors? A study of Dutch recipients' choices'. *Human Reproduction*, 20, 820–4.

Cook, R. and Golombok. S. (1995). 'A survey of semen donation: phase II – the view of the donors'. *Human Reproduction*, 10, 951–9.

Cook, R., Golombok, S., Bish, A. and Murray, C. (1995). 'Disclosure of donor insemination: parental attitudes'. *American Journal of Orthopsychiatry*, 65, 549–59.

Crawshaw, M. (2002). 'Lessons from a recent adoption study to identify some of the service needs of, and issues for, donor offspring wanting to know about their donors'. *Human Fertilization*, 5, 6–12.

Daniels, K. and Lewis, G. M. (1996). 'Openness of information in the use of donor gametes: developments in New Zealand'. *Journal of Reproductive and Infant Psychology*, 14, 57–68.

Department of Health and Social Security (1984). 'Report of the Committee of Inquiry into Human Fertilization and Embryology'. London: HMSO (Comnd. 9314).

Erikson, E. H. (1968). *Identity: Youth and Crisis*. New York: Norton.

Fielding, D., Handley, S., Duqueno, L., Weaver, S., *et al.* (1998). 'Motivation, attitudes and experience of donation: a follow-up of women donating eggs in assisted conception treatment'. *Journal of Community and Applied Social Psychology*, 8, 273–87.

Finkler, K. (2001). 'The kin in the gene: the medicalization of family and kinship in American society'. *Current Anthropology*, 42, 235.

Freeman, T. and Richards, M. (2006). 'DNA Testing and Kinship: Paternity, Genealogy and the Search for the "Truth" of our Genetic Origins', in F. Ebtehaj, B. Lindley and M. Richards (eds.), *Kinship Matters*. Oxford: Hart.

Freeman, T., Jadva, V., Kramer, W. and Golombok, S. (2009). 'Gamete dona-tion: parents' experiences of searching for their child's donor siblings and donor'. *Human Reproduction*, 24, 505–16.

Frith, L. (2001). 'Beneath the rhetoric: the role of rights in the practice of non-anonymous gamete donation'. *Bioethics*, 15, 473–84.

Godman, K. M., Sanders, K., Rosenberg, M. and Burton, P. (2006). 'Potential sperm donors', recipients' and their partners' opinions towards the release of identifying information in Western Australia'. *Human Reproduction*, 21, 3022–6.

Gollancz, D. (2001). 'Donor insemination: a question of rights'. *Human Fertility*, 4, 164–7.

Golombok, S., Brewaeys, A., Cook, R., Giavazzi. M. T., *et al.* (1996). 'Children: the European study of assisted reproduction families: family functioning and child development'. *Human Reproduction*, 11, 2324–31.

Golombok, S., MacCallum, F., Goodman, E. and Rutter, M. (2002). 'Families with children conceived by donor insemination: a follow-up at age twelve'. *Child Development*, 73, 952–68.

Golombok, S., Lycett, E., MacCallum, F., Jadva, V., *et al.* (2004). 'Parenting infants conceived by gamete donation'. *Journal of Family Psychology*, 18, 443–52.

Gottlieb, C., Lalos, O. and Lindblad, F. (2000). 'Disclosure of donor insemi-nation to the child: the impact of Swedish legislation on couples' attitudes'. *Human Reproduction*, 15, 2052–6.

Greenfeld, D. A. and Klock, S. C. (2004). 'Disclosure decisions among known and anonymous oocyte donation recipients'. *Fertility and Sterility*, 81, 1565–71.

Greenfeld, D. A., Greenfeld, D. G., Mazure, C. M., Keefe, D. L., *et al.* (1998). 'Do attitudes towards disclosure in donor oocyte recipients predict the use of anonymous versus direct donation?' *Fertility and Sterility*, 70, 1009–14.

Hunter, M., Salter-Ling, N. and Glover, L. (2000). 'Donor insemination: telling children about their origins'. *Psychology and Psychiatry Review*, 5, 157–63.

Jadva, V., Freeman, T., Kramer, W. and Golombok, S. (2009). 'The experi-ences of adolescents and adults conceived by sperm donation: comparisons by age of disclosure and family type'. *Human Reproduction*, 24, 1909–19.

Jadva, V. (2010a). 'Sperm and oocyte donors' experiences of anonymous donation and subsequent contact with their donor offspring'. *Human Reproduction*, 26, 638–645.

(2010b). 'Offsprings' experiences of searching for and contacting their donor siblings and donor'. *Reproductive BioMedicine Online*, 20 523–532.

Janssens, P. M. W., Simons, A. H. M., van Kooij, R. J., Blokzijl, E., *et al.* (2006). 'A new Dutch law regulating provision of identifying informa-tion of donors to offspring: background, content and impact'. *Human Reproduction*, 21, 852–6.

Kenney, N. J. and McGowan, M. L. (2010). 'Looking back: egg donors' retrospective evaluations of their motivations, expectations, and expe-riences during their first donation cycle'. *Fertility and Sterility*, 93, 455–66.

Kirkman, M. (2004). 'Genetic connection and relationships in narratives of donor-assisted conception'. *Australian Journal of Emerging Technologies and Society*, 2, 1–20.

Laruelle, C., Place, I., Demeestrere, I., Englert, Y., *et al.* (2011). 'Anonymity and secrecy options of recipient couples and donors, and ethnic origins influence in three types of oocyte donation'. *Human Reproduction*, 26, 382–90.

Leeb-Lundberg, S., Kjellberg, S. and Sydsjo, G. (2006). 'Helping parents to tell their children about the use of donor insemination (DI) and determining their opinions about open-identity sperm donation'. *Acta Obstetricia et Gynecologica Scandinavica*, 85, 78–81.

Lindblad, F., Gottlieb, C. and Lalos, O. (2000). 'To tell or not to tell: what parents think about telling their children that they were born following donor insemination'. *Journal Psychosomatic Obstetrics and Gynecology*, 21, 193–203.

Lycett, E., Daniels, K., Curson, R. and Golombok, S. (2004). 'Offspring created as a result of donor insemination: a study of family relationships, child adjustment, and disclosure'. *Fertility and Sterility*, 82, 172–9.

Lycett, E. (2005). 'School-aged children of donor insemination: a study of parents' disclosure patterns'. *Human Reproduction*, 20, 810–19.

Nachtigall, R. D., Pitcher, L., Tschann, J. M., Becker, G., *et al.* (1998). 'The disclosure decision: concerns and issues of parents and children conceived through donor insemination'. *American Journal of Obstetrics and Gynecology*, 178, 1165–70.

Purewal, S. and van den Akker, O. B. A. (2009). 'Systematic review of oocyte donation: investigating attitudes, motivations and experiences'. *Human Reproduction*, 5, 499–515.

Rumball, A. and Adair, V. (1999). 'Telling the story: parents' scripts for donor offspring'. *Human Reproduction*, 14, 1392–9.

Sauer, M. V., Gorrill, M. J., Zeffer, K. B. and Bustillo, M. (1989). 'Attitudinal survey of sperm donors to an artificial insemination clinic'. *Journal of Reproductive Medicine*, 34, 362–4.

Sawyer, N. (2010). 'Sperm donor limits that control for the "relative" risk associated with the use of open-identity donors'. *Human Reproduction*, 5, 1089–96.

Scheib, J. E. and Ruby, A. (2008). 'Contact among families who share the same sperm donor'. *Fertility and Sterility*, 90, 33–43.

Scheib, J. and Cushing, R. A. (2007). 'Open-identity donor insemination in United States: is it on the rise?' *Fertility and Sterility*, 88, 231–2.

Scheib, J. E., Riordan, M. and Rubin, S. (2003). 'Choosing identity-release sperm donors: the parents' perspective 13–18 years later'. *Human Reproduction*, 18, 1115–27.

Scheib, J. E. (2005). 'Adolescents with open-identity sperm donors: reports from 12–17 year olds'. *Human Reproduction*, 20, 239–52.

Schover, L. R., Rothman, S. A. and Collins, R. L. (1992). 'The personality and motivation of semen donors: a comparison with oocyte donors'. *Human Reproduction*, 7, 575–9.

Smart, C. (2010). 'Family secrets: law and understandings of openness in everyday relationships'. *Journal of Social Policy*, 38, 551–67.

Snowden, R. (1990). 'The Family and Artificial Reproduction', in D. R. Bromham, M. E. Dalton and J. C. Jack (eds.), *Philosophical Ethics in Reproductive Medicine*. Manchester University Press.

Steinberg, L. and Silk, J. S. (2002). 'Parenting Adolescents', in M. H. Bornstein (ed.), *Handbook of Parenting*, Vol. 1, Mahwah: Lawrence Erlbaum Associates.

Thorn, P., Katzorke, T. and Daniels, K. (2008). 'Human semen donors in Germany: a study exploring motivations and attitudes'. *Human Reproduction*, 23, 2415–20.

Turner, A. J. and Coyle, A. (2000). 'What does it mean to be a donor offspring? The identity experiences of adults conceived by donor insemination and the implications for counselling and therapy'. *Human Reproduction*, 15, 2041–51.

Vanfraussen, K., Ponjaert-Kristoffersen, I. and Brewaeys, A. (2001). 'An attempt to reconstruct children's donor concept: a comparison between children's and lesbian parents' attitudes towards donor anonymity'. *Human Reproduction*, 16, 2019–25.

(2003). 'Why do children want to know more about the donor? The experiences of youngsters raised in lesbian families'. *Journal of Psychosomatic Obstetrics and Gynecology*, 24, 31–8.

Velleman, J. D. (2005). 'Family history'. *Philosophical Papers*, 34, 357–78.

(2008). 'Persons in prospect: II. the gift of life'. *Philosophy and Public Affairs*, 36, 245–66.

Wilson, S. (1997). 'Identity, genealogy and the social family: the case of donor insemination'. *International Journal of Law, Policy and the Family*, 11, 270–97.

LEGISLATION

The Human Fertilisation and Embryology Act 1990, as amended 2008

15 Ethical issues in embryo donation

Fiona MacCallum and Heather Widdows

Introduction

The use of a donated embryo in assisted conception was first reported by Trounson *et al.* in 1983, when a female patient was successfully treated using an embryo created from a donor egg and donor sperm. It was deemed by the clinicians involved to be no different from egg or sperm donation, and indeed they postulated that it could be less problematic in that there would be no inequality in the genetic contributions of the parents[1] (Trounson *et al.*, 1983). However, embryo donation (strictly defined as treatment using donated embryos) raises distinctive ethical concerns and questions. In this chapter we will focus on three areas which we consider key to debating these concerns, covering regulatory issues, the structure of the practice of embryo donation and ARTs generally, and the individual perspectives of recipients and donors. The first topic to be examined is the disparity in parenting selection criteria between embryo donation and adoption, two processes that share a structure whereby both result in a couple parenting a genetically unrelated child. In 2002 we examined the size of this disparity and concluded that it was not justified (Widdows and MacCallum, 2002). Here we revisit and update the debate, in the light of changing laws regarding donor anonymity and changing social attitudes towards donor conception. The second key area relates to the decision whether to donate embryos in the first place. We investigate the extent to which the moral status of the embryo, as frequently debated in ethical analyses, has any influence on decisions of potential donors, and the need for consent to donation to be truly fully informed. In addition, there are ethical issues relating to the exploitation of donors (or 'vendors'), particularly poor vendors, which are unlikely to be addressed by improving informed consent. Finally, we address matters relating to the way

[1] Parents, when used without a qualifying prefix (such as 'genetic') indicates the social parents who have responsibility for the child's upbringing.

in which embryo donation impacts upon society's perceptions of children. Developments in the ability to choose characteristics of donors, and the varying laws existing in different jurisdictions worldwide, have produced structural changes in the practice of ARTs. Increasingly, the ethical debate has focused on 'reproductive tourism' and the ethical disquiet arising from this global market.[2] Central to this argument are increasing concerns about the commercialization of reproductive treatment, and the commodification which may result for the 'products' of this trade: the children created using these technologies.

Parenting selection criteria for embryo donation compared with adoption

If treatment using donated embryos is successful, the recipient couple will rear a child that is genetically unrelated to them and who may have full genetic siblings elsewhere. It has been contended, therefore, by some that embryo donation strongly resembles adoption, and should 'receive the same safeguards' (Bernstein et al., 1996). In the UK the two procedures are regulated in very dissimilar ways, particularly with respect to the criteria applied to embryo donation recipients as compared with adoptive parents. The primary difference is that in adoption the selection process is lengthy and detailed and focuses on social and emotional factors, whereas in embryo donation the process is less involved and focuses on medical criteria. It should be noted that this analysis is primarily focused on the UK, and while similar issues apply elsewhere, there may also be places where they do not, for example in the USA where 'embryo adoption' agencies exist which do apply similar parental selection approaches to traditional adoption.

In order to be approved for adoption in the UK, a social worker is assigned to the family and begins an assessment procedure which takes about eight months, and involves several home visits. Following this, the social worker writes a report detailing the family circumstances, both factual but also descriptive information, focusing on areas such as the prospective adopters' personalities, their relationship history, the stability of the family structure, their feelings about adopting, and their reasons for wanting to do so. Although the aim is to fully prepare and educate prospective adopters, it can be perceived as an intrusive

---

[2] We recognize that reproductive tourism is a contentious term; however, we feel it is appropriate in at least some instances (although arguably not all), particularly where the aim is to subvert the legislation of the home country to meet certain preferences rather than simply to access any treatment which will result in a successful live birth: e.g. the case of UK couples travelling to Spain to seek anonymous donors.

procedure and is certainly time-consuming. However, the focus of the adoption services is on the needs of the adopted child, so this intensive process is deemed essential to protect the child's best interests.

In contrast, the primary criterion for parent selection in embryo donation is whether the mother is 'medically suitable', not whether the couple are socially and emotionally suitable to be parents. The only national social requirement is found in the Human Fertilisation and Embryology (HFE) Act 2008, which states that a woman 'shall not be provided with treatment services unless account has been taken of the welfare of any child who may be born as a result of the treatment (including the need of that child for supportive parenting)'. The HFEA guidance (HFEA, n.d.) on how to conduct the welfare of the child assessment suggests taking a medical and social history from each patient and their partner, and interviewing the couple separately if necessary. In cases where these assessments raise concerns that the couples may not provide supportive parenting, clinics are advised to seek further information from relevant sources, e.g. GPs or social services. Consent to seek this information must be sought from the prospective patients, and refusal to allow information disclosure can be taken into account when deciding whether to provide treatment.

The instruction to consider the welfare of the child does add a small moral and social dimension to the decision-making process. However, clinics are advised by the HFEA (HFEA, n.d) only to refuse treatment if they consider that 'any child who may be born or any existing child of the family is likely to be at risk of *significant* harm or neglect' (emphasis added). In practice, therefore, only those who are regarded as potentially physically harming their future children are likely to be refused for social reasons. Furthermore, since the decision regarding treatment is seen primarily as medical, it is likely to be made by a medical practitioner, rather than a professional trained in considering social and psychological factors. Most likely to be refused embryo donation treatment are thus those who are medically unfit, particularly when the HFEA publishes clinic success rates on its websites as a guide to patients. Given the disparity between embryo donation and adoption, there are three possible justificatory reasons which should be examined (Widdows and MacCallum, 2002): parent intentionality, the gestational experience and the technological imperative.

Parent intentionality is considered primary by some when it comes to founding a family. A distinction is made between family creation methods which actually cause a child to come into existence and those which embrace already existing children into a new family structure. On this model children who are adopted are different from those created by embryo donation (and indeed all ARTs) because adoptive children do not come into being because of parent intention. The significance of the intentionality argument when deciding parental rights and status of children conceived through ARTs is seen by its use as the main line of reasoning in some landmark legal judgments. In the US state of California, for example, courts have consistently sided with the rights of the intended parents in cases of surrogacy or gamete donation disputes. In *Johnson* v. *Calvert* (1993), the genetic mother rather than the gestational surrogate was ruled to be the legal mother, with the court stating that the woman who arranged to 'bring about the birth of a child she intended to raise as her own – is the natural mother'. A later case extended this reasoning to a situation where the intended parents were not genetically related to the child, but were still ruled to be legal parents by dint of their intention at the beginning of the surrogacy arrangement (*In re. Marriage of Buzzancz* (1998)). This has been described as the 'but for' test (Douglas, 1994). 'But for' the parents initiating the surrogacy arrangement, there would be no pregnancy; thus the parents' intent is causal in the child's creation.[3] UK law does not recognize intention as being of significance to the same degree (the birth mother is always the legal mother). However, intentions do play a role with gamete donors, for example, where it is their lack of intention to become a social parent that allows them to waive legal or moral responsibilities for their genetic offspring. Following the intentionality argument, 'but for' the wishes of the embryo donation parents the child would not exist, whereas in adoption the child exists regardless of parental intent. Thus, it could be argued that although the would-be adoptive parents have become such by acting upon their desire to parent, their desire has not caused the child to come into existence. Hence, the argument is that intentionality is a 'causal' difference between embryo donation and adoption.[4]

Although this 'causal' difference is obviously present, we argue that it is not as significant as the intention to parent (Widdows and MacCallum, 2002). The underlying intention of adoptive and embryo donation parents is the same – to be parents. The fact that the means

---

[3] Equally, it is true to say that without the intention of the surrogate, the child would not exist.

[4] There are different methods of creating 'donor embryos'; either they are created using a donor egg and donor sperm or they are 'donated embryos' (usually created but then not used by another couple). If the embryos are donated as embryos – rather than created by the commissioning couple from donor egg and sperm – then the force of the intentionality argument is reduced. These embryos did exist prior to the intention of these parents and thus the situation is arguably more similar to adoption.

used to achieve this differs is less important than the fact that the end goal is equivalent. With similar intention in both cases, the intentionality argument does not carry enough weight to justify the disparities in parenting criteria.

The second potential reason for the divergence is that in embryo donation there is a biological link to one parent, through gestation. This has a number of consequences: legal, emotional, social and practical. From a legal perspective, the embryo donation mother (and her partner) has parental status from birth, whereas in adoption parental rights and responsibilities have to be transferred after birth. This creates a clear difference between the processes, but once again it could be argued that it is a difference in means rather than ends. Once the adoption procedure is completed, adoptive parents' legal status is identical to that of embryo donation parents.

Emotionally, the gestational link is said to be important as it allows the opportunity for the mother to form a prenatal relationship to the foetus, thus conferring and reinforcing through pregnancy the perception of self as mother. This experience of pregnancy and birth can be as important as the genetic link, with findings that 'for some, the inability to gestate and give birth represents a greater loss than the inability to have a child whose genetic complement comprises 50% of their own genes' (Mahowald, 2000: 129). A study comparing embryo donation and adoptive parents found evidence of this feeling; one mother with two children conceived via embryo donation said: 'I mean, I'm sure people who adopt children feel the same eventually ... but when you actually give birth, I'm sure there is a stronger initial bond' (MacCallum, 2009). However, this reason is not compelling, for while gestation is incredibly significant for some women, it does not by itself guarantee bonding between mother and child. Even in 'natural' conceptions there are occasions when the mother fails to bond immediately with their child. Moreover, the comparison study found that there were no differences in the quality of parent–child relationships between adoptive and embryo donation parents when the children were of preschool age (MacCallum *et al.*, 2007). Thus, while gestation may give the embryo donation mother an initial advantage, it does not follow that adoptive mothers cannot bond as effectively, or that this will have a long-term effect on the parent–child relationship.

The third consequence of the gestational link is social in that it enables the couple to experience pregnancy, birth and childrearing as if they were a 'normal' couple who had conceived 'naturally', and to present it as such to others, with no need to disclose their use of donor treatment. In contrast, adoptive parents would find it difficult to keep private the reasons for the arrival of a child who will already be possibly a year or more in age. More importantly perhaps, the gestational link allows the prospect of not telling the child about the donor conception. In the previously mentioned comparison study, only one-third of the embryo donation mothers had told or planned to tell the child about the donor conception (MacCallum and Golombok, 2007). One of the most common justifications for this non-disclosure was the gestational link, with many subscribing to the views of this embryo donation mother: 'You're going to be carrying them for 9 months, you're going to be feeding them for 9 months, to all intents and purposes, you are their mother.' In comparison, 80 per cent of the adoptive mothers had told the child about the adoption by the age of 3, and the remainder planned to begin sharing the information with the child soon.

To cite this social consequence as a justification for the disparity would be to assume that keeping the child's genetic origins secret can be desirable. Although this was the case historically, and donor recipients were encouraged to keep the information private, many years of debate (Daniels and Taylor, 1993; Widdows, 2002) have led to a change in climate towards openness and an acknowledgment of the right of individuals to know their genetic heritage. This is reflected in the policies of several countries, including the UK, which in 2005 changed the law to allow future donor offspring access to identity of donors at age 18. Since the law is not retrospectively applied, the process of giving donor information to offspring will not occur until 2023, but when it does it will require careful handling and counselling to involved parties, similar to the care needed when considering contact between adoptees and birth families. From this perspective, the differences between the two processes seem to be diminishing, rendering the social reason even less significant.

Finally, gestation means that embryo donation parents do not have to face the same practical complications as can arise in adoption. The emphasis in contemporary adoption is on finding a 'home for a child', with applicants assessed not just on parenting per se, but on providing the right environment for a specific child with an established personality and specific needs. Part of understanding the needs of the child means taking into account the separation from, and relinquishment by, the birth parents, leading to the assumption that adoptive children have a 'significant wound' (albeit one which can heal). To support the child in recovering, and establishing a stable sense of self, adoptive parents 'need to be ... extraordinary parents – with an emphasis on the "extra"' (Campion, 1995: 38). It has been argued that there are parallels to this 'history of rejection' in embryo donation (Bernstein et al., 1996) with children viewing themselves as rejected by their genetic parent. However, such a comparison seems extreme – placing a child for adoption does not equate to donating an embryo (Widdows and MacCallum 2002). From a practical perspective, adoptive parents have to meet the child's needs and demonstrate very skilled parenting abilities. Embryo donation parents merely have to meet the 'welfare of the child requirements', that is not suggest significant risk to a child, since at the time of parent selection their child has no specific needs. As a justification for approaching the two processes in distinct ways, the practical reason is irreducible and equating embryo donation and adoption would not seem to be sensible. This said, it does not follow that it justifies maintaining the *scale* of the current disparity.

The third reason, the technological imperative, is concerned with structural differences in the two procedures, and arises from the way in which they originated, and the nature of the way they are perceived. Adoption is the oldest form of creating families other than natural conception. It evolved as a social solution to the problems of housing abandoned and orphaned children and providing heirs for childless couples. Over the last ~150 years, adoption laws have been passed, regulation has been formalized, and social criteria for adoptive parents have been set. By contrast embryo donation is a relatively new procedure which has been implemented as the technology required to perform it has become available, combining the techniques of IVF and gamete donation.[5] Thus, embryo donation is driven by the technological imperative – the assumption that scientific progress is good in itself and should be pursued. As a result, embryo donation and adoption have been conceived of in different ways – one is social and subject to social analysis and criteria and the other 'medical', and thus legitimized in a manner similar to other medical procedures. Although this viewpoint accounts for how the disparity in selection criteria has developed, it is explanatory rather than justificatory and does not provide grounds for maintaining the current procedures.

Embryo donation and adoption are not equivalent, particularly taking into account the potentially difficult background of many adopted children, so it seems appropriate to apply different levels of parenting criteria. Evidence on the psychological development of embryo donation children has found that they show no problems during the early and middle childhood years, suggesting that the current system is not

---

[5] Embryos become available for donation in two ways: they are donated by couples or single women who have undergone IVF, or are created specifically for the recipient couple using donor egg and sperm.

having adverse effects (MacCallum and Keeley, 2008). However, from an ethical analysis, the three reasons discussed seem inadequate to support the status quo, and suggest that social factors should have more of a role to play in embryo donation, as they do in adoption, albeit in a proportional manner. This could include preparing and educating embryo donation parents regarding how they deal with the information about the child's genetic origins. Changing legislation regarding donor anonymity has if anything made the magnitude of the current disparity even less easy to justify ethically. The wider implication is that social criteria should also be applied to other ARTs, and we would agree, but crucially this should be in a proportional way dependent on the similarities between procedures. For example, the possibility of an embryo donation child having a genetic family elsewhere, including full genetic siblings, would result in embryo donation requiring more consideration than egg or sperm donation, where the child retains a genetic connection to one parent. Thus, this conclusion is consistent with the notion of not applying social screening to spontaneous conception where none of these features arise.

Donation and the disposition decision

Of course, embryo donation should not be examined only from the perspective of the recipients, and the question of who should be approved for treatment, but also from the perspective of those who can or do donate embryos, and what drives these decisions. During IVF treatment the number of embryos transplanted in one cycle is generally limited to two or three, resulting in surplus embryos which can then be cryopreserved. Large numbers of these cryopreserved embryos are stored in laboratories across the world, for example over 400,000 in the USA alone (Hoffman *et al.*, 2003). Of course, many couples will not be successful in their first IVF cycle, or will desire more children, so use their stored embryos in subsequent treatments. The period of time for which storage is permitted is often limited by legislation. Once this limit is reached, or prior to that if the couple have completed their family or decide not to pursue further treatment, they have to decide how their embryos should be utilized with three potential options: allow embryos to thaw and discard, donate to another infertile couple, or donate to medical research. There is also a fourth 'option', which is to refuse to decide and simply to fail to respond to the letter or enquiries about what you wish to do with embryos; an option which many find attractive. Although exact percentages differ, it is consistently found that few couples are actually willing to donate their embryos to others even when stating support for donation in principle (Newton *et al.*, 2003), and indeed that a higher proportion of couples prefer their embryos to be discarded than donated (Darlington and Matson, 1999). To what extent is the difficult decision of what to do with supernumerary embryos influenced by ethical considerations?

From an ethical perspective, one key issue identified in analysing embryo disposition is the moral status of the embryo, and thus the respect with which it should be treated. Those who maintain that personhood or moral status begins at fertilization, such as the Catholic Church, believe that the embryo should be regarded as a human being and treated as such. The opposite point of view is that embryos are like property, the ownership of which can be transferred. Currently the legal position in the large majority of jurisdictions is in the middle, treating embryos as somewhere between 'person' and 'property'. The consensus among those involved in assisted reproduction is in line with this, in that practitioners should be seen as 'showing respect' for the embryo, that is by not unnecessarily creating or manipulating embryos (ESHRE Task Force on Ethics and Law, 2001), but not the same level of respect as is shown to actual persons. As a result, most countries limit research on embryos to the time period up to fourteen days after creation (when fetal tissue differentiation commences), and to situations where there is no viable alternative research object (they do, however, also allow the discarding of embryos, which could be seen as not 'respectful'). The question then arises as to how potential donors view their embryos, and whether their perception of the embryo's status and nature play a major factor in their decision-making.

One might assume that viewing embryos as 'persons' or potential persons would make donation a more attractive proposition than allowing embryos to be discarded and thus wasting potential life. Interestingly, the opposite pattern is seen. Mohler-Kuo and colleagues (2009) administered questionnaires about disposition to IVF patients with cryopreserved embryos in Switzerland where donation to other couples is currently not legal. The strongest correlate of disposition preferences was the couples' position on the moral status of embryo. Of the roughly 900 participants, 89% felt that the embryo deserved some respect, and half felt that the rights accorded to the embryo should be the same as to a human being. Importantly, those who equated the embryo's rights with those of a human being were less likely to be in favour of donation to other couples (Mohler-Kuo *et al.*, 2009). Similar findings regarding the symbolic nature of the embryo were reported by de Lacey's qualitative study of IVF patients who had discarded unused embryos. Many reported thinking before treatment that they would donate the resulting embryos, but that parenthood had changed how they viewed the embryos, attributing to them a personhood (de Lacey, 2005). As a consequence, donation, which had previously been seen as a positive step to help others achieve pregnancy, became more akin to giving up a child for adoption. De Lacey expanded on this by comparing IVF patients who had discarded embryos with those who had donated embryos (de Lacey, 2007). For the 'Discard' group, embryo donation was again paralleled with relinquishing a child for adoption, whereas discarding was viewed as more natural, like miscarriage. The 'Donate' group on the other hand viewed embryos as the 'seed' for potential life but not as children, so donation preserved this potential, while discarding an embryo was compared to pregnancy termination. This highlights the paradox that those who view their embryos as more 'child-like' in status and nature are in fact more likely to discard them.

Therefore, the definition and moral conception of the embryo does seem to have some influence on couples' disposition decisions. However, Lyerly *et al.* (2006) found that this is not the whole story. Their participants considered the nature of the embryo, but placed more importance on their responsibility to their own embryos than on the abstract moral status (Lyerly *et al.*, 2006). Disposition decisions were affected more by personal values, such as feelings about what family means, than by the ethical question of the 'rights' of the embryo. Qualitative interviews of Belgian IVF patients support this view (Provoost *et al.*, 2009), where the most significant finding was that participants who perceived the embryo as being highly symbolic of the relationship between the couple were very reluctant to donate their cryopreserved embryos to others. Conceptualizing the embryo in this way is more likely to occur when the embryo has been created from the couples' own gametes than when donor eggs or sperm have been used, or the embryo has already been donated from another couple. Therefore, couples with their own genetic embryos may be less inclined to donate them since the personal symbolism of the embryos influences their decision more than the moral status of the embryo per se.

Due to the complex nature of the disposition decision, many couples find it intensely difficult to come to a resolution (hence the numbers of couple who take the 'fourth' option of simply refusing to make a decision). Combined with the requirement for clinicians and others to show 'respect' for embryos, this can give rise to ethical dilemmas. Over 70 per cent of couples have not made a definite decision about their embryos, even four or five years after their last IVF treatment (Nachtigall *et al.*, 2005). Many couples seem to actually actively avoid the decision by not keeping in contact with the clinic. The dilemma occurs when the storage limit is reached, if the couples' decision has not been recorded. Embryos can become 'blocked' in clinics if consideration of the status of the embryo leads to unwillingness to destroy them without explicit instructions. One Spanish clinic has caused controversy by allowing donation to other couples of embryos where disposition decisions have not been made (Blackburn-Starza, 2010), without the donors' permission, which flies in the face of the principle of 'fully informed consent' and does not seem to equate with treating embryos with respect (this is further evidence for the potential problems of medical tourism discussed below). In the UK, clinics may store embryos for a maximum of ten years, after which they should be discarded or donated according to decisions made by the patients at the outset, that is, before they know the treatment outcome, although patients can change their minds during the storage period. Since attitudes toward donation can change, particularly with experience of parenthood (de Lacey, 2005), a decision made before treatment may be considered not to be 'fully informed', and revisiting this decision at regular intervals should be strongly encouraged. Although many clinics report waiting lists for embryo donation treatment due to a lack of willing donors, couples must be able to make decisions about their embryos freely, without coercion, and in possession of all the relevant facts.

In addition to these issues there are additional concerns when 'donors' (or middle men) sell embryos or eggs. Increasingly, British women and couples are travelling (often to Spain) in order to obtain cheaper treatment and to avoid the anonymity laws of the UK. Couples then purchase eggs from vendors; usually the sources are Spanish women or Eastern European women. Embryo sale (or egg sale to create embryos) raises many additional and complex issues that do not apply in donation. Some of these ethical concerns will be addressed towards the end of this chapter.

Commodification

The final issue we wish to address is concerned not just with donors, although perhaps most relates to them. It is the question of whether increasing use of ARTs is likely to further commodify children – in other words to push them to the 'property' end of the person/property spectrum. This is clearly not just a problem for embryo donation but for all ARTs; however, it could be argued that embryo donation is potentially more commodifying than other ARTs in that both gametes come from donors, whether as a couple donating an embryo, or two separate egg and sperm donors, and therefore there is more potential to turn the embryo into a 'product' where certain 'parts' or 'traits' are selected. This is particularly ethically concerning when donors are chosen not to overcome infertility or for health reasons (i.e. to avoid X-linked disorders), but to have a child of a different 'type'. Such practices are rare, but not unknown.

ARTs are usually perceived in a relatively benign manner (by users of the technology and the wider public), in part because the results are valued by individuals and society.[6] One result of this acceptance is that the broader cultural and social consequences of ARTs are under-theorized and under-researched. In particular there is little research done into changing understanding of children and whether increased use of these technologies changes expectations of children and parenting in general. In other words, are there cultural and social effects that extend beyond the communities who use these technologies to general understandings of children?

Such incremental changes which develop as new technology becomes available and normalized would not be surprising – as our discussion of the technological imperative has shown. Increased use and awareness of 'new' procedures gradually normalizes them and makes them familiar and less 'new'. This happens in a progressive way, one procedure or technology after another. Indeed, a recent report suggests that ARTs could become the routine method of conception for older couples, overtaking sexual conception within a decade (Vatja et al., 2010). It is not hard to imagine that the increasing use of such technologies gradually normalizes them to the point where the 'technical fix', and all the options and choices this offers parents pre-birth, becomes regarded as a standard conception option. Such uses of the technologies as valid options for all in order to choose traits, characteristics or parts of the resulting child is a very different scenario from using the technology in order to have 'one's own' child (the way ARTs are currently usually considered). In such a scenario, technologies of reproduction do not mimic natural conception and merely replicate the 'normal' conception process but offer new reproductive possibilities and thus potentially change the ethos of reproduction and have cumulative social effects. In terms of this issue they might move us further along the spectrum from person to property or from 'gift' to 'contract' and so result in a more commodified view of children. Worries about the change from 'gift' to 'contract' feed into larger debates in bioethics and are particularly important at the current time in terms of organ sale as well as gamete sale. Early work on this topic, most particularly the classic study of

---

[6] For a more expansive version of this argument see Widdows (2009).

blood donation by Richard Titmuss, highlights that the benefits of the gift relationship extend to significant public goods and social capital (Titmuss, 1970). Moreover, the 'altruistic' market not only brings significant goods but is also more effective in terms of delivering, in this instance good-quality blood in the necessary quantities, than a commodity market. Given this, many argue that what we should be doing before permitting sale is exploring every possible way of encouraging an altruistic market, which if the blood parallel holds, may well deliver more and better quality gametes as well as stop the risk of commodifying the children produced by these technologies. At its most simple, commodification means turning a person into an object or a thing, about which the language of ownership and property can be used and, significantly, into objects which can be bought and sold.[7] Eggs, gametes and embryos fit this definition in jurisdictions where their sale is legal, but not in jurisdictions where altruistic donation is the model (as in the UK). One reason given for not allowing 'sale' even when 'expenses' are permitted is because it alters the status of the gamete and changes the relationship between the mother and the gametes from one of recipient to one of purchaser. Children are not 'things' (although some still regard surrogacy as 'baby-selling'); however, they can be treated as things and the relationships with parents can change accordingly. Radin's broad definition which 'includes *not only actual buying and selling, but also market rhetoric, the practice of thinking about interactions as if they were sale transactions*' (emphasis in original) (Radin, 1987: 1859) encompasses much of what is of concern here. Key features of 'commodification' are, first, objectification occurs – persons become things onto which desires can be projected, and second, contract and sale become the framework of the relationship. These are not insignificant particularly when one thinks about the high costs involved and what couples and women sacrifice to avail themselves of such technologies.

Clearly the risks of commodification are less in embryo donation when it is used simply to have a child, or for health reasons. Certainly it is less problematic than when a type of child is chosen, for instance a deaf child, a 'saviour sibling' or a child of a certain sex for non-medical reasons.[8] At the more extreme end, parents are selecting gametes to

---

[7] A narrow understanding of commodification, defined by Radin as the '*actual buying and selling (or legally permitted buying and selling) of something*' (emphasis in original) (Radin, 1987: 1859).

[8] Some deaf couples have argued they should be able to choose a child for social and cultural reasons not for medical reasons. Parents argue that 'deafness is not a disability but a culture which they should be permitted to pass on' (Häyry, 2004: 510) with 'distinct language, activities, and institutions of that culture' (Anstey, 2002: 287). Saviour siblings are created as a 'match' for an earlier child. In other words they are

create embryos in an attempt to influence intelligence and appearance. It is now possible to purchase gametes from a website exclusively limited to attractive people if one is seeking a beautiful girl and from intellectually successful donors if one is seeking a clever boy (the uptake suggests that it is this combination that is sought).[9] Thus, while not mainstream, ARTs are already being used not to ensure a healthy child or a genetically related child but a particular type of child or a child with particular characteristics.

In all these instances the essential worry is the same: that as expectations are increased regarding what types of child can be created, if the resulting child is not the way the parents expect, will they be disappointed in a way that pre-ARTs they would not be? In other words, does the ability to choose – to technologically fix – particular parts of children or types of children, in this case to choose deafness or sex, change our expectations of children and commodify them? Does it make them more 'product' than person?

To suggest that we move from person to something which can be commodified is more or less likely depending on the technology and the motive for using it. For instance if one is using ARTs simply to experience as near as possible one's own child, then charges of commodification are weakened. If one is seeking to have a child of a particular type or a child with certain characteristics, then they are strengthened. There are many reasons for having a certain 'type' of child; the least controversial are for health reasons, for instance to avoid a genetic disorder. In such instances, although there might be some general risk that the increased use of such technologies normalizes intervention per se, as long as the intervention is only to have a healthy child then the risk of commodity seems small.

However, if we pay for certain characteristics, what happens to children who do not meet them? There are instances where children have been refused in surrogacy when the resulting child was disabled, or even because they were twins rather than the requested singleton (Taylor, 2001). In this case it does seem that at least some element of commodification is at work. It may be that the gestational experience mitigates this element, and that those who carry their ART-conceived child through pregnancy will be less likely to be disappointed with any

---

'designed' specifically to be a donor (although it may be the umbilical cord which is actually used) (Sheldon and Wilkinson, 2004).

[9] Beautifulpeople.com, which is primarily a dating website only for those rated as attractive, announced it was setting up a 'virtual egg and sperm bank', open to all purchasers. The site founder stated that 'everyone, including ugly people, would like to bring good-looking children into the world'.

result. Gestation though, as discussed earlier, while important to some is less so to others.

Concerns about commodification are compounded when we consider trade in gametes and embryos to be global. The term 'medical tourism' is used to define the movement of people from one legislative area to another to obtain treatment and procedures which are not available (or less easily available) within the country or state of their origin.[10] Medical tourism includes 'reproductive tourism'. Reproductive tourism denotes practices such as Irish women travelling to the UK for abortions; German couples travelling to Belgium for Pre-Implantation Genetic Diagnosis (PGD); and women travelling from Northern Europe and the USA to Eastern Europe, Spain and Greece for donor eggs for reproductive treatments or to India for 'surrogacy services'. Medical tourism is an important ethical issue because it is a market in which the relatively rich take advantage of the relatively poor. If there were not global inequities of wealth and differences in laws and standards in different jurisdictions, medical tourism would be impossible. Accordingly there are possibilities of coercion and exploitation for both vendors and purchasers/donors and recipients, as reflected in the example above of donation without express consent in one Spanish clinic.

However, the term 'medical tourism' does not take seriously the importance of the process for either side. The market for reproductive tourism – where richer women buy eggs and embryos from poorer, younger, more needy women – has increased over the last decade to the point of normalization. It is perfectly common for women from Western Europe, particularly the UK and Northern Europe, to travel to Spain or Eastern Europe for 'treatment'.[11] Women travel for different reasons; for some it is for cheaper treatment or to obtain procedures which are illegal in the home country.[12] A small number of UK couples travelling abroad for treatment cited a desire to use anonymous donors (Culley *et al.*, 2011), raising concerns about equity for the offspring who will not have the rights to donor identity now granted to those conceived in the UK. Prices paid for eggs differ; Spanish students are paid 600

---

[10] This issue is the focus of Chapter 8 in this volume, on transnational donation. For the purposes of the current chapter, what is key is the travelling to different jurisdictions where laws that are different from the laws in the home country apply, as well as the issue of 'paying' for the components of one's future child.

[11] Gupta cites that 'Dutch infertile women are travelling to Spain for eggs donated by University students' (Gupta, 2006: 31).

[12] Costs of treatment differ in different countries, hence fertility specialists are establishing clinics in cheaper countries; 'for example, private IVF centres in Russia, Portugal and Spain have been established by Finnish fertility specialists' (Aarnio, cited in Blyth and Farrand, 2005: 102).

euros, while US women are paid $6,000–$10,000 (Gupta, 2006), and Romanian women who donate in their own country are paid around $200 to $250. At the lower end of the market, there are issues about exploitation and coercion of donors which are ethically important. For instance, in one study it was reported that Romanian women who sold their eggs were paid a fraction of the price that the resulting embryos were sold for in Spanish clinics. Moreover, they returned for numerous harvestings, with all the risks to fertility and health this entails, simply to attain a living wage (Beeson and Lippman, 2006). Commodification is therefore an issue for donors, for recipients and for society more broadly.

If commodification and the wider trade in gametes, suggested by practices of reproductive tourism, are of ethical concern, then we should beware of an uncritical expansion of ARTs, perhaps particularly embryo donation. In particular we should beware of allowing parental preference to dominate to the extent where selection of parts or types of children are normalized, in order to ensure that such practices do not become more prevalent and ultimately result in a collectively more commodified attitude, not only to particular children but to all children. Accordingly, it is ethically important what type of ARTs are being practised and how they are regulated. It is not the technology that is ethically right or wrong but how it is used and the type of family dynamics it creates.

Conclusion

We first considered the ethical issues relating to embryo donation in 2002, when we surmised that there were not grounds sufficient to justify the extreme disparities in parenting criteria between this process and adoption. Revisiting this analysis, the same conclusions apply, and in fact the shift in attitudes and legislation towards openness about children's genetic origins has created more similarities between the two processes, weakening the reasons for the disparity still further. While not advocating implementing the same procedure for both, we would suggest that there should be consistency in whose interests are taken into account and the mechanisms used to do so. Thus, we argue for various levels of parenting criteria proportional to the similarities between procedures.

This conclusion is further supported by the additional discussions regarding donor perspectives and concerns about the growing global trade in sperm, eggs and embryos, which raise issues about commercialization and commodification. The uneasiness that donors experience with regard to donating their 'spare embryos' shows that there is something ethically significant at stake here. What is being donated has meaning for them and is connected to them, just as it is for the Romanian vendors. This suggests that gametes are not products like any others to be bought and sold; at least not without robust criteria, including social criteria, to help all parties negotiate the psychological, emotional and ethical aspects of these procedures.

Finally, and perhaps most importantly, insisting on some social criteria – however minimal – will give at least a modicum of recognition to the rights and interests of the children who are the products of the procedure. The comparison with adoption shows clearly just how much the interests of the future child (and adult) are neglected in debates about ARTs. While, as we have pointed out, there are good reasons for giving the future child less attention in embryo donation than in adoption, there are no good reasons for ignoring the interests of the future child altogether. The 'right of the future child' to know their genetic origins underpins the changes to anonymity of the practice. These rights are being systematically violated if couples are permitted to travel in order to attain embryos from anonymous donors. Likewise, concerns about commodification and commercialization are not just about the rights of donors. If knowing 'one's story' is important – as is presumed in adoption and in ART practices which rely on identifiable donors – then it matters what this story is. For instance, is it not as potentially damaging for a person to discover their gametes were purchased from an exploited vendor as to discover they were 'rejected' by their birth parents? In regulating such issues, the silent voice of the future child should be taken into consideration, as well as the loud voices of recipients and the somewhat quieter voices of donors and vendors.

REFERENCES

Anstey, K. W. (2002). 'Are attempts to have impaired children justifiable?' *Journal of Medical Ethics*, 28, 286–8.
Beeson, D. and Lippman, A. (2006). 'Egg harvesting for stem cell research: medical risks and ethical problems'. *Reproductive BioMedicine Online*, 13, 573–9.
Bernstein, J., Berson, A., Brill, M., Cooper, S. S., *et al.* (1996). 'Safeguards in embryo donation'. *Fertility and Sterility*, 65, 1262–3.
Blackburn-Starza, A. (2010). 'Spanish clinic allows IVF embryo donation "without consent"'. *BioNews*. Available at: www.bionews.org.uk/page_67168.asp.
Blyth, E. and Farrand, A. (2005). 'Reproductive tourism – a price worth paying for reproductive autonomy?' *Critical Social Policy*, 25, 91–114.

Campion, M. J. (1995). *Who's fit to be a parent?* London: Routledge.
Culley, L., Hudson, N., Blyth, E., Norton, W., Rapport, F., and Pacey, A. (2011). 'Crossing borders for fertility treatment: motivations and destinations of UK fertility travellers'. *Human Reproduction*, 26(9), 2373–81.
Daniels, K. and Taylor, K. (1993). 'Secrecy and openness in donor insemination'. *Politics and Life Sciences*, 12, 155–70.
Darlington, N. and Matson, P. (1999). 'The fate of cryopreserved human embryos approaching their legal limit of storage within a West Australian in-vitro fertilization clinic'. *Human Reproduction*, 14, 2343–4.
de Lacey, S. (2005). 'Parent identity and "virtual" children: why patients discard rather than donate unused embryos'. *Human Reproduction*, 20, 1661–9.
   (2007). 'Decisions for the fate of frozen embryos: fresh insights into patients' thinking and their rationales for donating or discarding embryos'. *Human Reproduction*, 22, 1751–8.
Douglas, G. (1994). 'The intention to be a parent and the making of mothers'. *Modern Law Review*, 57, 636–41.
ESHRE Task Force on Ethics and Law (2001). 'I. The moral status of the pre-implantation embryo'. *Human Reproduction*, 16, 1046–8.
Gupta, J. (2006). 'Towards transnational feminisms: some reflections and concerns in relation to the globalisation of reproductive technologies'. *European Women's Studies*, 13, 23–38.
Häyry, M. (2004). 'There is a difference between selecting a deaf embryo and deafening a hearing child'. *Journal of Medical Ethics*, 30, 510–12.
Hoffman, D. I., Zellman, G. L., Fair, C. C., Mayer, J. F., *et al.* (2003). 'Cryopreserved embryos in the United States and their availability for research'. *Fertility and Sterility*, 79, 1063–9.
Human Fertilisation and Embryology Authority (HFEA) (n.d.). Code of Practice 'The welfare of the child assessment process'. Available at: www.hfea.gov.uk/5473.html#guidanceSection5485 (accessed 30 January 2012).
Lyerly, A. D., Steinhauser, K., Namey, E., Tulsky, J. A., *et al.* (2006). 'Factors that affect infertility patients' decisions about disposition of frozen embryos'. *Fertility and Sterility*, 85, 1623–30.
MacCallum, F. (2009). 'Embryo donation parents' attitudes towards donors: comparison with adoption'. *Human Reproduction*, 25, 517–23.
MacCallum, F. and Golombok, S. (2007). 'Embryo donation families: mothers' decisions regarding disclosure of donor conception'. *Human Reproduction*, 22, 2888–95.
MacCallum, F. and Keeley, S. (2008). 'Embryo donation families: a follow-up in middle childhood'. *Journal of Family Psychology*, 22, 799–808.
MacCallum, F., Golombok, S. and Brinsden, P. (2007). 'Parenting and child development in families with a child conceived by embryo donation'. *Journal of Family Psychology*, 21, 278–87.
Mahowald, M. B. (2000). *Genes, Women and Equality*. Oxford University Press.

Mohler-Kuo, M., Zellweger, U., Duran, A., Hohl, M., *et al.* (2009). 'Attitudes of couples towards the destination of surplus embryos: results among couples with cryopreserved embryos in Switzerland'. *Human Reproduction*, 24, 1930–8.

Nachtigall, R., Becker, G., Friese, C., Butler, A., *et al.* (2005). 'Parents' conceptualization of their frozen embryos complicates the disposition decision'. *Fertility and Sterility*, 84, 431–5.

Newton, C. R., McDermid, A., Tekpety, F. and Tummon, I. S. (2003). 'Embryo donation: attitudes toward donation procedures and factors predicting willingness to donate'. *Human Reproduction*, 18, 878–84.

Provoost, V., Pennings, G., de Sutter, P., Gerris, J., *et al.* (2009). 'Infertility patients' beliefs about their embryos and their disposition preferences'. *Human Reproduction*, 24, 896–905.

Radin, M. (1987). 'Market-inalienability'. *Harvard Law Review*, 100, 1849–937.

Sheldon, S. and Wilkinson, S. (2004). 'Should selecting saviour siblings be banned?' *Journal of Medical Ethics*, 30, 533–7.

Taylor, C. (2001). 'One baby too many'. *TIME*, San Francisco.

Titmuss, R. M. (1970). *The Gift Relationship*. London: George Allen and Unwin.

Trounson, A., Leeton, J., Besanka, M., Wood, C., *et al.* (1983). 'Pregnancy established in an infertile patient after transfer of a donated embryo fertilized in vitro'. *British Medical Journal*, 286, 835–8.

Vatja, G., Rienzi, L., Cobo, A. and Yovich, J. (2010). 'Embryo culture: can we perform better than nature?' *Reproductive Biomedicine Online*, 20, 453–69.

Widdows, H. (2002). 'The Ethics of Secrecy in Donor Insemination', in D. Dickenson (ed.), *Ethical Issues in Maternal-Fetal Medicine*. Cambridge University Press.

(2009). 'Persons and their parts: new reproductive technologies and risks of commodification'. *Health Care Analysis* 17, 36–46.

Widdows, H. and MacCallum, F. (2002). 'Disparities in parenting criteria: an exploration of the issues, focusing on adoption and embryo donation'. *Journal of Medical Ethics*, 28, 139–42.

CASES

Johnson v. Calvert (1993) P2d. California Supreme Court
In re. Marriage of Buzzancz (1998) Rptr2d. Cal.

LEGISLATION

The Human Fertilisation and Embryology Act 1990, as amended 2008

16   Reproduction through surrogacy: the UK and US experience

Andrea Braverman, Polly Casey and Vasanti Jadva

Introduction

From its beginnings, surrogacy has been dogged by controversy. Even the terminology has been met with controversy (English *et al.*, 1991). In the United Kingdom arrangements where the surrogate is also the genetic mother of the child have been defined as 'partial', 'straight' or 'genetic' surrogacy, and arrangements where the surrogate is not genetically related to the child have been called 'full', 'host' or 'gestational' surrogacy.

In the United States surrogacy originally described an arrangement in which intended parents attempted conception through the use of a woman's egg, and that woman underwent inseminations with the intended father's sperm. In this case the surrogate was providing both the genetics and the gestation. As in vitro fertilization emerged as a viable treatment option, another surrogacy option emerged wherein a couple or individual worked with a woman who would carry a genetically unrelated embryo that was transferred to her. In this scenario the surrogate contributes only the gestation. In 2006 1 per cent of all fresh ART cycles in the United States involved a gestational surrogate (for a total of 1,042 cycles); additional cycles were performed involving donor eggs (CDC, 2006). In the UK the number of surrogate births, although rising, is harder to estimate due to a number of more informal home-insemination arrangements. In this case IVF is not required and so the surrogate birth goes unregistered as such.

The medical community struggled to define IVF surrogacy, and terms such as 'host uterus' were suggested. In the United States two terms have ultimately emerged. 'Traditional surrogacy' denotes the situation where the surrogate is both the genetic and gestational contributor. 'Gestational carrier' or 'gestational surrogacy' are the terms used to denote a situation where the surrogate is contributing only the gestation. To further complicate the terminology, the term 'surrogate' and 'gestational carrier' (or simply 'carrier') are used interchangeably. Finally, the terminology 'intended parent(s)' has come to characterize the individual or couple who wish to parent the resulting child. Since intended parents are not necessarily the genetic parents (as is the case with the use of a gamete donor in a gestational carrier arrangement), the broader term of 'intended parents' emerged as an appropriate umbrella term. As the Internet made access to information about surrogacy easily available, the terminology shifted again, and use of the term 'surrogacy' became established in chat rooms and on websites. In this chapter we will use the terms gestational and genetic surrogacy to describe the two types of surrogacy arrangements, as they are the most prevalently used terms.

Surrogacy in the United States and the United Kingdom

In this section we will explore surrogacy through the experience in the United States and the United Kingdom.

In the United States commercial surrogacy emerged in the 1980s, offered by a handful of brokers (Spar, 2006). Ethical debates centred on the question of whether a woman had the right to contract and receive compensation for her pregnancy and delivery, or whether payment for such services simply constituted baby-selling. As IVF became a viable option, the two components of surrogacy separated and women could truly provide only the labour, apart from the gestation. This separation of eggs and gestation also allowed the industry to grow (Spar, 2006) as women could now carry a pregnancy without the long-term implications of a genetic child being raised by another family. Feminists are divided on what surrogacy represents for women. One group argues that women should have complete autonomy over their bodies whereas another group argues that women should not be 'breeders' and their value based on the commodification of their bodies falling into three categories: 'the symbolic harm to society of allowing paid surrogacy, the potential risks to the woman of allowing paid surrogacy, and the potential risks to the potential child of allowing paid surrogacy' (Andrews, 1990: 169).

In the United States commercial gestational surrogacy arrangements take place despite the lack of formal guidelines from the American Society for Reproductive Medicine (Teman, 2010). An agency will match intended parents with prospective gestational surrogates. Alternatively, intended parents can search for their own candidate via websites that allow for advertisements from both parents and surrogates. Most brokers will have requirements for the surrogates, informed by the IVF centre's emphasis on medical safety for the surrogate, for example age limits, parity and body mass index. Surrogates are then screened by both the physician and the mental health professionals. Intended parents are usually required to have counselling regarding managing the gestational surrogacy experience. Finally, a legal contract is negotiated and treatment begins after all parties have signed. Often, compensation is put into a trust fund and compensation is paid monthly. Surrogacy is addressed separately in the United States on a state-by-state basis whereby in some states surrogacy is strictly forbidden and in others it is regulated by legislation (Crockin and Jones, 2010). In the UK, on the other hand, it is illegal for individuals to advertise that they are in need of, or are willing to act as, a surrogate. A number of small, voluntary organizations guide couples and surrogates through the surrogacy process and offer counselling services. They can also help with drawing up an informal contract which, although not legally binding, does prepare those involved for various eventualities: for example, fetal abnormalities or multiple births. Such support groups offer a valuable service to couples and surrogates; however, their involvement is not mandatory, and some couples may choose not to access them.

Surrogacy remains legal in the UK on an altruistic and non-commercial basis. That surrogacy is legal at all in the UK stands in contrast to many other European countries including France, Germany, Italy and Spain, where it is illegal. In France, for example, surrogacy is prohibited based on the belief that it entails the deliberate abandonment of the child by the gestational mother. The judgment to outlaw surrogacy in France was also based on the belief that another principle was in breach; that the body is *res extra commercio*, it cannot be sold, rented, or be the subject of a contract (Code (Nouveau) de Procedure Civile Français, 1977).

In fact, surrogacy law in the UK has changed very little from the initial legislation laid out in the Surrogacy Arrangements Act 1985. The Act was hastily drafted after the 'Baby Cotton' case hit the headlines in 1985. The concerns over payment to surrogate Kim Cotton prompted the prohibition of commercially arranged surrogacy. Indeed it is still prohibited to pay surrogates more than 'reasonable expenses', and the acquisition of a parental order following the birth of the child is dependent on this. However, exactly what is considered acceptable expenses has not been explicitly defined and high levels of 'expenses' often changes hands. In the United States, in states where surrogacy is permitted, financial compensation is independently negotiated; surrogates are autonomous and can negotiate their own compensation.

Placing limitations on financial compensation can be construed as arbitrary and paternalistic.

Another important feature of UK surrogacy law is that any contracts agreed upon by parties involved are not enforceable in law (HFE Act 1990) and given that the surrogate is considered the legal mother at birth, this creates a possibility that the surrogate will not relinquish the child to the intending parents. The situation in the UK, where no commercial brokers exist to mediate relationships between the surrogate and the couple, means that often very close and trusting relationships develop between the different individuals involved. While it may be beneficial for the intending couples to have some form of guarantee, in the form of legal support, that the child will be handed over to them following the birth, in practice this would be difficult to implement. However, most UK surrogacy arrangements are successful, with only a very small number of published reports of cases in which the surrogacy arrangement has gone wrong. In such cases, however, it would seem that the overriding concern of the English courts is the welfare of the child, making judicial decisions on a case-by-case basis and supported by facts. Two recent cases of disputed custody of a surrogacy child saw the English court make clear that the child's welfare is considered priority over public policy. In the case of *re L*, the High Court granted legal parenthood to an English couple who had entered into a commercial surrogacy arrangement with a surrogate in the USA (Ghevaert, 2011), thereby overlooking the couple's breach of the position of UK law on commercial surrogacy in favour of the interests of the child. In another case, *re TT*, the English court awarded legal parenthood to the surrogate mother, who had refused to hand the child over to the intended parents. The surrogate had entered into an informal surrogacy arrangement with the intended couple, in which the surrogate was inseminated with the sperm of the intended father. However, the relationship between the two parties had subsequently broken down during the pregnancy. The Court's decision to award care to the surrogate mother was, again, based on consideration for the child's welfare, and it was decided that the attachment already formed between the surrogate and the child was such that it would cause significant harm to the child to remove her into the care of the intended parents (Cameron, 2011).

In the United States most arrangements where the surrogate is not providing her genetic material have seen that the genetic mother will be deemed the legal mother and courts continue to struggle with nuanced situations involving multiple donors (Crockin and Jones, 2010).

That UK surrogacy law is still largely unchanged (with notable exceptions) since the hurried Surrogacy Arrangements Act 1985 is both frustrating and indicative of a reluctance to fully embrace surrogacy as an acceptable means of creating a family. It is especially frustrating in light of the recommendations of two government-commissioned inquiries into the ethical implications of human reproduction, including surrogacy; the Warnock Committee produced recommendations in 1984, as did the Brazier Committee in 1998. The recommendations of neither Committee were acted upon, either at the time, or since. In the years since the Brazier Report (1998), the Human Fertilisation and Embryology (HFE) Act 2008 has come into force. The major change as a result of the new legislation is that surrogacy is now an available option for unmarried and same-sex couples, thanks to the eligibility for parental orders being extended to include such families. However, single parents remain ineligible for parental orders, despite them being eligible now for adoption and donor insemination.

Despite the slow pace of change within UK surrogacy law, currently the law does, in fact, often enable successful surrogacy arrangements to take place. In order to make the process easier for those involved, there are areas in which the law could be amended. For example, currently the surrogate is the legal mother of the child until she signs the parental order to transfer parentage. In the USA parentage is transferred immediately at birth, meaning that if there are any issues over the child's health, it is the intended parents who are consulted about treatment. Currently in the UK, intending parents have no legal right to make decisions for their child for the first few months of the child's life, that is until the parental order has been granted. A move to a system closer to that in the USA in this sense may, as mentioned above, facilitate the surrogacy process for those involved.

Surrogacy raises the question as to who is the patient? Or rather, whose wishes should carry more weight in making decisions over the pregnancy? Is it the couple who are being treated for infertility? Or is it the surrogate, who risks her health by carrying the baby? In the USA and the UK, as for women in typical pregnancies, the surrogate is considered the patient. She receives all information about the pregnancy and it is her responsibility to share this with the intended couple (if they are not present at medical appointments). In Israel, on the other hand, all medical information about the surrogacy, including whether or not the surrogate is pregnant, is given to the intending mother (Teman, 2010). While such situations mean that intending couples may feel highly involved in the birth of their child, the surrogate could feel frustrated over not being able to access medical information that directly concerns her health (Teman, 2010). Similarly, it is unclear how much control the intended parents should have over the surrogate's conduct during pregnancy (e.g. smoking, alcohol, exercise, and even driving). Should the surrogate maintain complete autonomy over her body, or does the fact that she is carrying a child intended for another couple grant the couple a degree of control? Without any legal contract, there are certainly no concrete consequences for the surrogate. The power balance between intending parents and surrogates is a delicate one in surrogacy arrangements, as is the degree of control belonging to each in decision-making during the pregnancy. As a recent case in Canada has shown, even with a legal contract drawn up prior to the pregnancy, it can be hard to decide whose voice matters most. A couple had engaged in a gestational surrogacy arrangement with a surrogate, and discovered during an ultrasound in the first trimester of the pregnancy that the fetus was likely to have Down's syndrome (Hyder, 2010). The parties had entered into a contract, which meant that when the surrogate refused the couple's request for an abortion, the couple would be absolved of all further responsibility of the child. In the end, the surrogate eventually agreed to the abortion, but the case demonstrates the potential uncertainty in surrogacy arrangements.

Recent years have seen a rise in the number of British couples seeking surrogacy treatment abroad, in India or the USA for example. Travelling abroad for surrogacy arrangements is often cheaper than treatment in the UK, and the fact that other countries permit payment to surrogates sometimes means increased availability and numbers of women willing to act as surrogates, not to mention increased access to surrogates since advertising surrogacy services is not permitted in the UK but may be permitted elsewhere. Also, the shortage of surrogates belonging to ethnic minority groups in the UK means that couples from certain backgrounds looking for genetic surrogates may look abroad. However, by travelling abroad for their surrogacy arrangement, intended parents are vulnerable to complicated legal challenges where surrogacy laws differ to those in the UK (Gamble, 2009), including their legal status as parents of the child, if they are unaware of these differences. The United States have also found that cross-border fertility care is raising novel legal issues and some intended parents have encountered problems getting permission to take children home (Crockin and Jones, 2010).

A recent example of one such case is *Re X and Y* in 2008 (Ghevaert, 2011). Here, a couple had travelled to Ukraine in order to engage in a surrogacy arrangement. Although in the UK the surrogate mother is considered the legal mother of the child until parentage is transferred, in Ukraine the intended couple are considered the legal parents. Therefore, the twins born from this arrangement had no right to enter the UK because the Ukrainian surrogate and her husband were considered the legal parents, despite their being conceived with the British man's sperm; and yet, under Ukrainian law, the Ukrainian couple had no parental obligation towards them. The High Court eventually awarded the intended couple a parental order, after recognizing that the twins had been left 'marooned, stateless, and parentless' in Ukraine, and faced being brought up in a Ukrainian orphanage. The judge also described the case as a 'cautionary tale' for anyone considering a foreign surrogacy arrangement.

Considerations for the surrogates

Gestational surrogates need to consider both the medical risks and the emotional/psychosocial risks to themselves as well as to their children, partners, family, friends, and their community. In the USA a mental health professional will raise these issues with the gestational surrogate and her partner. In the absence of formal guidelines, a standard of care has emerged to include an individual assessment and, frequently, assessment of the surrogate's partner. The evaluation looks to establish that the surrogate engages in a stable and healthy lifestyle and can make an informed decision weighing all the potential risks and demands. The psychological evaluation can include psychological testing in addition to the clinical interview.

The counselling for the surrogate should encompass all aspects of the experience. This includes helping the surrogate anticipate the impact of surrogacy, including the potential for attachment to the developing child, and what her expectations are from the experience. A major factor to be explored is her expectations of her relationship with the intended parent(s), both during the pregnancy and after, to determine whether they are congruent with those of the intended parent(s). The counselling should also explore what support or objections she anticipates to the surrogacy pregnancy.

In commercial surrogacy the surrogate's compensation is negotiated prior to the pregnancy. In the United States surrogates can set their own compensation either by advertising on the Internet or through a surrogacy broker. Some surrogacy broker programmes set their own compensation. Experienced surrogates frequently receive higher compensation than a woman who has never been a surrogate. Additional considerations regarding compensation may include whether a surrogate has other desirable attributes, such as having health insurance or residency in a geographically desirable location (in respect of surrogacy laws). The most common consideration for additional compensation is in the case of a multiple pregnancy and invasive procedures like amniocentesis or a Caesarean section. Most surrogates receive additional reimbursement for any costs incurred as a result of the pregnancy, for example maternity clothes, childcare, lost wages, and so on. Many practices in the United States limit the number of pregnancies and duration of time between pregnancies based on obstetrical risks, but there are no agreed limits.

Historically, the criticism of compensation has been that payment for such services is the commodification of childbearing and is tantamount to baby-selling or prostitution. Steinbock (1990: 129) outlined the four main moral objections stated in the 1984 Warnock Report:

1. It is inconsistent with human dignity that a woman should use her uterus for financial profit.
2. To deliberately become pregnant with the intention of giving up the child distorts the relationship between mother and child.
3. Surrogacy is degrading because it amounts to selling a child.
4. Since there are some risks attached to pregnancy, no woman ought to be asked to undertake pregnancy for another in order to earn money.

Should compensation reflexively engender feelings of exploitation? A woman has the ability to independently analyse the physical, emotional and social costs of a pregnancy. It can be argued that compensation reflects the time demands, physical inconveniences, time management burdens of appointments and other tasks associated with the pregnancy, just as it is argued that payment reflects an undue inducement. Who determines whether this is autonomy or coercion? In the United Kingdom, where compensation is prohibited but compensation for expenses is allowed, often the amount of money the surrogate ultimately receives may not be that different to the amount a surrogate in the United States receives from the 'commercial' surrogacy.

Criticisms continue to the present and include concerns about the exploitation of 'vulnerable populations'. These populations are deemed vulnerable due to economic deprivation, limited education or lack of access to employment. These concerns are now amplified with the availability of cross-border reproduction, and concerns about 'outsourcing' pregnancy to India renew these criticisms (see Pennings and B. Gürtin, Chapter 8). Concerns about the exploitation of women in economically deprived areas must take into consideration the particular context of that country. At first glance, differences in payments to surrogates between India and the USA, for example, suggest that intended parents and agencies are capitalizing on a vulnerable population, who are offering their services for comparatively lower payment. However, the question of whether surrogates of lower socioeconomic status are being exploited is not as straightforward as simply comparing amounts of payment received. One must also look to the value of that amount of money relative to a particular country and economy. Objectively, US surrogates are paid more than Indian surrogates; however, when taking into account the worth of that payment in real terms, an Indian surrogate would receive the equivalent of almost ten years' worth of family income (Pande, 2009). Therefore, in terms of 'real' value, payment offered to Indian surrogates may constitute a *greater* amount than that offered to US surrogates. However, this too may be considered morally questionable by some. By offering 'vulnerable' populations the opportunity to earn vast sums of money, are we applying increased coercion? The issue of contention may not be differences in payments to surrogates (real or perceived) between countries, but, once again, simply the issue of commercial surrogacy itself.

In the West many surrogates state that they wish to carry another pregnancy to help others, and because they enjoy pregnancy. Surrogates may carry for intended parents who are opposite-sex couples, same-sex couples or single parents. An ethical quandary arises around the reasons for needing a surrogate. One argument is that the medical and emotional risk of a surrogacy pregnancy is justified only when undertaken to help someone else have a baby who cannot do so on their own. In this analysis, it is argued that the risk of a pregnancy by a surrogate must be less than the risk (or absolute need) on the part of the other woman. Same-sex couples or single men or women would not be seen to meet the ethical criteria in this analysis. Should a medical practitioner refuse to treat a same-sex couple or a single man or woman, legal arguments in some countries (such as in the United States) would suggest that the intended father(s) or mother(s) should not be refused because 'any refusal to treat cannot be based on a categorical refusal to treat a patient because he or she is part of a legally protected class of persons' (Crockin and Jones, 2010: 211). As discussed in the chapter on single parents by choice (Graham and Braverman, Chapter 11), a counter-argument to this 'protected class' position is whether the perceived harm to the child of deliberately not providing a mother or father trumps the individual's or couple's right to procreate. Still, an issue remains whether it is ethical to ask a woman to take on the risks of pregnancy for reasons of the sex of the intending parent(s) rather than the infertility of a couple.

So long as informed consent is obtained from the surrogate, is the desire to become a parent sufficient grounds for entry into a surrogacy arrangement? If the gestational surrogate is fully informed of the status and relationship of the intending parents, should the surrogate be free to make her own decision and decide whether or not she wishes to act as a surrogate for these people?

Surrogates may have different feelings and desires depending on the circumstances of the need for a surrogate, for example medical need due to illness, because neither partner has a uterus, psychological needs or other particular circumstances. The question is whether the surrogate should be able to decide whether or not to go ahead with a particular couple or individual knowing their circumstances or whether regulations should be imposed which might restrict the use of a surrogate to certain intending parent(s) who meet particular criteria.

A gestational surrogate does not intend to be a parent to the child she carries, but rather portrays herself as being 'the oven' or fulfilling the role of the very first 'babysitter'. In other words, they will give great care to the developing baby and will do everything they can to keep that child healthy and well, but they do not see themselves in the role of a parent. Surrogates do not plan to take on the tasks of loving, protecting, nurturing, teaching, guiding and bonding with a child. A parent is the person who intends to be the emotional and psychological caregiver to the child, as one who devotes themselves to the well-being of that child. It is not that the surrogate does not have the emotional capacity to be a parent but rather understands that her intentions are not to engage in and promote herself in a parenting role. Surrogates provide a very essential and valued service to the intended parents and feel they are making a substantial contribution and difference in their community. Surrogates contextualize the risks of pregnancy into broader risks such as choosing to drive a car. Surrogates do not assess pregnancy risks as substantial and, therefore, are willing to take on this reasonable risk. To include only surrogates who have children is thus substantiated, as a nulliparous woman cannot have the information to assess the emotional risks or the physical challenges of a pregnancy.

Feminists have argued that surrogacy is the ultimate exploitation of women; the intrinsic value of a woman is reduced to being a 'breeder' and the poor will be exploited by the rich (Andrews, 1989: 222–3). Others have argued that women should have complete control over their body and this is represented in the choice to become pregnant for someone else. To ban surrogacy would be paternalistic – with others 'knowing' better than the surrogate herself about what she is able to manage and choose to do. In his discussion of the legalities of surrogacy, Gostin makes the civil liberties argument and states 'those who would ban or criminalize surrogacy have a heavy burden to explain why they would allow the state to stifle an activity that fulfils a human need without imposing any tangible harm on others' (Gostin, 1990: 7)

Relationship between the couple and surrogate

British surrogacy arrangements enable a strong relationship to develop between the surrogate mother and the intended parents during the surrogacy arrangement (van den Akker, 2000). In cases where couples may have met their surrogate through a third party, couples have been found to have known their surrogate for an average of seventeen weeks before going ahead with the first attempt to conceive (MacCallum *et al.*, 2003). This initial period of contact can be viewed to be important for ensuring that both parties develop a good relationship that will help ensure a successful surrogacy arrangement. The relationship that is typically maintained between the intending mother and surrogate (MacCallum *et al.*, 2003; Ragoné, 1994) continues during the pregnancy with intending mothers often attending antenatal appointments and scans. Such a close relationship is viewed by some as essential for allowing the surrogate mother to take her moral obligations to the unborn child seriously (van Zyl and van Niekerk, 2000).

Surrogates who were previously known, that is friends or relatives of the intending couple, have been found to maintain more frequent contact during the pregnancy compared to previously unknown surrogates (MacCallum *et al.*, 2003), and given that such relationships are already established, it is possible that such arrangements could result in better experiences. However, the use of known surrogates raises concerns over whether such women might be pressured into being surrogates. Findings from a UK study found that 77 per cent of intending mothers who had used a known surrogate stated that the decision that she act as the surrogate was made by the surrogate herself (MacCallum *et al.*, 2003). However, some have questioned whether known surrogates can enter into a surrogacy relationship free from coercion (Tieu, 2009). Also, given that known surrogates are more likely to maintain contact with the intended parents as the child grows up, this could place undue strain on an existing relationship. The role of the known surrogate would also need to be defined. MacCallum *et al.* (2003) found that most couples and known surrogates (77 per cent) agree that the surrogate would play no special role in the child's life beyond that appropriate to her relationship status with the child, for example as aunt or family friend.

Whereas contact with the surrogate mother is thought to give the child a better understanding of his or her origins, it has also been suggested that this may undermine the relationship between the intended mother and the child. However, some couples may desire a less involved surrogate mother so as not to feel threatened or undermined in their parental role. Studies of surrogacy families have revealed that contact with surrogates lessens over time, but that parents who were still in contact with the surrogate mother reported a positive relationship with them (Jadva *et al.*, 2012). It has been suggested that as contact with the couple diminishes, surrogates may feel more dissatisfied with the surrogacy arrangement (Ciccarelli and Beckman, 2005). The desired level of contact by couples may also depend on whether or not the surrogate is the genetic parent of the child; intended mothers who are not genetically related to their child may feel less secure in their mothering role if the genetic surrogate remained in close proximity to the family. Findings from Jadva *et al.* (2012) shows that mothers, fathers and children in genetic surrogacy families do have less frequent contact with the surrogate mother than those in gestational surrogacy families when the child is age 10, but that contact also depended on whether the surrogate was previously known (i.e. family member or friend) to the intended parents or previously unknown (met through a third party, i.e. surrogacy organization). Contact between the child and the surrogate was most frequent when the surrogate was a previously known gestational carrier and least frequent when the surrogate was a previously unknown genetic carrier.

The relationship between the couple and the surrogate, particularly when the child is still young, will determine the level of contact the surrogate has with the child. A UK study of 34 surrogate mothers found that surrogates varied in the degree of contact they maintained with families from having no subsequent contact, having some contact with the couples only, and others making regular visits to see each other's families (Jadva *et al.*, 2003). In the UK and the USA, no laws exist to ensure that children conceived using surrogacy will have access to the identity of their surrogate. This seems particularly surprising given that the UK has chosen to remove donor anonymity and has brought in legislation to enable offspring conceived by gamete donation to have access to identifying information about their donor. As with informal donor insemination arrangements that take place outside of a regulated clinic, in cases of surrogacy that bypass clinics, that is self-insemination of the intended father's sperm by the surrogate, it is not clear if children born through surrogacy will have these same rights or access to donor information.

Considerations for the children born through surrogacy

The two types of surrogacy, genetic and gestational, may give rise to differing levels of importance for the child. A child who is genetically related to the surrogate may place more importance on knowing her identity and wanting contact with her either for social or medical reasons. In contrast, a child who has a gestational surrogate may not place as much importance on contact. However, it is important to note that gestational surrogacy provides a new type of phenomenon where IVF enables a woman to carry a child to whom she is not related. We do not know how important this gestational relationship will prove to be for the child and the surrogate. Will a child want to know who their gestational carrier is? And more so, will they feel that they would want to meet her and have ongoing contact with her? Or will gestational surrogates be viewed by the child as one of the many medical components that were needed to bring about a birth using assisted conception? There is little research addressing these questions; however, a follow-up study by Jadva *et al.* (2012) found that around two-thirds of surrogacy children had seen their surrogate mother during the past year at the time of interview (when the child was age 10), and of these children the majority reported that they liked their surrogate mother, with only 1 child feeling ambivalent towards her.

If gestational surrogates do prove to be of importance for a child's identity, then surrogacy in cases where the surrogate lives in a different country, or where she does not speak the same language as the surrogacy child, may have a future impact on the child. For example, would families who have accessed Indian surrogates maintain contact with their surrogate, and if so, how would the surrogate child feel about having a gestational carrier who comes from a different cultural, religious or socio-economic background to themselves?

The issue of commodification of surrogates can also raise potentially difficult questions for the child's relationship with the surrogate. We do not know how a child will feel if they find out that their surrogate was paid, in some cases vast amounts of money, to carry them. But when surrogates come from a different socio-economic background to the intended families, in particular in cases where they may be perceived to be facing financial hardships, then what moral obligations might the family feel towards the surrogate during the pregnancy and into the future? More importantly, what moral obligations might the resultant child feel if he or she chooses to make contact with her?

Follow-up studies on the psychological and socio-emotional development of surrogacy children have found that they do well and do not appear to be negatively affected as a result of their surrogacy birth (Golombok *et al.*, 2004, 2006a, 2006b). However, little is known about another group of children who are also affected by surrogacy: the existing children of the surrogate. Concerns over the surrogate's children include how they may feel about having a close relationship with the intending couple which, following the birth of the child, lessens or stops altogether. Furthermore, it is not known how the surrogate's children feel about seeing their mother pregnant with a child (a genetic half-sibling in genetic surrogacy) who she then hands over to someone else to raise. Such situations could lead to potential difficulties in the relationships that exist within the surrogate's family, yet little empirical data exists on how the surrogate's own family is affected by surrogacy.

Telling the child about their surrogacy conception

A fundamental question that has appeared in much of the literature about conception involving a third party is that of disclosure: should parents tell their child that there was a third party involved in their conception, be it through donor gametes or a surrogate mother? For a more detailed discussion of this issue, see Appleby, Blake, and Freeman, Chapter 13.

With regard to disclosure within surrogacy families, research has found greater openness with regard to the circumstances of the child's conception than in gamete donation families. Surrogacy families tend to be more like adoptive families in their readiness to disclose their child's origins to their friends, families and to the child (MacCallum *et al.*, 2003), often referring to the surrogacy in terms of 'broken tummies' and 'tummy-mummies'. This readiness may be due to the fact that, unlike gamete donation parents, they must explain the arrival of a child in the absence of a pregnancy. Although surrogacy parents appear more comfortable about disclosing, it must be borne in mind that the genetic surrogacy arrangements create the opportunity for two levels of disclosure. In other words, parents may decide to be open with their child about the gestational role of the surrogate mother, and keep her additional genetic contribution secret. Indeed, Raoul-Duval and colleagues (1992) reported that when egg donation mothers were asked what they will tell their children, the majority responded that they will 'tell the truth'. In fact, on closer inspection, the authors found that to most mothers this meant telling what the authors describe as a 'white lie': merely informing the child that they were conceived using IVF, with no mention of the donated egg. Similarly, in a study looking at intra-family egg donation, Jadva *et al.* (2011) found that almost half

(44%) of mothers had been open with others about the use of IVF but not the egg donation, and 22% reported that they had not told others that they had used a known donor.

A similar pattern of incomplete disclosure has emerged among the genetic surrogacy families. Readings *et al.* (2011) described a situation wherein all of the surrogacy families in the study reported having been open to their child about the surrogacy, but only 24% of genetic surrogacy families had told their child about the use of the surrogate's egg (i.e. that the surrogate mother is also their genetic mother). This is more surprising still when considered alongside a disclosure rate of 41% among egg donation families in the same study (Readings *et al.*, 2011). What exactly prevents these genetic surrogacy families from disclosing all the facts relating to their child's conception is unknown.

In cases where parents are not open about all details of the child's conception, the possibility of the child working it out for themselves is also heightened. This leads to a potentially complicated scenario, where parents feel that they have been open with their child about surrogacy, but where their child may still feel betrayed or lied to.

Partial disclosure may be an attractive option to surrogacy parents because it explains the child's presence in the absence of a pregnancy and alleviates some of the guilt or tension that may arise from secret-keeping. Parents in genetic surrogacy arrangements may also regard the amount of sensitive information too great to share with their child all at once. However, although these parents have not completely concealed the involvement of the surrogate mother, they have failed to disclose the information that may be of most significance to children born of genetic surrogacy arrangements, that is that the woman who they regard as their mother is not, in fact, their genetic mother. A reason cited by parents for not having disclosed this information to their child is that the child is still too young to understand. However, this claim is questionable when almost half of the egg donation families in the same study have been completely open with their child (Readings *et al.*, 2011).

It has been suggested that where there is secrecy surrounding the circumstances of the child's birth, not only does this obstruct the rights of the child, but it will be detrimental to family relationships because it may create boundaries between those who 'know' the secret (the parents) and those who do not (the child) (Karpel, 1980). Some have even raised the possibility that this may interfere with the attachment process (Lycett *et al.*, 2005) and thus may have damaging consequences for the child's psychological well-being and development. In discussions of secrecy, perhaps the most important voices to listen to are those of adult adoptees and donor insemination offspring themselves. On this subject they are fairly consistent in their reproach of secrecy, which has prohibited adoptees from constructing a coherent sense of self and identity, and from answering questions about their biological family (Triseliotis, 1973; Turner and Coyle, 2000). Although surrogacy families appear to be more forthcoming than donor insemination families in this respect, for those children who have not been told about their surrogate conception (gestational surrogacy), it is unknown as to whether this information is of equivalent significance to knowing or not knowing one's genetic origins. It may be that knowledge that their *birth* mother, as opposed to their *genetic* mother, is not the same woman who has brought them up, is of less importance or value.

Some have questioned whether parents should be forced to be open with their children where a third party has been involved in their conception (Wallbank, 2002; McGee *et al.*, 2001). Wallbank (2002) argues that if the interests of the child are truly held to be paramount, current UK legislation does not go far enough to ensure that the children's interests in knowing their birth origins are provided for. She suggests that a general welfare principle alone is not sufficient to guarantee that children's rights in this area are respected, and that nothing less than a change in the law to make openness mandatory will do so.

Conclusions

Surrogacy continues to create much legal, ethical and social debate as it enters its fourth decade of widespread existence. Further complicating the debate is the cross-border care that has brought surrogacy to countries such as India. Identifying the issues for all the stakeholders in a surrogacy arrangement – surrogates, children born from surrogacy arrangements, intended parents and other family members such as the surrogate's children – is critical in sorting through the suppositions of each stakeholder's needs versus the facts. There is a thin line between paternalism and exploitation when considering the surrogate's needs. Similarly, there is a thin line for the intended parents between reproductive autonomy and accountability. Surrogacy is a viable parenting option if all rights, responsibilities and considerations are explored for each stakeholder.

REFERENCES

Andrews, L. B. (1989). *Between Strangers: Surrogate Mothers, Expectant Fathers, and Brave New Babies*. New York: Harper & Row.

(1990). 'Surrogate Motherhood: The Challenge for Feminists', in L. Gostin (ed.), *Surrogate Motherhood: Politics and Privacy*. Indianapolis: Indiana University Press.

Brazier, M., Campbell, A. and Golombok, S. (1998). *Surrogacy: Review for Health Ministers of Current Arrangements for Payments and Regulation*. Report of the Review Team. Cm. 4068. Department of Health, London.

Cameron, G. (2011). *CW* v. *NT and another* [2011] EWHC 33, *Family Law Week*.

Centers for Disease Control and Prevention (CDC), statistics available from www.cdc.gov/ART/ART2006/section2c.htm#f40. Accessed. June. 30, 2009.

Ciccarelli, J. C. and Beckman, L. J. (2005). 'Navigating rough waters: an overview of psychological aspects of surrogacy'. *Journal of Social Issues*, 61, 21–43.

Crockin, S. L. and Jones Jr., H. W. (2010). *Legal Conceptions: The Evolving Law and Policy of Assisted Reproductive Technologies*. Baltimore: The Johns Hopkins University Press.

English, M. E., Mechanick-Braverman, A. and Corson, S. L. (1991). 'Semantics and science: the distinction between gestational carrier and traditional surrogacy programs'. *Women's Health Issues*, 1, 155–7.

Gamble, N. (2009). 'Crossing the line: the legal and ethical problems of foreign surrogacy'. *Reproductive Biomedicine Online*, 19, 151–2.

Ghevaert, L. (2011). 'International surrogacy: progress or media hype?' *BioNews*, 590.

Golombok, S., Murray, C., Jadva, V., MacCallum, F., *et al.* (2004). 'Families created through surrogacy arrangement: parent-child relationships in the 1st year of life'. *Developmental Psychology*, 40, 400–11.

Golombok, S., MacCallum, F., Murray, C., Lycett, E., *et al.* (2006a). 'Surrogacy families: parental functioning, parent-child relationships and children's psychological development at age 2'. *Journal of Child Psychology and Psychiatry*, 47, 213–22.

Golombok, S., Murray, C., Jadva, V., Lycett, E., *et al.* (2006b). 'Non-genetic and non-gestational parenting: consequences for parent-child relationships and the psychological well-being of mothers, fathers and children at age 3'. *Human Reproduction*, 21, 1918–24.

Gostin, L. (1990). *Surrogate Motherhood: Politics and Privacy*. Indianapolis: Indiana University Press.

Hyder, N. (2010). 'Couple request surrogate mum to abort over disability'. *Bionews*, 579.

Jadva, J., Murray, C., Lycett, E., MacCallum, F., *et al.* (2003). 'Surrogacy: the experiences of surrogate mother'. *Human Reproduction*, 18, 2196–204.

Jadva, V., Casey, P., Readings, J., Blake L. and Golombok, S. (2011). 'A longitudinal study of recipients' views and experiences of intra-family egg donation'. *Human Reproduction*. doi: 10.1093/humrep/der252.

Jadva, V., Blake, L., Casey, P. and Golombok, S. (2012). 'Surrogacy families ten years on: relationship with the surrogate, decisions over disclosure and children's understanding of their surrogacy origins'. *Human Reproduction*.

Karpel, M. (1980). 'Family secrets'. *Family Process*, 19, 295–306.

Lycett, E., Daniels, K., Curson, R. and Golombok, S. (2005). 'School-aged children of donor insemination: a study of parents' disclosure patterns'. *Human Reproduction*, 20, 810–19.

MacCallum, F., Lycett, E., Murray, C., Jadva, V., *et al.* (2003). 'Surrogacy: the experience of commissioning couples'. *Human Reproduction*, 18, 1334–42.

McGee, G., Vaughan-Brakman, S. and Gurmankin, A. D. (2001). 'Disclosure to children conceived with donor gametes should not be optional'. *Human Reproduction*, 16, 2033–8.

Pande, A. (2009). '"It may be her eggs but it's my blood": surrogates and everyday forms of kinship in India'. *Qualitative Sociology*, 32, 379–97.

Ragoné, H. (1994). *Surrogate Motherhood: Conception in the Heart*. Oxford: Westview Press.

Raoul-Duval, A., Letur-Konirsch, H. and Frydman, R. (1992). 'Anonymous oocyte donation: a psychological study of recipients, donors and children'. *Human Reproduction*, 7, 51–4.

Readings, J., Blake, L., Casey, P., Jadva, V., *et al.* (2011). 'Secrecy, disclosure, and everything in between: decisions of parents of children conceived by donor insemination, egg donation, and surrogacy'. *Reproductive Biomedicine Online*, 22, 485–95.

Spar, D. L. (2006). *The Baby Business: How Money, Science and Politics Drive the Commerce of Conception*. Boston: Harvard Business School Press.

Steinbock, B. (1990). 'Surrogate Motherhood as Prenatal Adoption', in L. Gostin (ed.), *Surrogate Motherhood: Politics and Privacy*. Indianapolis: Indiana University Press.

Teman, E. (2010). *Birthing a Mother*. Berkley: University of California Press.

Tieu, M. M. (2009). 'Altruistic surrogacy: the necessary objectification of surrogate mothers'. *Journal of Medical Ethics*, 35, 171–5.

Triseliotis, J. (1973). *In Search of Origins: The Experiences of Adopted People*. London and Boston: Routledge and Kegan Paul.

Turner, A. J. and Coyle, A. (2000). 'What does it mean to be a donor offspring? The identity experiences of adults conceived by donor insemination and the implications for counselling and therapy'. *Human Reproduction*, 15, 2041–51.

Van den Akker, O. (2000). 'The importance of a genetic link in mothers commissioning a surrogate baby in the UK'. *Human Reproduction*, 15, 1849–55.

Van Zyl, L. and van Niekerk, A. (2000). 'Interpretations, perspectives and intentions in surrogate motherhood'. *Journal of Medical Ethics*, 26, 404–9.

Wallbank, J. (2002). 'Too many mothers? Surrogacy, kinship and the welfare of the child'. *Medical Law Review*, 10, 271–94.

Warnock, M. (1984). *Report of the Committee of Inquiry into Human Fertilisation and Embryology*. London: Department of Health and Social Security.

LEGISLATION

FRANCE

Code (Nouveau) de Procedure Civile Français (1977). Art. 315, Art. 343, Art. 1128, *Jurisprudence*. Dalloz, 11 rue Soufflot, 75240 Paris Cedex 05

UK

Human Fertilisation and Embryology (HFE) Act (1990) Section 3(5)
Human Fertilisation and Embryology (HFE) Act 1990, as amended 2008 Sections 35–54
Surrogacy Arrangements Act 1985

17 Some conclusions regarding the interaction of normative and descriptive elements in reproductive donation

Guido Pennings

If one message jumps out of this book, it is the complexity of reproductive donation. There is a huge variety of cultural, legal and moral rules regarding third-party reproduction. The regulatory systems constantly evolve as the world in which they function evolves. This evolution can be seen in changes as diverse as modifications in value hierarchies (children's rights versus parental rights), techno-scientific developments (egg banking after vitrification), expansion of the world wide web (donor offspring looking for their donor siblings) and low-cost airlines (reproductive tourism). Moreover, due to globalization and internationalization, systems infect each other across large distances. The abolition of donor anonymity in Sweden was picked up by Australian states and returned to Western Europe. Continually legislators are setting up social experiments by modifying the legislation of assisted reproduction. However, we will only learn from these experiments if we spend time and effort analysing and interpreting them. The wealth of information to be gathered from the different systems worldwide should enable us to better rule our own practice, to better predict what will happen if we alter things and to better reach the moral goals we have set.

The proximate endeavour of this book was to provide a state of the art of the scientific information on donation. The ultimate goal was to use this information to help with the adaptation of the normative systems that currently regulate the practice. Many legislations are not (or not always) based on the scientific evidence. As a consequence, the laws may have unforeseen, unwanted and/or unintended consequences. The introduction of the identification requirement for donors can illustrate this point. Donors who know that they will become identifiable to their donor children are reluctant to accept the current maximum limit on donor offspring. A considerable number of them limit their donation to one or two families. So while a reduction in the number of donors was predicted, the overall effect on the availability of gametes for use in the clinic is greater than predicted.

Still, not all applications of medically assisted reproduction can be based on scientific evidence. This may be because there are few cases with highly specific characteristics, as in intrafamilial donation, or simply because we have to wait for the long-term developments, as in donor identifiability and contact. It is important to realize that the precautionary principle does not work in the field of medically assisted reproduction; we cannot wait for scientific evidence before accepting new requests and new systems. The main reason for this is that it would lead to a 'catch-22': we can only accept certain forms of reproductive donation when we have shown that they are safe and sound but we cannot prove this because we have to reject these applications as long as we do not have this proof. This problem does not release us from the duty to thoroughly think through the situation and to try to predict possible problems with these requests and systems. In fact, it implies that our first duty is to organize the scientific research in order to get feedback so that we can make informed decisions about future applications of a similar kind.

The complexity of the practice of donation also increases because one should not only take into account the system one imposes but also the reaction by people who disagree. More than ever before, we see that the people involved no longer blindly abide by the rules and accept them as given. Patients who are excluded by law from access to treatment look for salvation abroad. Donor offspring groups, parents and so on take initiatives and organize their own solutions. The voluntary donor registries are a good example here. Also the web searches by parents of donor offspring or donor offspring themselves show that they do not accept the limitation on information regarding the donor. Although they might not get access to the donor directly, they can obtain at least bits of information about the donor and his/her contribution by looking at their half-siblings. This example also shows the far-reaching impact of the procedures. Children who come to know their donor, their donor siblings and their families have to reorganize their concept of 'family'. In itself this is nothing new since there are numerous instances of 'deviations' from the genetic family for which people have to create their own interpretation of the situation. The 'donor family' may be special nevertheless because of the donation setting (with its own rules and regulations) and the specificity of the relationships (with a time gap, spatial distance and possibly high number of half-siblings). This social experiment should not frighten us, but it is important for future policy-making that we gather information on the well-being of the people living the experience.

While this book helps to contextualize the moral rules regarding reproductive donation, it also clearly demonstrates the limitations of scientific evidence in guiding normative structures. The main reason for this lies in the deontological nature of some of the basic positions in this debate. Views on responsible parenthood, acceptable reproduction and family planning, virtuous medicine, rights of individuals and society in the regulation of private life and so on are based on broad clusters of ideas that are dispersed in society through cultural and legal institutions and rooted in long histories. These views are specified in rights, rules, duties and obligations that are not grounded in considerations about the welfare of children, parents, surrogates or donors. One may be opposed to payment for surrogacy, not because one believes that this is bad for the people involved, but because one believes that human reproduction should not be commercialized. One may favour telling the children about their donor conception, not because one believes that this increases the children's well-being, but because one believes that parents should not lie to their children. Scientific evidence is powerless against such deontological rules in the sense that it cannot directly refute or corroborate these rules. This point is important because one of the reactions from consequentialists, when they have presented 'irrefutable' evidence about a certain procedure, is that everyone should agree with their conclusion. People who are not convinced by the evidence must be of bad faith or unreasonably stubborn. However, deontologists can maintain their position without being inconsistent.

This finding should not lead to a bleak picture of the interaction between the ethical rules and the evidence from the humanities, however. First, most Western societies tend to adopt a predominantly consequentialist position when designing policy measures and regulation. Consequentialists, who ground their moral positions mainly on the effects of actions and laws, should take into account the scientific findings regarding these effects. Second, instead of looking for a direct proof or refutation of deontological rules, one may try to construct a wide reflective equilibrium in which normative and descriptive elements are brought together. The scientific evidence is not directly placed against certain rules and rights but becomes part of a global moral position. The task then becomes to construct a coherent framework that avoids outright contradictions as much as possible. This is a vast enterprise that will never end. A definitive moral system could only be built if the world were to stop ... And we don't want that, do we?

Index

abusive parents, 64
access to treatment, 145
Act No. 20/1966 Coll., on Public Health
    Care, 127
Act of 5 December 2003 No. 100, 128
Acts on Assisted Fertility Treatments
    (1237/2006), 127
adoption, 65
adoption and embryo donation, 276–7
Advisory Committee on Assisted
    Reproductive Technology (ACART),
    169
altruism, 100, 101
altruistic donation, *see* trivialis[ing]
    altruistic donation
American Bar Association (ABA), 93
American Society for Reproductive
    Medicine (ASRM), 78, 93, 134
    compensation for egg donors,
        compensation of, 157
    Ethics Committee, 100, 101, 169, 206
    guidelines for oocyte donation, 153
    surrogacy guidelines, 290
anonymity of donors, 308
    gamete donation, 151–2
    personalised, 162
    in Spain, 116–17, 122
anonymous sperm donation, 4, 58
anthropology and ARTs, 71–3
Archbishop of Canterbury, 6
Aristotle, 35
artificial gametes, 24–5
artificial insemination (AI), 5
    eighteenth century, 5
    legal status, 8
artificial insemination by husband
    (AIH), 7
Assisted Human Reproduction Act
    (2004), 127
Assisted Human Reproduction Act
    (2006), 116
assisted reproduction, 2

communitarian approach to, 94
ethical orientation of, 93–4
individualistic, market-based approach
    to, 94
informed consent and, 95–6
UK and US regulations of, 94
UK communitarian autonomy
    approach to, 94
US individualistic autonomy approach
    to, 94
assisted reproductive technologies
    (ARTs), 16, 112, 189
anthropology, 71
benefits, 20, 52
British South Asians and, 83
CBRC in, 130
in China, 72
Christianity and, 80
cultural embeddedness of, 72
cultural relevance of, 71
in Egypt, 72
ethical dilemmas, 30, 31–7
ethical obligations of providers, 43
family structure and, 192
for gays and lesbians, 44
globalization impact, 70
heterosexual couples and, 198
IFFS Surveillance 07 of, 74
influence of Internet, 144
Islamic view, 80–1
Judaism and, 81
legislation of different countries,
    127–9
lived experiences of, 46
localization processes of, 70
questions related to, 36
religious perspectives, 79–82
single persons and, 206
social use of, 198–9
in Spain, *see* Spain
usage in foreign country, 45
within societies, 84

Assisted Reproductive Technology Act
    (2007), 128
autonomy
    disclosure issues, 236
    issues, with CBRC, 143–4
autosomal recessive gene mutations, 23

'Baby Cotton' case, 291
Barton, Dr Mary, 232
Belmont Report, 34
    concepts involved in implementing
        principles, 33
    key principles, 32
beneficence, 33, 94, 184
Bentham, Jeremy, 35
bioethics, 37, 46, 94
BioLaw rights, 119
biological father, 1
biological kinship, 54, 58
biological mother, 1
biologically effective cryoprotectants, 15
biologically related child, reasons for
    having, 65–8
blastocyst development, 19
blastomeres, 14
blood-relationships, moral failing of
    non-provision of, 62
British Medical Association (BMA), 225
British South Asians and ARTs, 83
brother-to-sister donation, 175
Brown, Louise, 71
Browne v. D'Alleva, 105

Carter, C. O., 5
Catholic Church, 5
child, rights of, 38
child-bearing, analogy of, 66
childlessness, 72
children
    anonymity of donor and, 118
    biological kinship and, 58
    biological parents vs. non-biological
        parents, 58, 60, 62
    consanguinity and, 58
    disclosing of donor details and, 236
    effect of abusive parents, 64
    genetic endowment and, 58
    homophobic victimization by peers,
        215
    identity formation in, 59–61
    impact of resemblance, 59–61
    need for a father, 193–4
    negative outcome of single parent
        fostered, 193
    open-identity donation and, 258–61

parenthood perspective of, 57–65
    of same-sex parents, welfare of, 212–18
    victimization of, 215
Christianity and ARTs, 80
chromosomal anomalies, 19
cloning, 22
collaborative reproduction, 1
    involvement of third parties, 3
    reasons for choosing, 1
commercial surrogacy, see surrogacy
commercialisation, 3
    of CBRC, 143
commodification, 3, 39
    of embryo donation, 284–5
compensation, of gamete donors, 98–102,
    115
confidentiality, 117
congenital abnormalities, 19
consanguinity, 58, 61
    genetic risks of, 23–4
    intrafamilial donation and, 173
'conscription of the virgins', 5
Conservation, management and provision
    of data of donors in artificial
    insemination Act (2002), 128
Convention for the Protection of Human
    Rights and Dignity of the Human
    Being with regard to the Application of
    Biology and Medicine: Convention on
    Human Rights and Biomedicine, 154
Courtship of Eddie's Father, the, 194
criminalisation of AID, 6
cross-border reproductive care (CBRC),
    79, 130
    access to treatment, 145
    arguments against, 142
    ARTs and, 130
    autonomy issues, 143–4
    coerced conformity of, 137–9
    communication problems, 143
    different causes of, 131
    empirical evidence of, 131
    equality issue, 145
    ESHRE study, 132–4
    gamete procurement and
        transportation, 135–7
    harmonization of, 139–40
    heterogeneity factors, 132
    intending parents and, 132–5
    issues with, 141–6
    justice factor, 145–6
    moral pluralism of, 140–1
    potential destinations, 139
    regulation of, 137
    in Romanian clinics, 141

safety issues, 142
cryobanking of sperm, 8
cryopreservation, 14–15
 approaches for use, 15
 biologically effective cryoprotectants, 15
 clinical storage temperture, 14
 cryopreserved (frozen) donated material, 14
 cryopreserved spermatozoa, 21
 effect of toxicity, 15
 of eggs, 18
 long-term follow-up, 21
 problems with, 14
 rationale for use, 16
 storage duration, 15
cryoprotectants, 18
Cryos, 135
CryoShip TM Global Service, 136
cytoplasmic transfer, 23

Daniels, Norman, 220
daughter-to-mother donation, 175
Davis v. *Davis*, 97
deontology, 35, 235
developing world and egg donation, 45
diethylstilboestrol tragedies, 21
dimethylsulphoxide (DMSO), 15
disclosing donation, idea of, 78, 106–8
 comparitive studies of disclosing and non-disclosing families, 240–1
 deontological reasoning, 235
 disclosing-families, 239–40
 disclosure rates, 234
 ethical issues, 241–5
 ethical overview, 235–6
 family welfare and, 243
 heterosexual couples and, 234
 medical welfare of donor and, 242–3
 non-disclosing families and, 237–8
 practicalities of, 233–5
 rights, 244–5
 surrogacy, 302–4
Disclosure of Donor Information Regulations, 118
disposition of stored embryos, 96
diversity
 ARTs and, 71–3, 79
 in egg donation practice, 73–6
 in ethical deliberations of donation, 76–9
 in gamete donation practice, 75
 of government regulations, 79
 reproductive donation and, 73–6
 in sperm donation practice, 73–6

in surrogacy practice, 75
DNA paternity testing, 4
Doe v. *Blue Cross Blue Shield of Massachusetts*, 93
Doe v. *XYZ Co.*, 107
donated gametes, legal status of, 96–8
donated tissues, forms of, 14
donation contract, 117
Donor Conception Network, 141
donor gamete screening, 136
donor identification, 252
donor identity, disclosure of, 106–8, 113, *see also* disclosing donation, idea of
 experiences of parents making contact with child's donor relations, 256–8
 open-identity donation and, 254–5, 258–61
 parent-child relationship, 256
donor insemination (DI), 75, 189, 205, 232, 234, 237, 252
Donor Registry, 113
Donor Sibling Link, 253
Donor Sibling Registry (DSR), 39, 253, 256
donor siblings, identification of, 253
donor-conceived children, legal parentage of, 102–6
donors
 altruistic motivation of, 123
 educational level in Spain, 123
 gametes, 35, 36
 with psychiatric problems, in Spain, 123
 recruitment of, 38
 siblings, risk of marriage between, 5
 Spain, profile in, 123
 types of, 8
Down syndrome, 122
dyslexia, 60

ectogenesis, 6
egg donation, 2, 18–19
 cultural response of, 74
 disclosure and, 234
 diversity in, 73–6
 donors from developing world, issues with, 45
 empirical research of, 47
 ethics related to, 37–9
 in Germany, 65, 75
 as a gift exchange, 101
 in Italy, 77
 mother-child relation in terms of, 93
 overview of, 91
 programs, 101

egg donation (*cont.*)
  protection of donor, 77
  in Spain, 46, 122
  in UK clinics, 169
egg freezing, problems with, 18
egg recipient, rights of, 38
egg sharing, 39, 101, 159–61
  altruistic donation, 160
  commercial transaction and, 159
  ethical claims, 159
  problems with, 159
  related to payment, 160
egg vitrification, 19
embryo donation
  commodification of, 284–5
  disposition decision of, 277–80
  parenting selection criteria for,
    271–7
Embryo Protection Act, 77, 128
embryo transfer, ethico-legal status, 17
embryonic stem cells (ESCs), 14, 24
embryos
  donation, 17–18, 75
  ethical questions related to donation,
    40
  freezing of, 18
  legal status of, 96
  risk of miscarriage, 21
  selection of, 2
enucleated 'healthy' egg, 23
epididymis, 16
Equality Act (Sexual Orientation), 224
ESHRE Ethics and Law
    Task Force, 141, 154, 170
ethical questions
  disclosing of donor details, 241–5
  diversity in, 76–9
  egg donation, 38
  embryo donation, 40
  financial remuneration for donors, 78
  for formulating policies, 47–8
  infertility, 42–3
  open-identity donation, 253
  reproduction of gays and lesbians, 44
  single parents, 43
  for social science research, 46–7
  SPCs, 190–1
  sperm donation, 39–40
  surrogacy, 41
  transnational donation, 44–5
Eugenic Institute, 5
European Community treaty, 138
European Convention on Human Rights,
    98
European culture, 23

European Society for Human
    Reproduction and Embryology
    (ESHRE), 131, 144
  on direct payment, 154
  Task Force on Ethics and Law, 170
European Union Tissues and Cells
    Directive (2004), 3, 136, 140, 143,
    154
Europe-based ESHRE study on CBRC,
    132–4
eutelogenesis (AID), 6, 8
  criminilisation of, 6
  infertile couple and, 7
  moral acceptance, 9
  Piddington's views, 10
  reforms, 7
  in Spain, 113
  Wand Committee on, 10
Evans v. *UK*, 98
ex vivo reproductive cells, 131

Facebook, 38
'Facultative Motherhood without Offence
    to Moral Law: every woman's right
    to motherhood', 5
Family Law Reform Act
    (1987), 7, 232
family relationship and intrafamilial
    donation, 176–81
Family Tree DNA, 4
father/child relationships, in terms of
    sperm donation, 93
fatwa and ARTs, 80–1
fecundity, 13
fee-for-service, 78
Ferguson v. *McKiernan*, 105
fertility
  defined, 13
  tourism, 131
Fertility Clinic Success Rate and
    Certificate Act (1992), 93
fertility treatment
  in Britain, 92
  counselling, 95
  in US, 92
fetal growth restriction, 21
financial remuneration, for donors
  altruism argument, 156
  argument against, 154–6
  arguments for, 156–9
  in case of financially disadvantaged
    individuals, 155
  controversy related to, 152–4
  egg sharing, 160
  ethical questions related to, 78

gamete donors, 98–102
  human dignity argument, 155
  models for payment, 158–9
  psychological issues/abusive behaviour,
    155
  in Spain, 115
  wage model, 158
for-profit gamete banks, 92
French Law on Bioethics (2004), 116

gamete donation, 68, 107, 237
  anonymity, 151–2
  argument related to donors, 154–9
  Christianity views, 80
  ethical question, 77
  in Greece, 75
  Islamic view, 80
  legal regulations in UK and US,
    92–108
  overview of, 91–2
  parties involved in, 92
  reciprocity and, 161–4
  recruitment and payment of gamete
    donors, 98–102, 152–4
  religious perspective of, 80
  in UK, 232–3
Gamete Intra-Fallopian Transfer
  (GIFT), 15
gamete-like cells, 24
gays and lesbians, reproduction
  of, 44, 74
  assistance to, 225
  criticisms at research level, 215–18
  in France, 133
  homophobic victimization of children
    and, 215
  legal status of parentage, 103
  psychological wellbeing of child,
    213–14
  psychosexual development of child,
    214–15
  societal influence, 218–19
  welfare of child and, 212–18
generation without antecedent sexual
  union, 6
genetic fatherhood, 77
Genetic Integrity Act (2006:351), 129
genetic motherhood, 77
Germany, 128
  donor identity, disclosure of, 113
  egg donation, 75
  sperm donation, 75
germ-line stem cells, 24
gestational link and embryo donation,
  274–6

gestational surrogacy, 20, 21, 289,
  290, 292, 300, 301, 304,
  see also surrogacy
gift relationship, between donor and
  recipient, 3, 100
glycerol, 15
godmother, 177
Google, 38
grand misconception theory, 59

Halakha (Jewish religious law), 81
half-siblings, 38
harmonization of CBRC, 139–40
Hecht v. Superior Court, 97
Helsinki Declaration, 32, 34
Hermann J. Muller Repository for
  Germinal Choice, 6
heterologous insemination, 5
heteroplasmy, 22
Hippocratic Oath, 31, 34
HLA-C molecules, 21
HLA-C/KIR typing, 22
Holocaust, 32
homologous insemination, 5
Human Assisted Reproductive
  Technology Act (2004), 128
Human Fertilisation and Embryology Act
  (HFE Act, 1990), 7, 9, 92, 129
  Code of Practice for fertility clinics,
    159
  financial limit, 99
  HFEA Code of Practice, 8th edition,
    95
  HFEA-licensed provider, 102
Human Fertilisation and Embryology
  Authority, 7
  Disclosure of Donor Information
    Regulations (2004), 129
Human Reproductive Technology
  Amendment Act (2004), 129
Human Rights Act, 224

identifiable donors, types of, 250
identity formation and resemblance, 60
IFFS Surveillance 07, 74
illegitimate babies and adoption, 7
in vitro fertilisation (IVF), 13, 15,
    16, 17
  baby, 3
  global technology of, 72
  Islamic view, 80
  neonatal malformation and, 18
  in Spain, 114
induced stem cells (ISCs), 24
infertile heterosexual couples, 252

infertility, 13, 36, 72, 73, 199
  ethical questions, 42–3
  stigma associated with, 65
Infertility Consumer Support for
  Infertility (iCSi), 141
Infertility Treatment Act (1995), 129
informal insemination, legal
  consequences of, 103
informed consent and assisted
  reproduction, 95–6, 174
  egg sharing, 161
insurance coverage, for infertility, 42
International Committee Monitoring
  Assisted Reproductive Technologies
  (ICMART), 134, 145, 168
International Federation of Gynecology
  and Obstetrics (FIGO), 141
international transport of
  gametes, 135–7
Internet, influence on ARTs, 144
intimate relationships, between adult and
  child, 55–7
intra-cervical insemination (ICI), 15
intra-cytoplasmic sperm injection (ICSI),
  2, 15, 19, 73
intrafamilial donation, 6, 41–2
  disclosure issues, 182
  donor relative and, 173–6
  family relationship and, 176–81
  parent–offspring relationship and,
    181–4
  reasons for, 172–3
  regulation and professional guidelines,
    169–72
  secrecy issues, 181, 183
  in UK, 75
intra-uterine insemination (IUI), 15
involuntary childlessness, 73
Islamic view of ARTs, 80–1
IVF baby, 3

Janssen v. Alicea, 105
Johnson v. Superior Court, 97, 107
Johnson v. Clavert, 273
Judaism and ARTs, 81
justice, 33, 94

K.M. v. E.G., 105
Kant, Immanuel, 35
Kids are All Right, The, 108
killer Ig-like receptors (KIRs), 21
kinship revolution, 71
Kleinman, Arthur, 72
Kurchner v. State Farm Fire and
  Casualty, 96

Lafollette, Hugh, 51, 63
Lancet, the, 18
Law 32/2006 de Procriação medicamente
  assistida, Diário da República, 1.a
  série No.143–26 de Julho de 2006,
  128
Law 3089, 23 December 2002, 128
Law 3305/2005, 128
Law for the Protection of the Embryo, 65
Leckie v. Voorhies, 105
legal fatherhood, 102, 103
legal guardianship, 54
legal parentage of donor-conceived
  children, 102–6
Legge 19 febbraio 2004, n. 40 Norme in
  materia di procreazione medicalmente
  assistita. Gaceta Ufficiale n. 45, 24
  February 2004, 128
Legge federale concernente la
  procreazione con assistenza
  medica (Legge sulla medicina della
  procreazione, LPAM), (1998), 129
Ley 14/2006, de 26 de mayo, sobre
  técnicas de reproducción humana
  asistida, B.O.E. núm. 126, 27 May
  2006, 128
liquid phase storage of tissues, 14
Loi n°2004–800 du 6 août 2004, 128

McIntyre v. Crouch, 104
macroethics of donation, 76–9
major depression, 43
male infertility, treatment for, 2
male sexual dysfunction, 16
Marginalized Reproduction, 83
market inalienability, concept of, 3
Mattes, Jane, 196
medical infertility, 13
Micro-Epididymidal Sperm Aspiration
  (MESA), 16
microethics of donation, 76–9
microinsemination, 139
Mill, John Stuart, 35
Mintz v. Zoernig, 104
mitochondrial donation, 22
mitochondrial genetic disease, 22
mitochondrion DNA (mtDNA), 22, 23
Model Act on Assisted Reproductive
  Technology (ABA Model Act, 2008),
  93, 100, 104, 105
moral pluralism, 79
  of CBRC, 140–1
moral quality, of parent–child
  relationship, 56
moral theory

deontology, 35
utilitarianism, 35
virtue ethics, 35
Moses, 61
mother/child relationships, in terms of
    egg donation, 93
Muller, Hermann, 6
multi-ethnic societies and ARTs, 82–4
'My Three Sons', 194

National Commission on Assisted
    Human Reproduction, 114, 115
National Conference of Commissioners
    on Uniform State Laws, 93
National Ethics Committee on Assisted
    Reproductive Technology (ECART),
    170
National Health Service (NHS), 7, 9,
    92, 220
National Institute for Health and Clinical
    Excellence (NICE), 220
National Research Act, 32
neonatal malformation and IVF/ICSI
    cycles, 18
non-disclosing families, 237–8
    vs. disclosing families, 240–1
non-Jewish donors and Halakha, 82
non-maleficence principle, 33, 77
non-random mating patterns, 23
North American Christian-based
    culture, 23
novel treatment, in donation, 21
Nuremberg Code, 34
Nuremberg Tribunal and principles in
    medical research, 32
Nuremburg trials, 20

offspring of consanguineous unions, risk
    factors of, 23
oocyte donation, 139, 176
    ASRM guidelines for, 153
    donor anonymity, 162
oogenic stem cells, 24
open-identity donation, 251
    children's responses, 258–61
    donors, impact on, 262–4
    on parental disclosure
        decisions, 254–5
    social, policy and ethical context,
        251–4
    sperm donors, 256
ovarian hyperstimulation syndrome
    (OHSS), 17, 37, 142, 160

P.D. v. S.K., 105

parent selection, in embryo donation,
    271–7
parentage contests, in context of gamete
    donation, 96
parentage of donor-conceived children,
    102–6
parental disclosure, concerns
    of, 106–8
parent–child relationship, 55–7, 237
    intrafamilial donation and, 181–4
    in terms of donation, 93
parenthood, see also single parents by
    choice (SPCs)
    biological terms, 53
    children's perspective, 57–65
    forms of, 53–5
    good, 59
    legal terms, 54
    perspective of adults, 55–7
    social terms, 54
payment controversy, related to gamete
    donation, 152–4
percutaneous-epididymal sperm
    aspiration (PESA), 16
Piddington, Marion Louisa, 5, 10
Plato, 35
positive eugenics, 6
pre-eclampsia, 21
pre-implantation genetic diagnosis, 2
prenatal diagnosis, 2
progenitors, of child, 1
prohibitive policies, 76
psychological disorders, 123
psychological evaluation protocol, for
    donors, 121
psychopathology, 123

Ravitsky, Vardit, 106
reasonable compensation, for egg and
    sperm donation, 100
recognition theory, 60
recurrent miscarriage, 21
Regulation No. 568/1997 on
    Artificial Fertilisation eng.
    heilbrigdisraduneyti.is/laws-and-
    regulations/nr/686, 128
relatedness, 71
religious perspectives, on donation,
    79–82
Reproducing the Future: Anthropology,
    Kinship and the New Reproductive
    Technologies, 71
reproductive donation, 14, 222, 308
    diversity in, 73–6
Reproductive Medicine Act (1992), 127

reproductive tourism, 44–5, 131, 132, 139
resemblance, importance in identity formation, 59–61
respect for persons, 32
restrictive policies, 76
retrograde ejaculation, 16
right to know one's genetic origins, 106–8, *see also* disclosing donation, idea of
Roman Catholic Church, 40, 80
Roman v. Roman, 97

Sacred Congregation of the Holy Office of the Vatican, 5
scientific motherhood, 10
self-appraisal, 60
self-appreciation, 60
self-determination, 78, 244
self-insemination, 189
self-love, 60
self-renewing cells, 24
self-replicating body fluids, 100
semen donation, compensation issues related to, 153
Shenfield, Françoise, 132
single fathers by choice (SFCs), 189, 198
decision to become, 201
gender bias and, 194–5
single mother by choice (SMC), 189, 197
children of, 204
decision to become, 199–201
experiences of, 202
role of father and, 202–4
single parents and ethical issues, 43
single parents by choice (SPCs), 189, 199
children of, 204–5
ethical debate, 190–1
future prospects, 205–7
ideal family and, 192
need for a father, 193–4
routes to, 189–90
welfare of child and, 192
Skywalker, Luke, 60, 61
Sloan, Louise, 192
slow-freeze protocols for eggs, 19
Smith, Iain Duncan, 193
social fatherhood, 1, 77
social infertility, 13
social motherhood, 1, 77, 183
social order of sexual reproduction, 3
social science research, 38, 43, 45, 46–7
Sociedad Española de Fertilidad (SEF), 121

Society of Assisted Reproductive Technologies (SART), 134
somatic cell, 24
Spain, 128
act regulating ARTs, 113
alcoholics in donor samples of, 123
anonymity of donors, 116–17
CBRC laws, 133
children conceived by a donor, limit of, 115
donor recipients and children, 117–20
donor registry, legislation of, 120–1
donor selection process, 121–3
donor treatment, 114
egg donation business in, 46
family relationship in, 112
financial compensation, 115
IVF in, 114
law regarding ARTs in, 113–16
National Donor Registry of, 115
psychological disorder donors, 123
sperm donation in, 114
type of egg donors, 122
Spanish Act about Assisted Human Reproduction (14/2006), 118
Spanish Act about Assisted Human Reproduction Techniques (35/1988), 113
sperm bank, 6, 8
sperm donation, 2
cultural response of, 74
diversity in, 73–6
ethical questions, 39–40, 77
in Germany, 75
in Italy, 77
overview of, 91
parentage effects of, 104
sperm immotility, 73
spermatogenic stem cells, 24
spermatozoa, 15–17, 18
adverse medical outcome of donation, 16
spindle, 18
stem cells, 24–5
sterility, 13
Stichting Geertgen clinic, 162, 164
Stopes, Marie, 6
stored eggs, legal status of, 96–8
stored sperm, legal status of, 96–8
straight surrogacy, 20
Strathern, Marilyn, 71
sub-cellular 'donation', 14, 22–3
substance abuse, 43

surrogacy, 20
  compensation, 296
  considerations for children born
    through, 301–2
  considerations for surrogates,
    295–9
  counselling for surrogate, 295
  definitions, 289
  in Denmark, 75
  disclosure of, 302–4
  diversity in, 75
  ethical questions, 41
  in Finland, 75
  forms of, 2
  in Germany, 65
  informed consent and, 96
  money received for, 44
  mother–child relationship, 93
  payment regulations in UK, 99
  relationship between couple and
    surrogate, 299–300
  in Sweden, 75
  in United Kingdom, 291–5
  in United States, 289, 290–1
Surrogacy Arrangements
  Act (1985), 291
surrogate (gestational) mother, 1
Swan, Henry Waterman, 5
Swedish Act of Artificial Insemination
  1985, n. 1140/1984, 113
Swedish Law of Artificial Insemination,
  117
Switch, the, 108
systematic assessment of risks and
  benefits, 33

test tube babies, 6, 7
testicular sperm extraction (TESE), 16
thalidomide tragedies, 21
third-party reproductive assistance, 3, 71,
  74, 75, 76, 80, 81, 82
tort system, 95
transnational donation, 130
  empirical evidence on, 131
  ethical issues of, 44–5
  of gametes, 135–7
  harmonization of, 139–40
  moral pluralism in, 140–1
  regulation of, 137
  safety issues, 142
trisomy 21 pregnancy, 17
trivialis[ing] altruistic donation, 101,
  168, 176
trophoblast cells, 21

trophoblast HLA-C molecules, 21
Turkish Penal Code, 138
Tuskegee syphilis study, 32
'Two and a Half Men', 194

UK Archbishop's Committee, 7
UK Government Departmental
  Committee, 7
UK Human Fertilisation and Embryo
  (HFE) Act (2008), 192, 252, 293
UK Human Fertilisation and
  Embryology Act 1990 118, 198
UK law
  for CBRC, 132
  gamete donation, 232–3
  legal status, of frozen gametes, 96–8
  regarding donor identity, 107
  for surrogacy, 291–5
UK payment, for gametes, 98–102
UK's Human Fertilisation and
  Embryology Authority, 136
unfertilized eggs, ovulation of, 18
Uniform Parentage Act of 2000 (UPA,
  2000), 93
Universal Declaration of Human Rights,
  34
US law
  legal status, of frozen gametes, 96–8
  regarding donor identity, 107
  for surrogacy, 290–1
US sperm donation business, 101
USA National Research Foundation for
  Eugenic Alleviation, 5
uteri, 14, 15, 19
uterine natural killer (uNK) cells, 21
uterus donation, biological issues of, 20

Valencia Infertility Institute (IVI), 121
Velleman, David, 57
  on assisting a child, 58
  on belongingness, 61
  on biological kinship, 58
  on blood relation, 59
  on communal child raising, 58
  on consanguinity, 61
  example of Luke Skywalker, 60
  on growing up with biological parents,
    57
  on non-biological parents, 62, 64
  on procreation, 57
  on resemblance, 59–61
virtue ethics, 35
vitrification, 15
vitrified oocytes, 19

voluntariness of donors, 33, 163
voluntary consent, of human subject, 32
voluntary donor registries, 309

Wand, J. W. C., 8
  on AID, 9
  on AIH/D, 9
  pros and cons for AI, 9
Warnock, Mary, 8, 183
Warnock Report, 296
Warnock symbolism of gametes fusing, 9

websites, of donor families
  and donors, 4
Wells v. *Wells*, 104
World Health Organisation (WHO), 73
World Medical Association, 32

Yearworth v. *North Bristol NHS
  Trust*, 96

zina, 81
zona pellucida, 19